BEYOND PATIENT PATHWAYS

How Healthcare Systems Make Patients and Organise Care

Davina Allen

Routledge
Taylor & Francis Group
LONDON AND NEW YORK

Designed cover image: Getty Images

First published 2026
by Routledge
4 Park Square, Milton Park, Abingdon, Oxon OX14 4RN

and by Routledge
605 Third Avenue, New York, NY 10158

Routledge is an imprint of the Taylor & Francis Group, an informa business

British Library Cataloguing-in-Publication Data
A catalogue record for this book is available from the British Library

ISBN: 978-1-032-75653-0 (hbk)
ISBN: 978-1-032-75652-3 (pbk)
ISBN: 978-1-003-47501-9 (ebk)

DOI: 10.4324/9781003475019

Typeset in Times New Roman
by SPi Technologies India Pvt Ltd (Straive)

In memory of my friend and fellow Fellow,
Tim Draycott, whose brilliance, mischief, and company
shaped the research on which this book is based.

CONTENTS

Preface *x*
Acknowledgements *xiii*
List of Abbreviations *xv*
Glossary *xvii*
Fieldnote Conventions *xix*

PART 1
Reframing Coordination **1**

INTRODUCTION TO PART 1 3

1 The Trouble with Coordination: Organisational Challenges and the Seductions of Pathways 5

2 Reimagining Coordination: Sociological Perspectives 15

3 Studying Coordination in the Wild: Case, Methods, and Theoretical Framework 25

PART 2
The Provisional Patient – The Unscheduled Care Assemblage **37**

INTRODUCTION TO PART 2 39

4 Calls, Codes, Dispatch: Emergency Medical Services Control Centre Work 43

5 Between Crisis and Care: Emergency Medical Services Responder Work 60

6 From Arrival to Admission: Emergency Department Work 76

7 Evolving Objects: Unscheduled Care Transitions 100

Summary of Part 2 114

PART 3
The Definitive Patient – The Acute Care Assemblage 117

INTRODUCTION TO PART 3 119

8 Assessment and Alignment: Preoperative Orthogeriatric Work 123

9 Bodies and Materials: Operating Department Work 146

10 Conscripted Objects: Acute Care Transitions 167

Summary of Part 3 186

PART 4
The Distributed Patient – The Recovery Care Assemblage 189

INTRODUCTION TO PART 4 191

11 Recovery and Discharge Planning: Postoperative Orthogeriatric Work 195

12 Reablement and Infrastructures: Community Resource Team Work 230

13 Unstable Objects: Recovery Care Transitions 255

Summary of Part 4 284

PART 5
Conclusion: Trajectory Assemblage Synthesis and Implications for Service Improvement and Research **287**

14 Beyond Pathways: Making Coordination Work 289

Appendix 1 *313*
Index *316*

PREFACE

Over the past two decades, high-income countries have launched a wide range of initiatives to improve the integration of care systems. Many of these efforts have been shaped by the metaphor of care pathways – rational-linear models of organisation adapted from manufacturing. Yet, despite the widespread adoption of strategies to map and standardise the patient journey, coordination remains an intractable challenge and a persistent source of failures in quality and safety.

This book challenges the dominant logic of pathways thinking. Using hip fracture as an illustrative case, it draws on ethnographic research that traced the patient journey from initial contact with emergency services through diagnosis, surgery, recovery, and home discharge. Building on the sociology of patient trajectories (Strauss et al., 1985), translational mobilisation theory (Allen, 2018; Allen and May, 2017), and assemblage thinking (Deleuze and Guattari, 1987), new conceptual resources are introduced to describe and explain how patients, care, and treatment are organised and mobilised within and across services.

By moving beyond prescriptive models to examine real-world organising practices, the book critically examines which concerns are centred in care, the different requirements of coordination, and the variety of arrangements that make concerted action possible. In doing so, it invites a shift – from designing systems around imagined pathways to organising care around the realities of practice.

About This Book

This book is organised into four parts. Part 1 sets the scene by establishing the policy, conceptual, and practical foundations for what follows. It opens in Chapter 1 with a discussion of the persistent challenges of coordination in care systems and offers a critical examination of the promises and limitations of the care pathways metaphor. Chapter 2 introduces sociological perspectives that help reframe how organisational processes in healthcare are understood. Chapter 3 concludes the section with an account of the ethnographic study and the theoretical and conceptual resources that underpin the analysis.

Parts 2–4 examine three distinctive configurations of organisational arrangements in hip fracture care. Individual chapters describing and explaining specific services are complemented by dedicated chapters that explore the transitional arrangements between them.

Part 2 focuses on the *unscheduled care assemblage*. It examines the patient journey from the moment of first contact with emergency services, through the diagnostic process, and eventual referral to the specialist orthogeriatric service. The section comprises chapters on the emergency medical services control centre (Chapter 4), emergency medical services responders (Chapter 5), and the emergency department (Chapter 6), culminating in an analysis of transitional arrangements (Chapter 7). In this phase of the hip fracture trajectory, the clinical status of the patient is provisional, and attention focuses on those concerns necessary to permit a decision about entry into the system. Human actors play a central role in the mobilisation and alignment of activity in a fast-paced, resource-constrained environment.

Part 3 explores the *acute care* assemblage. It spans the period from admission to hospital, through surgery, post-anaesthetic recovery, and return to the ward. In this phase, the patient is configured as a definitive and clinically recognisable object of practice and enrolled within a structured and standardised framework of interventions and actions. Chapters examine preoperative ward activity (Chapter 8), the work of the operating department (Chapter 9), and the transition processes that connect services (Chapter 10). Here, the analysis foregrounds the divergent collective objects of practice of the orthogeriatric ward and the operating department, and the central role of formal artefacts in mediating this relationship. The mobilisation of activity during this phase of the trajectory depends on mechanisms of conscription, bracketing, and reconstruction.

Part 4 focuses on the *recovery care assemblage*. It encompasses postoperative ward care, discharge planning, and community-based services. This phase of the trajectory is marked by extended, distributed, and contested understandings of the patient and the emergence of more unstable and expansive forms of organisation. Chapters examine postoperative ward work (Chapter 11) and the role of a community resource team (Chapter 12). A final chapter (Chapter 13) analyses discharge processes and the transition from hospital to community care, revealing the challenges of organising integrated care at this interface.

Chapter 14 concludes the analysis. It synthesises the insights gained from adopting a unique trajectory-wide perspective and considers their implications for service improvement, theoretical development, and future research.

The book can be read in different ways.

- It can be read in its entirety as a descriptive ethnography of a whole trajectory of care.
- In conjunction with Chapter 3, individual empirical chapters can be read for ethnographic insights into the individual services comprising the hip fracture trajectory.
- In conjunction with Chapter 3, each part can be read to better understand how different assemblage configurations impact the organisation of care within and between services.
- Chapters 1, 2, 3, and 14 can be read as methodological and theoretical resources for research purposes.

However this book is read, my hope is that it will be of interest to health and social care practitioners, sociologists, health services researchers, and improvement scientists, and stimulate reconsideration of the challenges of coordination in practice, as well as further studies designed to better understand this organisational complexity.

References

Allen, D. and C. May (2017). 'Organizing practice and practising organization: an outline of translational mobilization theory'. *Sage Open* **7**: 2.

Allen, D. (2018). 'Analysing healthcare coordination using translational mobilisation theory'. *Journal of Health Organization and Management* **32**(3): 358–373.

Deleuze, G. and F. Guattari (1987). *A Thousand Plateaus: Capitalism and Schizophrenia*. Minneapolis, University of Minneapolis Press.

Strauss, A.L., S. Fagerhaugh, B. Suczet, and C. Wiener (1985). *Social Organization of Medical Work*. Chicago, IL, University of Chicago Press.

ACKNOWLEDGEMENTS

This research would not have been possible without the support of staff across the health and care services at the study site. I am deeply grateful to those who welcomed me into their social worlds, shared their insights into the system, and allowed me to observe their work. Numerous patients and families permitted me to witness their care and treatment. I cannot thank them enough for this generosity. The study was undertaken as part of an Improvement Science Fellowship, supported by The Health Foundation. This was a remarkable opportunity for which I remain immensely appreciative. Not only did it enable me to pursue a demanding and unpredictable programme of research, I was also fortunate to benefit from stimulating discussions with my fellow Fellows – Julie Reed, Carl Macrae, and the late Tim Draycott – as well as the guidance and expertise of our scheme coaches, Bill Lucas and Fiona Reed, and Director of Research, Professor Nick Barber.

Data generation was completed during the lifetime of the Fellowship, but analysis and writing had to be woven into my ongoing work and were significantly delayed by the additional demands brought about by the COVID-19 pandemic. The world I studied has changed considerably in the intervening period. Even so, I believe the value of this research lies more in its approach than in the specific empirical details. As we confront the far-reaching consequences of the pandemic – staff burnout, workforce shortages, care backlogs – and embrace new technologies and evolving roles, deepening our understanding of the complex organisational challenges within care systems has never been more urgent.

Aspects of this work have appeared in a different form elsewhere. Chapter 4 draws on: Allen, D. (2021). 'Prioritising the mobilisation of emergency services: patient making at the healthcare gateway'. *Journal of Health Organization and Management*, 35(2), 160–176. Reproduced with permission from Emerald Publishing.

The analysis of transitions in Chapters 7, 10, and 13 draws on: Allen, D. (2024). 'Why is hospital discharge so difficult? Reconsidering patient trajectories in theory and practice: insights from an ethnographic study of transitions in hip fracture care'. *Social Science & Medicine*, 347, 116769. This article is published open access under a CC BY license and is reused in accordance with the terms of that license.

ABBREVIATIONS

A&E	Accident and Emergency Department
ACU	Ambulatory Care Unit
AMPDS	Advanced Medical Priority Dispatch System
ANT	Actor Network Theory
APP	Advanced Paramedic Practitioner
AU	Assessment Unit
BM	Blood Glucose Monitoring
BMI	Body Mass Index
CAD	Computer-Aided Dispatch
CAS Card	Clinical Assessment Services Card (patient record in ED).
CDU	Clinical Decision Unit
COPD	Chronic Obstructive Pulmonary Disease
CRT	Community Resource Team
CT	Computed Tomography Scan
CTA	Computed Tomography Angiography
CPR	Cardiopulmonary Resuscitation
CVA	Cerebral Vascular Accident
DHS	Dynamic Hip Screw
DNAR	Do Not Attempt Resuscitation
DVT	Deep Vein Thrombosis
ECG	Electrocardiogram
ED	Emergency Department
EMI	Elderly Mentally Infirm
EMS PCR	Emergency Medical Services Patient Care Record
EMT	Emergency Medical Technician
GCS	Glasgow Coma Scale
GP	General Practitioner

GTN	Glyceryl Trinitrate
HB	Haemoglobin Level
INR	International Normalised Ratio
IV	Intravenous
MTS	Manchester Triage System
NEWS	National Early Warning Score
NHS	National Health Service
NMC	Nursing and Midwifery Council (UK regulator)
NOF	Neck of Femur
OD	Operating Department
ODPCR	Operating Department Patient Care Record.
PACU	Post-Anaesthetic Care Unit
PE	Pulmonary Embolism
PEG	Percutaneous Endoscopic Gastrostomy
POVA	Protection of Vulnerable Adults
RCN	Royal College of Nursing
SATS	Blood oxygen saturation
SBAR	Situation, Background, Assessment, Recommendation
T&O	Trauma and Orthopaedics
TIA	Transient Ischaemic Attack
TMT	Translational Mobilisation Theory
TTH	Tablets to Take Home
UA	Unified Assessment
UCS	Urgent Care Service
UK	United Kingdom
UTI	Urinary Tract Infection

GLOSSARY

Echocardiogram — an ultrasound scan which creates moving images of the heart structure and functions.

Electrocardiograph — a device used for measuring the electrical activity of the heart.

Glasgow Coma Scale — a tool used to determine a person's level of consciousness, by assessing eye-opening, verbal response, and motor response, each with a numerical score.

Health Board — a regional organisation responsible for planning and delivering healthcare services to people in a specific geographical area in Wales – including hospitals, primary care, community care, and mental health services.

Local Authority — an instrument of local government, which has a responsibility for public services and facilities in a particular area.

National Early Warning Score (NEWS) — a system for scoring the six physiological measurements that are routinely recorded at the patient's bedside – respiratory rate; oxygen saturation; temperature; systolic blood pressure; heart rate; and level of consciousness. Its purpose is to identify acutely ill patients. Each parameter scores nil to three, and individual scores are added together for an overall score. The higher the score, the greater the clinical risk, indicating the requirement for additional monitoring or possibly allocation of a space in intensive care.

Safeguarding	healthcare staff's responsibility for protecting individual's health, well-being, and human rights; enabling them to live free from harm, abuse, and neglect.
See and Treat Model	a service model which is part of a broader effort by the Welsh Ambulance Service to address increasing demand and improve patient outcomes. Paramedics use clinical guidelines and decision-support tools to determine whether a patient can be safely treated on-site, without transporting the patient to a hospital.
Stoma	a surgically created opening on the abdomen that allows waste – such as faeces or urine – to exit the body. The waste is typically collected in a bag attached to the skin, which must be emptied regularly.
Transient Ischaemic Attack	blood to the brain is temporarily interrupted, mimicking the conditions of a stroke.
Waterlow Score	a score developed in 1985 by Judy Waterlow to estimate the risk for the development of a pressure ulcer.
Welsh Clinical Portal	a national digital health record which includes GP records, diagnostic test results, radiography images, and certain medical documents (such as referral letters and clinical attendance).

FIELDNOTE CONVENTIONS

[…] words, phrases, or sentences omitted
(material added by the author to make the context/meaning clear)
Data have been edited to preserve anonymity
All names of people and places are pseudonyms
All data extracts are fieldnotes, unless otherwise specified

PART 1
Reframing Coordination

PART 1

Reframing Coordination

INTRODUCTION TO PART 1

Part 1 lays the groundwork for the book by examining the problem of coordination and developing the conceptual resources needed to analyse how healthcare is organised. Chapter 1 explores why coordination remains a persistent and unresolved challenge in health and social care. It critically examines both the appeal and the limitations of pathways thinking and calls for a deeper understanding of how care is organised in practice. Chapter 2 introduces sociological concepts and perspectives that help to illuminate the complexity, fluidity, and relational interdependence that characterise care settings. Chapter 3 sets out the ethnographic approach, research materials and theoretical framework that inform the analysis. Together, these chapters provide the foundation for the empirical enquiry that follows.

DOI: 10.4324/9781003475019-2

1

THE TROUBLE WITH COORDINATION

Organisational Challenges and the Seductions of Pathways

> Managers all go around with their spreadsheets, pretending that their department is doing well. But there is no pathway, it is not owned by anyone. It is a virtual reality that only exists in management-speak.
>
> (Senior Clinician - Interview)

Over the last 50 years, care systems in high-income countries have been transformed by advances in science and technology, in service organisation, and the impact of demographic trends and shifting disease patterns. While new medical technologies have revolutionised treatment, they have also contributed to a growing population with cumulatively complex needs (May et al., 2014; Shippee et al., 2012). Specialist services, professions, and support roles have proliferated, with activity increasingly distributed across multiple providers, departments, and organisations. Hospital in-patient populations now typically present with high acuity, complexity, and rapid turnover; while in the community, growing numbers of people depend on finely-balanced arrangements for long-term condition management and support (Bjornsdottir, 2018; Hughes et al., 2020; Melby et al., 2018).

These advances have brought significant benefits, but also major coordination challenges, with wide-ranging impacts on healthcare quality and safety (Leary et al., 2021).

> Western health care practices are far from effective, efficient, patient-centred, safe, timely, and equitable - however exactly defined - not so much because of the failings of individual health care workers, but because of a lack of coordination of their individual activities.
>
> *(Timmermans and Berg, 2003: 202)*

DOI: 10.4324/9781003475019-3

A WHO Europe (2012) report identified service fragmentation and lack of coherence as the main barriers to effective care. In North America, the Lucian Leape Institute (2012) linked poor service integration to adverse events, calling for service coordination to be a top priority for safe, effective, and efficient care. Similar observations are echoed in national patient safety reviews (Institute of Medicine, 2001; National Patient Safety Agency, 2007; The Health Foundation, 2011).

Pathways to Coordination

A wide range of initiatives have aimed to improve care organisation and integration over the past two decades (Ahgren and Axelsson, 2011). Targeted activities span time-critical interventions, through service transitions to complex needs support. Efforts have included structural realignments (Morris et al., 2014), development of coordinating technologies (Allen, 2009; Timmermans and Berg, 2003), re-engineering of service interfaces (AHRQ, 2013), creation of case manager and navigator roles (McMurray and Cooper, 2016), integrated care programmes for older adults (Johri et al., 2003; Wodchis et al., 2015), and financial incentives (Zutshi, Peikes and Smith, 2014).

Despite variations in strategies and technologies, activity has been significantly influenced by the 'care pathway' metaphor. While definitions vary, pathways thinking assumes care can be organised through structured processes that define the content and sequencing of activities. This is captured in the familiar phrase: 'The right person, in the right place, doing the right thing, at the right time, with the right outcome – while prioritising the patient experience' (Allen, 2010).

Care pathway models reflect the dominance of rational-linear approaches to healthcare improvement. Their roots lie in classical management theory (Fayol, 1949), with one of the most recognisable applications being Frederick Taylor's scientific management at Ford Motor Company in the 1920s, which led to the creation of assembly lines that made standardisation and mass production possible (Taylor, 1911).

Emerging in North America in the 1980s, care pathways were initially introduced to bring about efficiencies to meet requirements imposed by healthcare insurers, but soon became a cornerstone for addressing a diverse agenda (Pinder et al., 2005).

> From almost nowhere, apparently, they appear to have become the tool of choice for ensuring (or so it is claimed) quality of care, equity of treatment, optimal allocation of resources and a rational division of labour between healthcare professionals. Simultaneously, it is claimed that they respond even-handedly to concerns for patient safety, variable healthcare quality and spiralling health costs.
>
> *(Pinder et al., 2005: 3)*

Appealing to patients, providers, and planners alike, the pathway metaphor suggests a guided journey through care – implying coordination, direction, and clarity (Checkland et al., 2020). It reduces uncertainty for patients, helps planners comprehend service relationships, and offers a framework for improving care delivery and organisation. Over the last decade, professional bodies such as The European Pathways Association and dedicated journals like The International Journal of Care Coordination have emerged to promote best practices and scholarly discourse. National authorities – including NHS Improvement England, Health Education and Improvement Wales, Haute Autorité de Santé, and the Australian Commission on Safety and Quality in Healthcare – have endorsed pathways thinking, further institutionalising it as a strategy for optimising service outcomes.

Now ubiquitous in healthcare, the pathway metaphor has inspired a wide array of interventions: critical paths for evidence-based condition management (Woldrum, 1987); maps outlining individual care ecologies (Antonelli and Lind, 2012); integrated care pathways as coordinating artefacts (Allen, 2009); flow charts, checklists (Vanahecht et al., 2010); planning tools for visualising service relationships (Checkland et al., 2020; Pinder et al., 2005); frameworks for complex condition management (van der Feltz-Cornelis et al., 2023); and process technologies for managing unit activity (Schrijvers et al., 2012). This diversity of definitions, components, and interventions has made it challenging to draw general conclusions about effectiveness (Ouwens et al., 2005). Rather than dampening enthusiasm, however, this lack of precision may help to explain the widespread appeal and adoption of pathways thinking.

Contemporary healthcare systems are shaped by multiple, often contradictory, institutional logics – sets of assumptions, beliefs, and values that guide activity (Thorton and Ocasio, 2008). Logics are reflected in material practices, work cultures, and symbolic representations, steering practitioners' and decision-makers' attention. They are 'institutional' because they align with formal arrangements governing a field (e.g., health policy, legislation, regulation, markets).

Historically, professional logics dominated healthcare organisations, but shifts in regulation and policy have introduced managerial and market logics, reshaping formal structures. Whereas professional logics prioritise practitioner judgement and patient needs; managerial logics stress planning and efficiency; and market logics focus on customer satisfaction, standardisation, and performance. It is not uncommon for multiple logics to coexist within an organisational field, but this can produce ambiguous or conflicting messages and formats that must be reconciled in practice (Andersson and Liff, 2018; Goodrick and Reay, 2011; Vivier et al., 2024).

Traditionally, care organisations have separated professional and administrative activities (Ruef and Scott, 1998), but today, management, market, and professional work are increasingly intertwined (Noordegraaf, 2013, 2016).

In this context, pathways have acted as boundary concepts (Löwy, 1992), aligning clinicians, managers, planners, and users around improving healthcare quality (Allen, 2009). Boundary concepts are loosely defined yet cohesive, enabling cooperation across groups without erasing distinct identities. Their vagueness allows flexible translation and adaptation of ideas, and interventions open to local reinvention are more likely to spread (Greenhalgh et al., 2004; de Leat and Mol, 2000; Prout, 1996).

Pathways thinking serves diverse institutional logics. Coupled with management theories, it supports efficiency, cost containment, and service access (Schrijvers et al., 2012). As trust has shifted from professional expertise to auditable evidence-based standards (Power, 1997), pathways have enabled new clinical governance models (Ellis and Johnson, 1999). They also align with improvement logics, empowering staff to manage service quality (Allen, 2009), and are used by commissioners and insurers to define contracts (Checkland et al., 2020; Pinder et al., 2005). Though often promoted as tools for patient-centeredness (Seys et al., 2021), pathway activity has focused on specific diseases or processes (Grocott, 2019), limiting their reach to improved communication rather than outcomes. Recently, interest has grown in aligning pathways with customisation logics (Mannion and Exworthy, 2017), reflecting respect for individual values. This is seen in proposals for combining standardised and customised pathways for complex conditions (Smeds, 2019), developing new 'patient-centered' pathways (Olsen et al., 2021), and using experience-based co-design (Grocott, 2019).

Beyond their flexibility, pathways also help to create organisational legitimacy. Many organisational practices are not driven by efficiency or function, but the need to secure societal support by adopting structures and procedures that align with widely accepted cultural models (Meyer and Rowan, 1977). Organisations operate within institutional fields which generate distinctive pressures about the appropriate ways of acting which transcend any one organisation's control (DiMaggio and Powell, 1983; Suchman, 1995). This is why organisations increasingly come to resemble one another. While early adopters seek performance gains, over time, practices become 'infused with value beyond the technical requirements of the task at hand' (Selznick, 1957: 17; cited by DiMaggio and Powell, 1983). Meyer and Rowan (1977) argue that creating formal structures that align with institutional norms signals that an organisation is pursuing valued goals in an appropriate way. Nevertheless, structures that celebrate prescription myths in the institutionalised environment may differ from those that are necessary to act efficiently. Consequently, formal organisational structures may be only loosely coupled with everyday work processes.

The Challenges and Limitations of Pathways Thinking

Sociologically informed research has underscored the challenges and limitations of pathways thinking for driving improvement. Although the metaphor's

success can be partly attributed to its conceptual flexibility, this wide-ranging appeal also presents difficulties in reconciling the diverse interests involved in effective pathway interventions. For example, Olsen et al. (2021) describe tensions between rationalising and patient-centred logics in the development of a pathway to support older patients transitioning from hospital to home. Similarly, my research found that efforts to create a shared mental health safety pathway for providers and users failed due to the difficulty of integrating their needs into a single tool (Allen, 2009).

Pathways may have heralded new patterns of compromise between clinicians and managers, but studies reveal tensions between their prescriptive qualities and professional logics that value autonomy, judgement, and discretion. Local pathway projects, often led by nurses in quality roles, may struggle to enrol medical staff, resulting in stalled development or failed implementation (Allen, 2014). In a large randomised controlled trial, Martin et al. (2017) reported that while medical staff voiced concerns about an emergency laparotomy pathway's impact on professional judgement, this led not to resistance, but a 'nuancing of pathways-as-realised'. Implementers shifted from strict compliance to focusing on elements that supported, rather than replaced, professional judgement.

Pathways are not neutral tools. Their development involves choices about inclusion and exclusion. Drawing on cultural cartography, Pinder et al. (2005) analysed a cataract pathway in a UK Primary Care Trust, arguing that pathways, like maps, impose order rather than reflect reality. Despite intentions to be patient-centred, the pathway prioritised impairment and reduced care to a clinical disposal decision, excluding carers and ignoring the biographical disruption of chronic illness (Bury, 1982) and the task of rebuilding identity (Siegel and Krauss, 1991). The pathway also elevated some providers while marginalising others.

Metaphors are generative (Schon, 1993). They frame problems in ways that suggest certain solutions, and several commentators have highlighted the constraints of pathways thinking. Building on their critique of pathway content, Pinder et al. (2005) advocate the development of pathway 'maps' from various perspectives – patients, commissioners, and providers – rather than striving for a single, comprehensive depiction. Here, the intent is to offer a mechanism for mediating the logics of standardisation and patient-centredness inherent in pathway design. Checkland et al. (2020) found that pathways can constrain thinking, making some solutions seem obvious while obscuring others. In their study, which involved a population with variable needs, conceptualising care as a unidirectional pathway made it difficult to ensure that services were integrated. They propose the metaphor of a service map as more valuable for service commissioning. This recognises the diverse and unpredictable ways patients engage with services, and reframes commissioning as mapping the landscape and then coordinating activity.

Critical engagement with care pathways should not be mistaken for sociological cynicism. Many authors expressed sympathy for developers' efforts to improve services. Nor are these insights an argument against pathways or rational planning technologies. Nevertheless, it is clear that given the complexity of care systems, pathways are not a universal panacea (Bragato and Jacobs, 2003). Not only does the metaphor embody many of the tensions it is designed to resolve, the linearity, order, and formality associated with the image of a patient pathway is increasingly at odds with the reality of service delivery.

Care systems are turbulent. Many patients' needs do not align with standardised routes. Staff juggle growing workloads, workflow interruptions, and complex regulatory demands. The organisation of care and treatment is shaped by shifting relationships, competing priorities, and unforeseen contingencies. It is often responsive practices – those that adapt to variation and absorb disruption – that enable the system to function and remain resilient in the face of complexity (Allen, 2014; Hollnagel, 2014). In this context, the prescriptive qualities of pathways conflict with the inherent unpredictability of healthcare work. Some of the most persistent coordination challenges arise at care system interfaces (Aase and Waring, 2020), yet pathways have typically been confined to single domains. Their application across service boundaries – especially between hospital, community, and social care – remains limited.

Despite decades of quality initiatives and widespread pathways use, a recent review found only incremental progress in strengthening coordination, calling for new strategies to secure further gains (Gandhi et al., 2018). Past efforts have concentrated on designing and implementing models, rather than building foundational research (Scott et al., 2024). An important priority then is to develop a deeper understanding of organisational processes across the spectrum of care system activity. This is necessary to determine when coordination requires 'Tayloring' patients to the organisation, and when organisations must adapt to patients (Pinder et al., 2005). Such insight will clarify when rational planning technologies have value and how they should be applied, and when alternative approaches are needed and what strategic investments are required to support them (Timmermans and Berg, 2003).

References

Aase, K. and J. Waring (2020). 'Crossing boundaries: establishing a framework for researching quality and safety in care transitions'. *Applied Ergonomics* **89**: 103228.

Ahgren, B. and R. Axelsson (2011). 'A decade of integration and collaboration: the development of integrated health care in Sweden, 2000–2010'. *International Journal of Integrated Care* **11**(Spec Ed): e007.

AHRQ (2013). *Re-engineered Discharge (RED) Toolkit: Tool 1 Overview*. Rockville, MD, Agency for Healthcare Research and Quality.

Allen, D. (2009). 'From boundary concept to boundary object: the practice and politics of care pathways development'. *Social Science & Medicine* **69**(3): 354–361. https://doi.org/10.1016/j.socscimed.2009.05.002

Allen, D. (2010). 'Care pathways: an ethnographic description of the field'. *International Journal of Care Pathways* **14**(1): 4–9. https://doi.org/10.1258/jicp.2009.009015

Allen, D. (2014). 'Lost in translation? "Evidence" and the articulation of institutional logics in integrated care pathways: from positive to negative boundary object?' *Sociology of Health & Illness* **36**(6): 807–822. https://doi.org/10.1111/1467-9566.12111

Andersson, T. and R. Liff (2018). 'Co-optation as a response to competing institutional logics: professionals and managers in healthcare'. *Journal of Professions and Organization* **5**(2): 71–87. https://doi.org/10.1093/jpo/joy001

Antonelli, R. and C. Lind (2012). 'Care mapping: an innovative tool and process to support family-centered, comprehensive care coordination'. Poster session presented at the *Annual Primary Care Innovation Conference of the Harvard Medical School Primary Care Center*, Boston, MA.

Bjornsdottir, K. (2018). '"I try to make a net around each patient": home care nursing as relational practice'. *Scandinavian Journal of Caring Sciences* **32**(1): 177–185.

Bragato, L. and K. Jacobs (2003). 'Care pathways: the road to better care'. *Journal of Health Organization and Management* **17**(3):164–180. https://doi.org/10.1108/14777260310480721

Bury, M. (1982). 'Chronic illness as biographical disruption'. *Sociology of Health & Illness* **4**(2): 167–182.

Checkland, K., J. Hammond, P. Allen, A. Coleman, L. Warwick-Giles, A. Hall, N. Mays, and M. Sutton (2020) 'Road to nowhere? A critical consideration of the use of the metaphor "care pathway" in health services planning, organisation and delivery'. *Journal of Social Policy* **49**(2): 405–424. https://doi.org/10.1017/S0047279419000400

De Leat, M. and A. Mol (2000). 'The Zimbabwe bush pump: mechanisms of a fluid technology'. *Social Studies of Science* **30**(2): 225–263.

DiMaggio, P.J. and W.W. Powell (1983). 'The iron cage revisited: institutional isomorphism and collective rationality in organizational fields.' *American Sociological Review* **48**(April): 147–160.

Ellis, B.W. and S. Johnson (1999). 'The care pathway: a tool to enhance clinical governance'. *Health Organization and Management* **17**(3): 164–180.

Fayol, H. (1949). *General and Industrial Management*. London, Pitman.

Gandhi, T., G. Kaplan, L. Leape, D. Berwick, S. Edgman-Levitan, A. Edmondon, G. Meyer, D. Michaels, J.M. Morath, C. Vincent, and R. Wachter (2018). 'Transforming concepts in patient safety: a progress report'. *BMJ Quality & Safety* **27**: 1019–1026. https://doi.org/10.1136/bmjqs-2017-007756

Goodrick, E. and T. Reay (2011). 'Constellations of institutional logics: changes in the professional work of pharmacists'. *Work and Occupations* **38**(3): 372–416. https://doi.org/10.1177/0730888411406824 (Original work published 2011)

Greenhalgh, T., G. Robert, F. Macfarlane, P. Bate, and O. Kyriakidou (2004). 'Diffusion of innovations in service organizations: systematic review and recommendations'. *The Milbank Quarterly* **82**(4): 581–629. https://doi.org/10.1111/j.0887-378X.2004.00325.x

Grocott, M.P. (2019). 'Pathway redesign: putting patients ahead of professionals'. *Clinical Medicine* **19**(6): 468–472. https://doi.org/10.7861/clinmed.2019-0292

Hollnagel, E. (2014). *Safety-I and Safety-II: The Past and Future of Safety Management*. Boca Raton, FL, CRC Press.

Hughes, G., S.E. Shaw, and T. Greenhalgh (2020). 'Rethinking integrated care: a systematic hermeneutic review of the literature on integrated care strategies and concepts'. *The Milbank Quarterly* **98**(2): 446–492 https://doi.org/10.1111/1468-0009.12459

Institute of Medicine (2001). *Crossing the Quality Chasm: A New Health System for the 21st Century*. Washington, DC, Institute of Medicine.

Johri, M., F. Beland, and H. Bergman (2003) 'International experiments in integrated care for the elderly: a synthesis of the evidence'. *International Journal of Geriatric Psychiatry* **18**(3): 222–235.
Leary, A., D. Bushe, C. Oldman, J. Lawler, and G. Punshon (2021). 'A thematic analysis of the prevention of future deaths reports in healthcare from HM coroners in England and Wales 2016–2019'. *Journal of Patient Safety and Risk Management* **26**(1): 14–21. https://doi.org/10.1177/2516043521992651
Löwy, I. (1992). 'The strength of loose concepts - boundary concepts, federative experimental strategies and disciplinary growth: the case of immunology'. *History of Science* **30**(4): 371–396.
Lucian Leape Institute (2012). *Order from Chaos: Accelerating Care Integration.* Boston, MA, National Patient Safety Foundation.
Mannion, R. and M. Exworthy (2017). '(Re)making the Procrustean bed? Standardization and customization as competing logics in healthcare'. *International Journal of Health Policy and Management* **6**(6): 301–304. https://doi.org/10.15171/ijhpm.2017.35
Martin, G.P., D. Kocman, T. Stephens, C.J. Peden, and R.M. Pearse (2017). 'Pathways to professionalism? Quality improvement, care pathways, and the interplay of standardisation and clinical autonomy'. *Sociology of Health & Illness* **39**(8): 1214–1329.
May, C.R., D.T. Eton, K. Boehmer, K. Gallacher, K. Hunt, S. MacDonald, F.S. Mair, C.M. May, V.M. Montori, A. Richardson, A.E. Rogers, and N. Shippee (2014). 'Rethinking the patient: using burden of treatment theory to understand the changing dynamics of illness'. *BMC Health Services Research* **26**(14): 281. https://doi.org/10.1186/1472-6963-14-281
McMurray, A. and H. Cooper (2016). 'The nurse navigator: an evolving model of care'. *Collegian: The Australian Journal of Nursing Practice, Scholarship & Research* **24**(2): 205–212.
Melby, L., A. Obstfelder, and R. Hellesø (2018). '"We tie up the loose ends": homecare nursing in a changing health care landscape'. *Global Qualitative Nursing Research* **5** https://doi.org/10.1177/2333393618816780
Meyer, J.W. and B. Rowan (1977). 'Institutionalized organizations: formal structure as myth and ceremony'. *American Journal of Sociology* **83**(2): 340–363.
Morris, S., R. Hunter, A. Ramsay, R. Boaden, C. McKevitt, C. Perry, N. Pursani, A.G. Rudd, L.H. Schwamm, S.J. Turner, P.J. Tyrrell, C.D. Wolfe, and N.J. Fulop (2014). 'Impact of centralising acute stroke services in English metropolitan areas on mortality and length of stay: difference-in-differences analysis'. *British Medical Journal* **349**: g4757. https://doi.org/10.1136/bmj.g4757
National Patient Safety Agency (2007). *The Fifth Report from the Patient Safety Observatory. Safer Care for the Acutely Ill Patient: Learning from Serious Incidents.* London, National Patient Safety Agency.
Noordegraaf, M. (2013). 'Reconfiguring professional work: changing forms of professionalism in public'. *Administration and Society* **48**(7): 783–810 https://doi.org/10.1177/0095399713509242
Noordegraaf, M. (2016). 'Hybrid professionalism and beyond: (new) forms of public professionalism in changing organizational and societal contexts'. *Journal of Professions and Organization* **2**(2): 187–206.
Olsen, C.F., A. Bergland, J. Debesay, A. Bye, and A.G. Langaas (2021) 'Patient flow or the patient's journey? Exploring health care providers' experiences and understandings of implementing a care pathway to improve the quality of transitional care for older people'. *Qualitative Health Research* **31**(9): 1710–1723. https://doi.org/10.1177/10497323211003861

Ouwens, M., H. Wollersheim, R. Hermens, M. Hulscher, and R. Grol (2005). 'Integrated care programmes for chronically ill patients: a review of systematic reviews'. *International Journal for Quality in Health Care* **17**(2): 141–146. https://doi.org/10.1093/intqhc/mzi016

Pinder, R., R. Petchey, S. Shaw, and Y. Carter (2005). 'What's in a care pathway? Towards a cultural cartography of the new NHS'. *Sociology of Health & Illness* **27**(6): 759–779. https://doi.org/10.1111/j.1467-9566.2005.00473.x

Power, M. (1997). *The Audit Society: Rituals of Verification*. Oxford, Oxford University Press.

Prout, A. (1996). 'Actor-network theory, technology and medical sociology: an illustrative analysis of the metred dose inhaler'. *Sociology of Health & Illness* **18**(2):198–219.

Ruef, M. and W.R. Scott (1998). 'A multidimensional model of organizational legitimacy: hospital survival in changing institutional environments'. *Administrative Science Quarterly* **43**(4):877–904.

Schön, D.A. (1993). 'Generative metaphor: a perspective on problem-setting in social policy'. *Metaphor and Thought*. A. Ortony Cambridge, Cambridge University Press: 137–163.

Schrijvers, G., A. van Hoorn, and N. Huiskes (2012). 'The care pathway: concepts and theories: an introduction'. *International Journal of Integrated Care* **12**(Spec Ed Integrated Care Pathways): e192. https://doi.org/10.5334/ijic.812

Scott, J., J. Waring, A.A. Abuosi, Y. Adole Agada-Amade, J.M. Bashar, A. De Brún, H. Cann, P. Crowley, L.H. Dewa, S. Spanos, and S. Wiig (2024). 'International research priorities for integrated care and cross-boundary working: an electronic Delphi study'. *International Journal for Quality in Health Care* **36**(4): mzae095, https://doi.org/10.1093/intqhc/mzae095

Selznick, P. (1957). *Leadership in Administration*. New York, Harper & Row.

Seys, D., E. Coeckelberghs, W. Sermeus, R. Van Zelm, M. Panella, A.B. Payedimarri, and K. Vanhaecht (2021). 'Overview on the target population and methods used in care pathway projects: a narrative review'. *The International Journal of Clinical Practice* **75**(10): e14565. https://doi.org/10.1111/ijcp.14565

Shippee, N.D., N.D. Shah, C.R. May, F.S. Mair, and V.M. Montori (2012). 'Cumulative complexity: a functional, patient-centered model of patient complexity can improve research and practice'. *Journal of Clinical Epidemiology* **65**(10): 1041–1051. https://doi.org/10.1016/j.jclinepi.2012.05.005

Siegel, K. and B.J. Krauss (1991). 'Living with HIV infection: adaptive tasks of seropositive gay men'. *Journal of Health and Social Behavor* **32**: 17–32.

Smeds, M. (2019). 'Managing care pathways for patients with complex care needs'. Linköping Studies in Science and Technology Licentiate Thesis No. 1839. Logistics and Quality Management Department of Management and Engineering Linköping University, SE-581 83 Linköping, Sweden https://liu.diva-portal.org/smash/record.jsf?pid=diva2%3A1315587&dswid=-2168 (accessed 27/3/25)

Suchman, M.C. (1995). 'Managing legitimacy: strategic and institutional approaches'. *Academy of Management Review* **20**(3): 571–610.

Taylor, F.W. (1911). *Principles of Scientific Management*. New York, Harper.

The Health Foundation (2011). *Evidence Scan: Levels of Harm*. London, The Health Foundation. https://www.health.org.uk/sites/default/files/LevelsOfHarm_0.pdf (accessed 28/03/25)

Thorton, P.H. and W. Ocasio (2008). 'Institutional logics'. *The Sage Handbook of Organizational Institutionalism*. R Greenwood, C. Oliver, R. Suddaby, and K. Sahlin-Andersson. London, Sage: 99–129.

Timmermans, S. and M. Berg (2003). *The Gold Standard: The Challenge of Evidence-based Medicine and Standardization in Health Care*. Philadelphia, Templeton University Press.

van der Feltz-Cornelis, C., E. Attree M. Heightman, M. Gabbay, and G. Allsopp (2023). 'Integrated care pathways: a new approach for integrated care systems'. *British Journal of General Practice* **73**(734): 422. https://doi.org/10.3399/bjgp23X734925

Vanahecht, K., M. Panella, R. Van Zelm, and W. Sermeus (2010). An overview on the history and concept of care pathways as complex interventions. *International Journal of Care Pathways* **14**(3): 117–123. https://doi.org/10.1258/jicp.2010.010019

Viver, E., B. Robinson, L. Jenkins, and A. Smit (2024). 'Institutional logics and relational shifts: permeating hierarchies and silos in the healthcare sector'. *Public Management Review* **26**(10): 2943–2965.

WHO (2012). *Modern Health Care Delivery Systems: Care Coordination and the Role of Hospitals*. Copenhagen, Denmark, World Health Organisation Europe.

Wodchis, W.P., A. Dixon, G.M. Anderson, and N. Goodwin (2015). 'Integrating care for older people with complex needs: key insights and lessons from a seven-country cross-case analysis'. *International Journal of Integrated Care* **15**: e021.

Woldrum, K. (1987). Critical pathways: marking the course. *Definition* 2.3: 1–4

Zutshi, A., D. Peikes, and K. Smith (2014). *The Medical Home: What Do We Know, What Do We Need to Know?* Rockville, MD, Agency for Healthcare Research and Quality.

2

REIMAGINING COORDINATION

Sociological Perspectives

Growing recognition of the limitations of rational-linear models in addressing healthcare coordination challenges has prompted calls for approaches that better engage with care system complexity and frontline delivery realities (Hollnagel et al., 2013; Wears et al., 2011). While quality improvement research has largely focused on interventions, a rich tradition of sociological work examining the everyday organisation and delivery of care offers a platform for advancing this agenda (Allen and Pilnick, 2006; Waring et al., 2016). This book draws on and contributes to that body of work.

This chapter introduces ideas about care trajectories, negotiated orders, and sensemaking, to illuminate how professionals organise and coordinate care in everyday settings. It outlines concepts from social worlds and strategic action fields traditions, offering tools to analyse how institutional contexts and practice ecologies shape collective action. It discusses practice-based approaches and Actor Network Theory (ANT) to explore how work is distributed between human and non-human actors, and how patients are enacted through technologies, documents, and situated interactions. Finally, it introduces assemblage thinking to conceptualise care as a dynamic and contingent configuration of people, practices, concerns, technologies, and organisational structures. Together, these ideas establish the book's conceptual groundwork. Chapter 3 builds on this by showing how these theoretical resources inform the study's analytical framework.

Care Trajectories

As an alternative to pathways thinking, my point of departure is the care trajectory concept developed by Strauss et al. (1985). Derived from extensive

DOI: 10.4324/9781003475019-4

ethnographic research in North American hospitals, it was designed to capture the complexity of healthcare processes and encompasses the 'physiological unfolding of a patient's disease' and 'the total organization of work done over that course, plus the impact on those involved with that work and its organisation' (Strauss et al., 1985: 8).

Care trajectories are emergent. They are shaped by contingencies arising from disease progression, organisational and technological factors, and the dynamic interactions of patients, families and providers. In contrast to the linearity, order, and formality associated with the pathways metaphor, thinking about the organisation of care through the prism of trajectories directs attention to the provisional and unpredictable qualities of care processes, as well as the profoundly distributed (and decidedly non-linear) dimensions of service delivery. Much of healthcare work is focused on keeping trajectories aligned despite these instabilities. Reserving the term coordination to refer to the formal processes and mechanisms for ordering activity, Strauss (1985, 1988) introduced the concept of articulation work to capture the ongoing effort required to manage contingencies, resolve breakdowns, and adjust workflows to keep trajectories on track.

Organisation and Organising

Negotiated Orders

Ideas about the dynamic qualities of care trajectories stem from Strauss and colleagues' work on negotiated orders (Strauss et al., 1963, 1964). Organisational studies had previously been dominated by functional approaches that emphasised stable structures, formal rules and plans, over variability, emergence, and change. Drawing on symbolic interactionism, Strauss et al., developed the negotiated order perspective to conceptualise the 'ordered flux' of organisational processes observed in ethnographic studies of two North American psychiatric hospitals. Underlining the recursive relationship between social order and social interaction, the approach showed how negotiations create social orders, which in turn condition negotiation processes.

> The realm of rules could be usefully pictured as a tiny island of structured stability around which swirled and beat a vast ocean of negotiation.
>
> *(Strauss et al., 1964: 313)*

This perspective marked a significant effort to bridge micro and macro perspectives in sociological theory (Berger and Luckman, 1966). Critics, however, contended that by downplaying formal structure, it struggled to address the constraints on action in organisational environments (Benson, 1977a, 1977b, 1978; Day and Day, 1977, 1978; Dingwall and Strong, 1985). In response, Strauss introduced the concepts of 'negotiation context' and 'structural context' (Strauss, 1978a: 247–258) to draw attention to proximal and distal influences on negotiations. Despite these additions, debates about structural constraints and agent-driven negotiation processes persisted, indicating challenges in applying the framework.

Sensemaking

From within organisational studies and social psychology, Weick also advanced a process view of organisation. While Strauss et al. (1963, 1964) underscored negotiation processes, Weick foregrounded sensemaking (Weick, 1995). For Weick, organisations are fluid and require continual accomplishment. They gain collective meaning in the interactions between the raw data of experience and the shared interpretative resources through which actors make sense of these experiences. Not to be confused with interpretation, sensemaking is performative; it is located in the material and discursive activities through which members organise their work, account for their actions, and construct the objects of their practice (Mills, 1940; Scott and Lyman, 1968).

Sensemaking can be informal – embedded in everyday social interactions – or formal, as in meetings, assessment processes, and record creation. People constantly make sense of changing situations, revising their understandings as new information emerges. Sensemaking may start as an individual process, but it is inherently social and often collective. Like the negotiated order perspective, however, many remained uncomfortable about the displacement of the material reality of organisation engendered by an understanding founded on conceptual and symbolic phenomena (Robichaud and Cooren, 2013).

Contexts, Ecosystems, and Action Fields

To examine the relationship between action and context in this study, I draw on social worlds (Strauss, 1978b, 1982) and strategic action fields (Fligstein and McAdam, 2011) perspectives.

Social Worlds

Social worlds are collective actors organised around shared concerns and offer a useful framework for analysing individual services within the hip fracture trajectory. The approach focuses on the constellation of people, materials, technologies, ideas, representations, practices, and discourses that comprise such formations. Its analytic strength lies in situating an issue within this broader ecosystem, which gives it meaning (Dingwall, 1999; Star, 1995). Some studies treat the social world as the primary unit of analysis, while others have examined particular activities within or across them (Clarke and Star, 2008). Increasingly, attention has turned to the relationships and interactions between different social worlds, with boundaries becoming a central focus of inquiry.

Strategic Action Fields

Social worlds thinking helps illuminate the services involved in hip fracture care and their interfaces. To analyse trajectory mobilisation across services, I also draw on strategic action fields thinking (Fligstein and McAdam, 2011). A strategic action field refers to a domain where actors – individuals, organisations, or groups – engage in strategic interactions to achieve specific goals. Like social worlds, the concept is ecological, encompassing multiple actors who operate within an institutional context that shapes norms, rules, and power dynamics. But whereas social worlds are meso-level social orders constituted around collective interests, strategic action fields are constructed on a situational basis around a common goal and can transcend the boundaries of social worlds. This distinction is especially relevant in hip fracture care, where services accommodate a wide range of patients and conditions. Integrating strategic action fields into the social worlds framework enables analysis of the constellation of actors involved in the hip fracture trajectory – within and across social worlds – and accounts for the contextual conditions shaping care mobilisation and coordination. This combined approach offers a nuanced understanding of how individual trajectories intersect with multiple, sometimes competing, trajectories across services and how transitions between them are organised.

Patients

This book offers a new way of thinking about patients. Ideas about care pathways and patient trajectories assume patients are pre-given social entities who progress immutably through healthcare systems. Here I adopt a non-essentialist conceptualisation: people do not arrive in healthcare systems as ready-made patients – work is required to make them objects of practice for a range of purposes. While objectification is often criticised for its association with dehumanisation, this approach follows Berger and Luckman's (1966) more neutral interpretation, in which objectification is understood as a mechanism for enabling action. Viewed in this light, 'the patient' is an organisational artefact, an 'effect' of processes through which certain concerns – corporeal, material, psychological, social – are made visible and rendered meaningful for care work (Allen, 2015). Rather than focusing on how services are organised around patients, I focus on how patients are enacted in healthcare practices, how specific concerns come to the fore at different moments, shaping what is recognised as important, actionable, or problematic, and the consequences of these object formation processes for trajectory mobilisation.

In conceptualising patients as objects of practice, the analysis draws on Mol's (2002) insights on ontological multiplicity in medicine. In her study of atherosclerosis across labs, clinics, operating theatres, epidemiology, and research, she invites a conceptual shift from disease as a passive object to the practices that enact it in varied forms. This book builds on this framing but differs in several respects. First, it centres on the patient rather than the disease. The tests, investigations and representations that are central to Mol's analysis are considered only insofar as they are featured in different enactments of the patient. Second, whereas Mol's analysis is primarily topographical – it centres on the sites in which disease is enacted – the analysis in this book is temporal–spatial – it traces practices of object formation as care is mobilised over time and across services. Third, I consider the appropriateness or effectiveness of enactments, asking what can change for care to be safely coordinated and mobilised. This orients the analysis to how patients are constituted in care processes and how this impacts trajectory mobilisation.

Transitions

A central concern in this book is how transitions between social worlds are organised and coordinated. Research on care system transitions remains limited and conceptually underdeveloped (Aase and Waring, 2020). In professional and policy literature, boundary crossing at service interfaces is typically framed as the transfer of responsibility from one provider to another, with success hinging on role clarity and accurate information exchange. These assumptions are reflected in the title of a manual – 'Passing the Baton' – produced by the National Leadership and Innovation Agency for Health (2008) to guide 'seamless transfers of care' from the hospital.

> In a relay race, you cannot just throw the baton up in the air and hope the next person catches it. You must keep a firm hand on the baton until you are sure the next person catches it.
>
> *(p. 4)*

In this analogy, the patient is imagined as an immutable entity, passed unchanged from one provider to the next. In contrast, this study conceptualises transition as an institutional status passage (Glaser and Strauss, 1971): a process of translating the patient from one social world's collective object of practice into another's. This builds on earlier research showing how nurses mediate service relationships and parse patient identities in navigating interfaces (Allen, 2015: Chapter 5). While, that study aimed to make visible the skills and knowledge underpinning this significant – but often overlooked – aspect of nursing work, here, the focus shifts to the relationships between services at transition interfaces, the infrastructural arrangements through which patients are organised and enacted for the purposes of transition, the object qualities of these enactments, and their implications for trajectory mobilisation.

Work, Practices, and Technologies

At its core, this book is about everyday work practices. It centres on the division of labour in hip fracture care, the distribution of activity within and between teams, and the arrangements that enable concerted action. The analysis is informed by a practice-based approach (Nicolini, 2012), draws on insights from ANT (Latour, 2005), and engages with studies of visible and invisible work.

Founded on the shared orientations of praxeology (Bourdieu, 1990), ethnomethodology (Garfinkel, 1967), structuration theory (Giddens, 1984), and activity theory (Engeström, 2000), a practice-based approach attends to how agents engage with socio-material conditions to pursue objectives. It rests on four theoretical premises. First, social phenomena are practical accomplishments, continuously reproduced through human agency. Second, artefacts – material (tools, technologies, instruments), cognitive (categories, rules of thumb, scores), formal, or informal – mediate activity. Third, practices emerge from the dynamic interactions of people and the material and social world. Fourth, relationships within and across practice networks can serve particular interests (Ortner, 1984).

ANT complements a practice approach by drawing attention to the socio-material relationships shaping how action unfolds. Technologies are not merely tools used in practice; they are integral to how work is structured, coordinated, and made visible or invisible. Their design features – such as scripts (Akrich, 1992) and affordances (Gibson, 1979) – play a key role in shaping what practitioners do and how they do it. ANT's symmetrical treatment of human and non-human actors highlights how agency is distributed: technologies prescribe, constrain, and enable action, while also being adapted and shaped by users (Berg, 1999; Timmermans, 1988). In healthcare, technologies such as clinical pathways, electronic records, and protocols are central to organising care, and this study contributes to research examining their use in practice (e.g. Berg, 1997a, 1997b, 1999; Dodier, 1998; Greatbatch et al., 2006).

This book also builds on the sociology of invisible work (Allen, 2015; Star and Strauss, 1999; Suchman, 1995). No work is intrinsically visible. Visibility is contingent, shaped by various indicators that shift depending on context and standpoint (Muller, 1999; Star and Strauss, 1999). Formal technologies such as clinical pathways are not neutral: they are laced with interests, elevating the contributions of some actors while rendering others invisible (Pinder et al., 2005). My research has shown that nurses make a crucial contribution to the organisation and coordination of patient trajectories (Allen, 2015), sustaining coherence and supporting quality and safety. Yet it remains background work (Star and Strauss, 1999) – visible in principle but typically taken for granted.

Invisible work is especially hard to recognise because the better it is done, the less visible it becomes (Suchman, 1995). Articulation work (Strauss, 1985) restores order in the face of disruption but lies outside rationalised models of labour (Berg, 1997a; Strauss, 1985, 1988). Sociologists distinguish between

formal knowledge – codified and institutionally recognised – and 'working knowledge', which is practical, situated, and often improvised (Ellingsen and Monteiro, 2003; Gherardi, 2000). Working knowledge is vital to navigating the gaps, uncertainties, and contradictions of formal systems, relying on the invisible coordination of experiential, organisational, and relational knowledge.

Invisible work comes in many forms, but it is still work. It adds to the cognitive, emotional, and organisational load of practitioners and competes with formally recognised – and visible – roles and responsibilities. Attending to invisible work reveals not only what holds organisational life together, but also what formal systems routinely overlook.

Assemblage Thinking

While the foundational ideas and theoretical perspectives discussed have value for zooming in – to analyse the diverse practices and actors involved in enacting patients and mobilising the hip fracture trajectory – zooming out to conceptualise the whole trajectory requires a different lens. For this, I draw on assemblage thinking.

Originating from Deleuze and Guattari (1987), an assemblage is a configuration of diverse human and non-human elements that come together to form a provisional whole. Unlike structured unities, where interdependent parts function together like organs in the human body, assemblages are fluid and dynamic (Müller, 2015), shaped through processes of territorialisation (which stabilises relationships), de-territorialisation (which disrupts or unsettles them), and re-territorialisation (where new arrangements emerge). Assemblages derive agency from the interactions between components, rather than any individual part.

In medical sociology, assemblage theory has been applied to the networks surrounding bodies during ill-health (Fox, 2011); the relational nature of frailty at the intersection of ageing bodies and their environments (Cluley, Fox and Radnor, 2021); and how individuals connect disparate signs and events into patterns recognised as illness before diagnosis (Locock et al., 2016). Viewing trajectories through the lens of assemblages highlights the interrelations between social worlds and reveals how trajectory scale, qualities, and complexity evolve over time and space.

Summary

This chapter has outlined the intellectual traditions and the theoretical frameworks underpinning the analysis throughout this book. In contrast to the linearity of pathways thinking, sociology offers rich concepts for illuminating the complexity of health and social care organisations. Yet, systematically studying these processes is not easy. Building on these foundations, the next chapter describes the study's methods, materials, and analytic framework.

References

Aase, K. and J. Waring (2020). 'Crossing boundaries: establishing a framework for researching quality and safety in care transitions'. *Applied Ergonomics* **89**: 103228.

Akrich, M. (1992). 'The de-scription of technical objects'. *Shaping Technology/Building Society: Studies in Sociotechnical Change*. W.E. Bijker and J. Law Cambridge, MA, MIT Press: 205–224.

Allen, D. (2015). *The Invisible Work of Nurses: Hospitals, Organisation and Healthcare*, London and New York, Routledge.

Allen, D. and A. Pilnick (2006). 'Making connections: healthcare as a case study in the social organisation of work'. *The Social Organisation of Healthcare Work*. D. Allen and A. Pilnick. Oxford, Blackwell Publishing: 1–17.

Benson, J.K. (1977a). 'Innovation and crisis in organizational analysis'. *The Sociological Quarterly* **18**: 5–18.

Benson, J.K. (1977b). 'Organisations: a dialectical view'. *Administrative Science Quarterly* **22**: 1–21.

Benson, J.K. (1978). 'Reply to Maines'. *The Sociological Quarterly* **19**: 497–501.

Berg, M. (1997a). *Rationalizing Medical Work: Decision-support Techniques and Medical Practices*. Cambridge, Cambridge University Press.

Berg, M. (1997b). 'Of forms, containers and the electronic medical record: some tools for a sociology of the formal'. *Science, Technology and Human Values* **22**(4): 403–434. https://doi.org/10.1177/016224399702200401

Berg, M. (1999). 'Accumulating and coordinating: occasions for information technologies in medical work'. *Computer Supported Cooperative Work* **8**: 373–401.

Berger, P. and T. Luckman (1966). *The Social Construction of Reality: A Treatise in the Sociology of Knowledge*. London, Penguin Books Ltd.

Bourdieu, P. (1990). *The Logic of Practice*. Cambridge, Polity Press.

Clarke, A. and S.L. Star (2008). 'The social worlds framework: a theory/method package'. *Science and Technology Studies Handbook*. E.J. Hackett, O. Amsterdamska, M. Lynch, and J. Wajcman. Cambridge, MA, The MIT Press: 113–137. Available from: https://www.researchgate.net/publication/261948477_The_Social_Worlds_Framework_A_TheoryMethods_Package (accessed 31/3/25).

Cluley, V., N. Fox, and Z. Radnor (2021). '"Becoming frail": a more than human exploration'. *Health* **27**(3): 417–434. https://doi.org/10.1177/13634593211038460

Day, R.A. and J.V. Day (1977). 'A review of the current state of negotiated order theory: an appreciation and critique'. *The Sociological Quarterly* **18**: 126–142.

Day R.A. and J.V. Day (1978). 'Reply to Maines'. *The Sociological Quarterly* **19**: 499–501.

Deleuze, G. and F. Guattari (1987). *A Thousand Plateaus: Capitalism and Schizophrenia*. Minneapolis, University of Minneapolis Press.

Dingwall, R. (1999). 'On the non-negotiable in sociological life'. *Qualitative Sociology as Everyday Life*. B. Glassner and R. Hertz. Thousand Oaks, CA, Sage: 215–225.

Dingwall, R. and P.M. Strong (1985). 'The interactional study of organizations: a critique and reformulation'. *Journal of Contemporary Ethnography* **14**: 205–231.

Dodier, N. (1998). 'Clinical practice and procedures in occupational medicine: a study of the framing of individuals'. *Differences in Medicine: Unravelling Practices, Techniques, and Bodies*. M. Berg and A.M. Mol. Durham and London, Duke University Press: 53–85

Ellingsen, G. and E. Monteiro (2003). 'Mechanisms for producing a working knowledge: enacting, orchestrating, and organizing'. *Information and Organization* **13**: 203–229.

Engeström, Y. (2000). 'Activity Theory as a framework for analysing and redesigning work'. *Ergonomics* **43**(7): 960–972.

Fligstein N. and D. McAdam (2011). 'Toward a general theory of strategic action fields'. *Sociological Theory* **29**: 1–26. https://doi.org/10.1111/j.1467-9558.2010.01385.x

Fox, N. (2011). 'The ill-health assemblage: beyond the body-with organs'. *Health Sociology Review* **20**(4): 359–371.

Garfinkel, A. (1967). *Studies in Ethnomethodology*. New Jersey, Prentice Hill.

Gherardi, S. (2000). 'Practice-based theorizing on learning and knowing in organizations'. *Organization*, **7**(2): 211–223. https://doi.org/10.1177/135050840072001

Gibson, J.J. (1979). *The Senses Considered as Perceptual Systems*. London, Allen and Unwin.

Giddens, A. (1984). *The Constitution of Society: Outline of a Theory of Structuration*. Cambridge, Polity Press.

Glaser, B.G. and A.L. Strauss (1971). *Status Passage*. New Jersey, Aldine Transaction.

Greatbatch, D., J. Hanlon, A. Goode, T. O'Caithain, T. Strangleman, and D. Luff (2006). 'Telephone triage, expert systems and clinical expertise'. *The Social Organisation of Healthcare Work*. D. Allen and A. Pilnick. Oxford, Blackwell Publishing: 115–142.

Hollnagel, E., J. Braithwaite, and R. Wears (2013). 'Preface: on the need for resilience in health care'. *Resilient Health Care*. E. Hollnagel, J. Braithwaite, and R. Wears. Farnham, Surrey, Ashgate: xiv–xxvi.

Latour, B. (2005). *Reassembling the Social: An Introduction to Actor-Network-Theory*. Oxford, Oxford University Press.

Locock, L., S. Nettleton, S. Kirkpatrick, S. Ryan, and S. Ziebland (2016). '"I knew before I was told": breaches, cues and clues in the diagnostic assemblage'. *Social Science & Medicine* **154**: 85–92. https://doi.org/10.1016/j.socscimed.2016.02.037

Mills, C.W. (1940). 'Situated actions and vocabularies of motive.' *American Sociological Review* **5**(6): 904–913.

Mol, A.M. (2002). *The Body Multiple: Ontology in Medical Practice*. Durham, NC, Duke University Press.

Müller, M. (2015). 'Assemblage and actor-networks: rethinking socio-material power, politics and space'. *Geography Compass* **9**(1): 27–41. https://doi.org/10.1111/gec3.12192

Muller, M.J. (1999). 'Invisible work of telephone operators: an ethnocritical analysis'. *Computer Supported Cooperative Work* **8**: 31–61.

National Leadership and Innovation Agency for Healthcare (2008). *Passing the Baton*. Llanharan, Wales: National Leadership and Innovation Agency for Healthcare.

Nicolini, D. (2012). *Practice Theory, Work and Organization: An Introduction*. Oxford, Oxford University Press.

Ortner, S. (1984). 'Theory in anthropology since the sixties'. *Comparative Studies in Society and History* **26**(1): 126–166.

Pinder, R., R. Petchey, S. Shaw, and Y. Carter (2005). 'What's in a care pathway? Towards a cultural cartography of the new NHS.' *Sociology of Health & Illness* **27**(6): 759–779 https://doi.org/10.1111/j.1467-9566.2005.00473.x

Robichaud D. and F. Cooren (2013). *Organization and Organizing: Materiality, Agency and Discourse*. New York, NY: Routledge.

Scott, M.B. and S.M. Lyman (1968). 'Accounts'. *American Sociological Review* **33**(1): 46–62.

Star, S.L. (ed) (1995). *Ecologies of Knowledge: Work and Politics in Science and Technology*. Albany, State University of New York Press.

Star, S.L. and A.L. Strauss (1999). 'Layers of silence, arenas of voice: the ecology of visible and invisible work'. *Computer Supported Cooperative Work* **8**: 9–30.

Strauss, A. (1988). 'The articulation of project work: an organizational process'. *The Sociological Quarterly* **29**: 163–178.

Strauss, A.L. (1978a). *Negotiations: Varieties, Contexts, Processes, and Social Order*. San Francisco, Jossey-Bass.
Strauss, A.L. (1978b). 'A social world perspective'. *Studies in Symbolic Interaction* **1**: 119–128.
Strauss, A.L. (1982). 'Social worlds and legitimation processes'. *Studies in Symbolic Interaction* **4**: 171–190.
Strauss, A.L. (1985). 'Work and the division of labor'. *The Sociological Quarterly* **26**(1): 1–19.
Strauss, A.L., S. Fagerhaugh, B. Suczet, and C. Wiener (1985). *Social Organization of Medical Work*. Chicago, IL, University of Chicago Press.
Strauss, A.L., L. Schatzman, R. Bucher, D. Ehrlich, and M. Sabshin (1963). 'The hospital and its negotiated order'. *The Hospital in Modern Society*. E. Freidson. New York, Free Press: 147–169.
Strauss, A.L., L. Schatzman, R. Bucher, D. Ehrlich, and M. Sabshin (1964). *Psychiatric Ideologies and Institutions*. London, The Free Press of Glencoe Collier-Macmillan.
Suchman, L. (1995). 'Making work visible'. *Communications of the ACM* **38**(9): 56–64.
Timmermans, S. (1988). 'Mutual tuning of multiple trajectories'. *Symbolic Interaction* **21**(4): 425–440. https://doi.org/10.1525/si.1998.21.4.425.
Waring, J., D. Allen, J. Braithwaite, and J. Sandall (2016). 'Healthcare quality and safety: a review of policy, practice, and research'. *The Sociology of Healthcare Safety and Quality*. D. Allen, J. Braithwaite, J. Sandall, and J. Waring. Chichester, West Sussex, Wiley Blackwell: 2–17.
Wears, RL., E. Hollnagel, and J. Braithwaite (2011). *Resilient Health Care Volume 2: The Resilience of Everyday Clinical Work*. Farnham, Ashgate.
Weick, K.E. (1995). *Sensemaking in Organizations*. Thousand Oaks, CA, Sage.

3

STUDYING COORDINATION IN THE WILD

Case, Methods, and Theoretical Framework

This chapter introduces the research study at the heart of the book – a detailed ethnographic exploration of how patients, care, and treatment were organised and mobilised across the hip fracture trajectory. Conducted in a single region of Wales, the study followed the work of a large NHS organisation spanning acute, community, and primary healthcare services, alongside the Welsh Ambulance Service and several local authorities responsible for social care planning and commissioning. The hip fracture trajectory spans multiple service domains and professional groups, offering a rich site for examining coordination in front-line practice.

The chapter sets the scene by describing the organisation of hip fracture care in the region and outlining the study's research design, data collection methods, and analytical approach. It also introduces the key concepts that informed the analysis and those that emerged through it, laying the foundation for the chapters that follow.

Hip Fracture

Hip fractures are common. The hospital in the study admitted approximately 500 people annually. Most injuries occur in people over 60. Typically, the result of fall – owing to frailty, reduced vision, or mobility problems – hip fractures are often linked to osteoporosis, a loss of mineral density and tissue that weakens bones. The incidence of injury is higher in women, who are more prone to osteoporosis. An unscheduled event, hip fracture generally requires surgery and hospital admission, with rehabilitation continuing for several months. Recovery is variable; NHS guidance suggests hospital stays range from one to four weeks (https://www.nhs.uk/conditions/broken-hip, accessed 31/03/25).

DOI: 10.4324/9781003475019-5

The hip fracture trajectory was selected as an illustrative case because it spans the full spectrum of health and social care – from emergency response through hospital treatment to community rehabilitation and offered an opportunity to examine rational-linear and emergent organisational processes. Although guided by evidence-based guidelines and performance standards (NICE, 2011), trajectory management is often complicated by co-existing health conditions common in older patients. Recovery and rehabilitation must also be tailored to individuals' functional capacities, home environments, and the availability of caregivers. Progression along the trajectory involves coordinating care across multiple services and managing transitions between them, providing a valuable opportunity to examine how diverse coordination mechanisms – structured, linear, flexible, and emergent – intersect.

Methods

There is a substantial body of ethnographic research on contemporary care systems, and recent years have witnessed growing interest in ethnographic approaches for quality improvement (Dixon-Woods, 2003; Sutton et al., 2014; Taxis and Barber, 2003). While there exists a wealth of richly descriptive studies of individual care settings (e.g. Bruni, 2023; Featherstone and Northcott, 2018; Nugus et al., 2011; Strong and Dingwall, 1979), research on transition (*pace* Allen et al., 2012; Skovgaard et al., 2022; Waring et al., 2014) is less common. To my knowledge, no studies have comprehensively explored the social–material organisation of an entire patient trajectory.

A distinctive contribution of this book is its focus on object formation as the central analytic lens. Building on ideas introduced in the previous chapter, this approach examines how patients are enacted – actively constructed, negotiated, and transformed – through organisational practices, technologies, documentation, and interactions across multiple settings. By tracing how the 'object' of care is differently constituted at different sites and moments, the analysis reveals how coordination is shaped by what is centred, foregrounded, or excluded. Object formation is not merely descriptive, but performative – a practical mechanism through which care work is ordered, enabled, and rendered actionable in complex systems (Mol, 2002). Placing object formation at the heart of the study makes visible the shifting logics and practical compromises that underpin the delivery of hip fracture care.

This singular focus was inspired by two classic ethnographies. First, *Social Organization of Medical Work* by Strauss et al. (1985) marked a shift from studies of professions, roles, and the division of labour to a comprehensive analysis of healthcare *work*. This distinctive lens led to the development of foundational concepts – safety work, machine work, sentimental work, articulation work, patient work, and comfort work. Second, *Patterns of Time in Hospital Work* (Zerubavel, 1979) examined how time is structured in hospitals, revealing tensions between organisational efficiency and patient-centeredness.

Both texts exemplify how detailed description and a focused analytical framework can illuminate overlooked dimensions of a familiar field. I encountered these works early in my academic career. They resonated with my everyday experiences as a nurse and revealed aspects of healthcare I had previously taken for granted.

This study was conducted as part of a three-year Improvement Science Fellowship funded by The Health Foundation. The Fellowship not only provided the time and resources to undertake this research – an uncommon privilege for senior academics – but also afforded the agility and freedom essential for advancing the work. The flexibility that traditionally characterises ethnographic research is increasingly difficult to sustain in today's research environment, where externally funded projects are governed by restrictive accountability frameworks.

Fieldwork extended over two years. I sat alongside call handlers in the Emergency Medical Services Control Centre and the Community Resources Hub, which coordinated community care referrals. I went on ride-outs with ambulance crews and rapid responders, accompanied hospital porters moving patients between the ward and Operating Department, and joined St John Ambulance Cymru personnel transporting patients home. I shadowed key individuals and events in the Emergency Department, Orthogeriatric Ward, Anaesthetics Room, Post-Anaesthetic Care Unit, Discharge Lounge, Community Rehabilitation Service, Community Nursing Service, and Trauma and Orthopaedic Outpatient Clinic. I also observed surgical work in the trauma and orthopaedic operating theatre. My focus was on front-stage activity. Time constraints precluded observation of backstage workers: radiographers conducting scans, radiologists interpreting results, laboratory staff processing tests, and the administrative, technical, and data analytics staff who maintained the information systems underpinning front-stage work.

Despite developments in rapid approaches (Vindrola-Padros and Vindrola-Padros, 2018), traditional ethnography involves extended immersion in a setting. In this study, the time spent in individual services was more limited. To mitigate this, I sought out enthusiastic participants willing to be shadowed and used this as my point of entry into the field. Data generation was focused from the outset on the management, organisation and mobilisation of care. I also benefitted from being able to draw on previous experience of studying the same healthcare setting (albeit for different purposes) and a clinical background, allowing me to quickly orient to the field and concentrate on core concerns.

For practical reasons, I could not follow individual patients through their full trajectory. Occasionally, the organisation of fieldwork led me to meet the same people at different stages of their care. These occurrences were welcome, but entirely serendipitous. While hip fracture was the focus of the research, the services observed managed a range of trajectories. Whenever possible, I have deployed data related to hip fractures in progressing the analysis marshalled in this book. On occasion, however, I have included fieldnotes from other patient trajectories where these illustrate important analytic insights.

Materials

Primary data sources included fieldwork-based observations and informal interviews with health and social care providers, alongside a large volume of formal and informal documents and artefacts (protocols, care record proforma, referral documents, checklists). A small number of audio-recorded interviews were also conducted (n = 13). Observations and informal interviews were recorded as low-inference fieldnotes – documenting what was observed and said without interpretation. Fieldnotes were word-processed, interviews were transcribed, and documents were catalogued by service and transition interface.

A total of 108 participants were enrolled in the research – either by consenting to being shadowed or participating in interviews. Patients and families were not formally recruited but were informed of the study and could opt out of observation. In some cases, where individuals lacked the capacity to consent, I withdrew from the field. The study received ethics and research governance approvals (IRAS ID: 94593). Further details of fieldwork data are provided in the introductory sections of Parts 2–4. Appendix 1 summarises data sources.

Fieldnotes and interview data were anonymised and uploaded into ATLAS.ti for coding and data management. Documents and artefacts were manually analysed. I approached documents and artefacts not just as sources of information, but as topics – examining how they were implicated in everyday practice. I observed participants interacting with both digital and paper systems, recognising that documents do not simply carry information but participate in making, structuring, and validating it (Berg, 1996; Berg and Bowker, 1997). These materials were also used as a resource to explore how professional and organisational concerns were formalised for trajectory mobilisation.

Theoretical Framework

Strauss et al. (1985) introduced the care trajectory concept to highlight the complexity and unpredictability of healthcare organisations, inspiring studies on patient experiences (Pescosolido, 2014), illness careers (Glaser and Strauss, 2007), life-course dynamics (Pavalko, 1997), inter-professional tensions (Allen et al., 2004a), and the interplay of multiple trajectories, including technology use (Timmermans, 1988). Yet having brought the fluidity of healthcare processes to the fore, the concept remained insufficiently theorised for analysing the network of relations and organisational contingencies shaping trajectories (Allen et al., 2004a; Strauss et al., 1985). While routinely deployed to denote care processes, few studies have exploited the concept as 'a means of analytically ordering the immense variety of events' (Strauss et al., 1985) through which trajectories evolve (Allen, 2024). Developed through an abductive approach (Timmermans and Tavory, 2012), the theoretical framework outlined in this book seeks to address this gap.

Translational Mobilisation Theory (TMT) (Allen, 2018; Allen and May, 2017) informed data generation and provided an initial lens to examine the socio-material arrangements mobilising hip fracture care. The constant comparative method (Glaser, 1965) was used to refine and extend the framework, leading to the development of new conceptual tools to account for (a) the coordination and organisation of transitions, and (b) how patients were enacted as objects of professional practice. Assemblage thinking (Deleuze and Guattari, 1987) was incorporated to conceptualise the trajectory as an emergent and dynamic whole.

Translational Mobilisation Theory

TMT is a mid-range sociological theory of organisation, designed to support the analysis of collective action which cannot be organised through bureaucratic or linear models (Hernes, 2014). Advancing understanding of such organisational forms is both a sociological and practical concern (Farjoun, 2010; Tsoukas & Chia, 2002), but investigating these processes is challenging (Allen and May, 2017).

Originating from research on the work of nurses (Allen, 2015a), a substantial body of ethnographic studies of healthcare work (Allen, 1997, 2000, 2001, 2009, 2015b; Allen et al., 2004a, 2004b), and conceptual insights from Normalisation Process Theory (May, 2013a, 2013b; May and Finch, 2009), TMT integrates the negotiated order perspective (Strauss et al., 1964), sensemaking (Weick, 1995), and strategic action fields theory (Fligstein and McAdam, 2011) with insights from Actor-Network Theory (Latour, 2005). It rests on four broad theoretical assumptions:

- **An ecological view of work systems** that attends to the interrelations between people, materials, and technologies and how these are shaped by – and shape – the context of action (Fligstein & McAdam, 2011; Strauss, 1978, 1982)
- **A process-oriented understanding of organisation**, in which human action and formal structures are conceptualised as operating in a dynamic, recursive relationship (Strauss et al., 1963, 1964; Weick, 1995)
- **A practice-based approach** that emphasises how actors make sense of, and respond to, everyday challenges, with particular attention to the mediating role of artefacts and technologies (Bourdieu, 1990; Engeström, 2000; Garfinkel, 1967; Giddens, 1984; Nicolini, 2012)
- **A socio-material perspective** which entails an analytic sensitivity to the distribution of activity between human and non-human actors, which are afforded symmetrical treatment in the analysis (Latour, 2005).

TMT comprises three core components:

- **Projects**: The units of analysis in TMT, projects are goal-oriented enterprises involving a network of actors, tools, practices, and conventions (Allen and May, 2017). In this study, the hip fracture trajectory was analysed as interrelated projects involving (a) the organisation of care and treatment within discrete social worlds and (b) the management of transitions between them.
- **Strategic Action Fields**: The institutional contexts in which projects are mobilised. These fields shape action through:
  - *Organising logics*: Shared normative conventions that define the scope and purpose of action;
  - *Interpretative repertoires*: Formal and informal cognitive artefacts and sensemaking resources;
  - *Materials*: Physical infrastructure, technologies, and other concrete resources;
  - *Structures*: Roles, entities, positions, policies, and interfaces that shape collective action.

In this study, the strategic action fields that conditioned the hip fracture trajectory were both embedded in, and extended beyond, individual social worlds.

- **Mechanisms**: The processes through which actors mobilise and sustain projects within a strategic action field:
  - *Object formation* – the creation of objects of practice through the use of available interpretative resources.
  - *Reflexive monitoring* – the evaluation of a field of action to generate awareness of project trajectories.
  - *Articulation* – the responsive coordination of people, tasks, and materials.
  - *Translation* – the mediation of perspectives and transfer of practice objects across settings.
  - *Sensemaking* – the use of interpretative resources to create meaning from unmediated experiences, order activity, and account for action.

By examining the relationships between projects, strategic action fields, and mechanisms, TMT offers a framework for understanding how action is shaped by, and in turn shapes, organisational context (Allen and May, 2017).

Transitions

In this study, transitions are conceptualised as discrete projects of collective action aimed at institutional status passages between social worlds (Glaser and Strauss, 1971). To examine these systematically, two additional concepts were introduced.

- **Transition Interface**: the boundaries between services and how their respective social worlds and strategic action fields give rise to, and create the conditions for, transitions.
- **Transition Infrastructure**: the socio-material arrangements and mechanisms of action that mediate collective action across transition interfaces.

Object Formation and the Enactment of Patients

The constitution of patients is a major driver in the organisation of care, and the fieldwork attended closely to these activities. In the initial phase of analysis, I coded significant quantities of data as examples of object formation, but it became clear that more granular conceptualisation was necessary. Not only were patients enacted in different ways around distinctive constellations of concerns, but these enactments also reflected different organising logics and had different object qualities.

- **Clinical logics** enacted patients as:
  - *Professional objects* aligned with specialist ontologies
  - *Intra-professional objects* supporting continuity of care
  - *Interdisciplinary objects* enabling collective decision-making
- **Administrative logics** produced patients as:
  - *Triage objects* for prioritising care
  - *Allocative objects* for resource distribution
  - *Referral objects* for accessing services
- **Mobilisation logics** generated patients as:
  - *Trajectory objects* for managing care progression
  - *Transition objects* for coordinating movement between services
- **Service logics** enacted patients as:
  - *Contractual objects* for managing risk and responsibility
  - *Collective objects* aligned with shared institutional goals—where the patient is 'more than one but less than many' *(Strathern, 1991).*

These enactments coexisted in practice, reflecting the interweaving of clinical, administrative, and mobilisation logics in everyday work. Coexistence was both formal, inscribed in coordinating documents, and informal, embedded in everyday routines. Transition objects are distinctive objects of practice, temporary stabilisations, that translate the patient from one collective object of practice to another, playing a central role in mediating status passages and coordinating activity across social worlds.

As well as reflecting different organising logics, patients had different object qualities. In some circumstances, they were enacted as *narrative objects*. Typically summative, and loosely formulated, narrative objects exhibited flexible stability, providing a temporary holding ground to enable cooperation. On other occasions, patients were enacted as *technical objects* (Rheinberger, 1997). Derived from studies of the history of science, technical objects are established, well understood and have reliable properties. They simplify and render invisible much of the complex work that underpins them, a process which is referred to as black boxing in actor network theory (Latour, 2005). Typically inscribed in formal documentation, in contrast to narrative objects, *technical objects* were concrete, specific, fixed, stable, and ready-to-hand. Patients were also constituted as *epistemic objects* (Knorr Cetina, 1997). In the philosophy of science and knowledge, the concept of epistemic objects, refers to objects or entities that are not fully understood or known, yet they drive inquiry and serve as focal points for interdisciplinary collaboration. Poorly defined, engagement with epistemic objects can lead to changes in understanding, allowing them to evolve. Accordingly, epistemic objects are characterised by multiple instantiations, open-endedness, flux, and emergence. Finally, patients were enacted as situated objects. Centred on local care arrangements and individual need, situated objects were formed through embodied engagement with patients in context. Provisional and adaptive, they reflected the requirements of tinkering and the logic of care (Mol, 2008), holding together the practical coordination of relations through responsiveness rather than mobilisation.

Tracing object-formation processes across the evolving trajectory highlighted how services enacted patients at different stages of care and treatment and how these enactments impacted the mobilisation and organisation of activity.

The Trajectory Assemblage

Both TMT and assemblage thinking conceptualise agency as arising from networks of socio-material relations. While TMT provides conceptual resources for the relational analysis of individual projects, assemblage thinking offers a complementary heuristic for adopting a wider perspective – one which conceptualises the trajectory as an emergent whole. By comparing the evolving configurations of practice across the hip fracture pathway, three distinctive care assemblages were identified: unscheduled care, acute care, and recovery care. Characterised by different forms of coordination, object formation, and institutional concern, these assemblages provide the organising structure for the empirical sections of this book.

The overall theoretical framework is summarised in Figure 3.1. The empirical chapters follow a structured, systematic approach. In each of the social worlds chapters, strategic action fields are described in detail, followed by an analysis of object formation and organisational processes. Chapters 7, 10, and

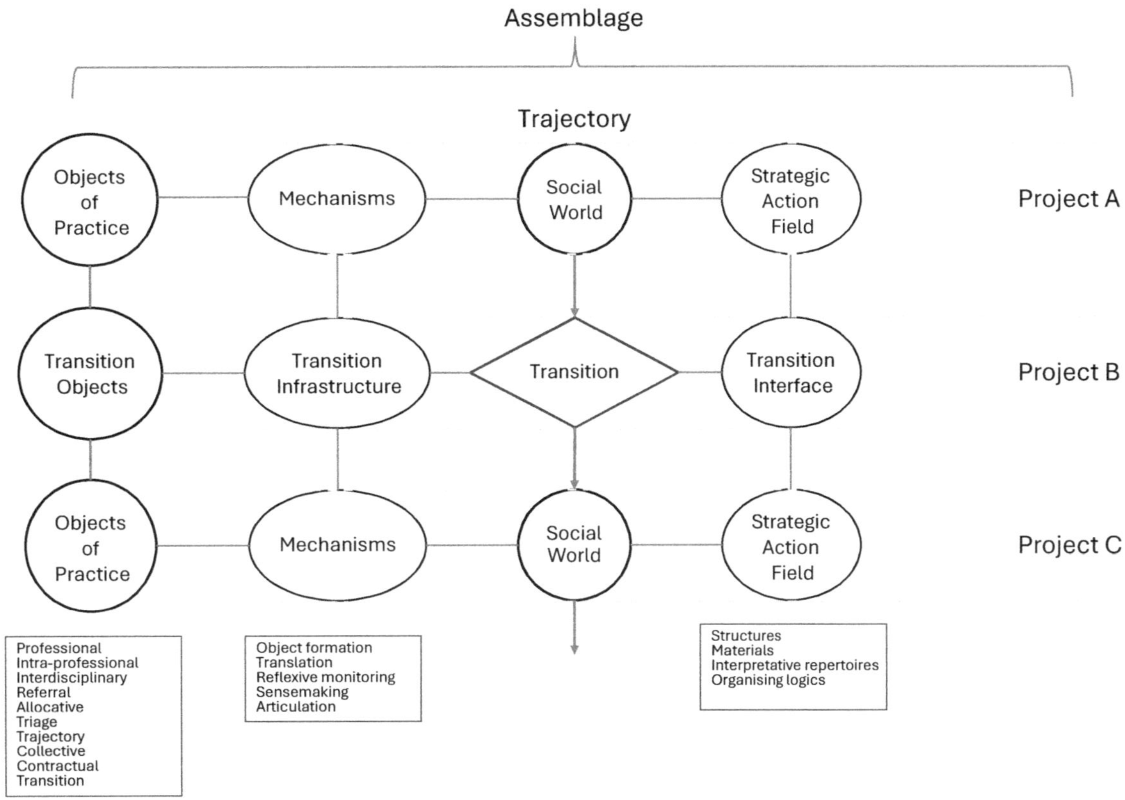

FIGURE 3.1 Patient trajectory assemblage theoretical framework.

13, which focus on transition, follow a consistent format: each begins with a description of the relevant transition interface, infrastructure, and transition objects, before examining transition management in depth. Ethnography allows for a range of expressive styles (Atkinson, 2020), but my aim here is clarity and transparency. Studying complex organisational processes is inherently challenging. By adopting a structured approach, I hope to make the analytical process visible and accessible to others pursuing similar inquiries, and in doing so, contribute to more systematic ways of researching – and ultimately improving – the organisation of care.

Summary

This chapter has introduced the hip fracture trajectory as an illustrative case for examining the organisation of care over time and across settings. It has outlined the study's methodological approach, data collection methods, and the key theoretical concepts that guided the analysis. With the scene now set, the book turns to the empirical investigation, beginning with an analysis of the unscheduled care assemblage.

References

Allen, D. (1997). 'The nursing-medical boundary: a negotiated order?' *Sociology of Health & Illness* **19**(4): 498–520. https://doi.org/10.1111/j.1467-9566.1997.tb00415.x

Allen, D. (2000). 'Negotiating the role of expert carers on an adult hospital ward'. *Sociology of Health & Illness* **22**(2): 149–171. https://doi.org/10.1111/1467-9566.00197

Allen, D. (2001). *The Changing Shape of Nursing Practice: The Role of Nurses in the Hospital Division of Labour*. London, Routledge.

Allen, D. (2009). 'From boundary concept to boundary object: the practice and politics of care pathways development'. *Social Science & Medicine* **69**(3): 354–361. https://doi.org/10.1016/j.socscimed.2009.05.002

Allen, D. (2015a). *The Invisible Work of Nurses: Hospitals, Organisation and Healthcare*. London and New York, Routledge.

Allen, D. (2015b). 'Inside "bed management": ethnographic insights from the vantage point of UK hospital nurses'. *Sociology of Health & Illness* **37**(3): 370–384. https://doi.org/10.1111/1467-9566.12195

Allen, D. (2018). 'Analysing healthcare coordination using translational mobilisation theory'. *Journal of Health Organization and Management* **32**(3): 358–373. https://doi.org/10.1108/JHOM-05-2017-0116

Allen, D. (2024). 'Why is hospital discharge so difficult? Reconsidering patient trajectories in theory and practice: insights from an ethnographic study of transitions in hip fracture care'. *Social Science & Medicine* **347**: 116769. https://doi.org/10.1016/j.socscimed.2024.116769

Allen, D., D. Cohen, K. Hood, M. Robling, C. Atwell, C. Lane, L. Lowes, S. Channon, D. Gillespie, S. Groves, J. Harvey, and J. Gregory (2012). 'Continuity of care in the transition from child to adult diabetes services: a realistic evaluation study'. *Journal of Health Services Research & Policy* **17**(3): 140–148. https://doi.org/10.1258/JHSRP.2011.011044

Allen, D., L. Griffiths, and P. Lyne (2004a). 'Understanding complex trajectories in health and social care provision'. *Sociology of Health & Illness* **26**(7): 1008–1030.

Allen, D., L. Griffiths, and P.A. Lyne (2004b). 'Accommodating health and social care need: routine resource allocation processes in stroke rehabilitation'. *Sociology of Health & Illness* **26**(4): 411–432. https://doi.org/10.1111/j.0141-9889.2004.00397.x

Allen, D. and C. May (2017). 'Organizing practice and practising organization: an outline of translational mobilization theory'. *Sage Open* **7**:2. https://doi.org/10.1016/j.socscimed.2009.05.002

Atkinson, P. (2020). *Writing Ethnographically*. London, Sage.

Berg, M. (1996). 'Practices of reading and writing: the constitutive role of the patient record in medical work'. *Sociology of Health & Illness* **18**(4): 499–524.

Berg, M. and G. Bowker (1997). 'The multiple bodies of the medical record: towards a sociology of an artifact'. *The Sociological Quarterly* **38**(3): 513–537.

Bourdieu, P. (1990). *The Logic of Practice*. Cambridge, Cambridge University Press.

Bruni, A. (2023). *Sociomaterial Practices in Medical Work: An Ethnography in the Operating Room*. London, Palgrave Macmillan.

Deleuze, G. and F. Guattari (1987). *A Thousand Plateaus: Capitalism and Schizophrenia*. Minneapolis, University of Minneapolis Press.

Dixon-Woods, M. (2003). 'What can ethnography do for quality and safety in health care?' *BMJ Quality & Safety* **12**: 326–327.

Engeström, Y. (2000). 'Activity theory as a framework for analysing and redesigning work'. *Ergonomics* **43**(7): 960–972.

Farjoun, M. (2010). 'Beyond dualism: stability and change as a duality'. *Academy of Management Review* **35**: 202–225.

Featherstone, K. and A. Northcott (2018). *Wandering the Wards: An Ethnography of Hospital Care and Its Consequences for People Living with Dementia*. London, Routledge.

Fligstein, N. and D. McAdam (2011). 'Toward a general theory of strategic action fields'. *Sociological Theory* **29**: 1–26. https://doi.org/10.1111/j.1467-9558.2010.01385.x

Garfinkel, H. (1967). *Studies in Ethnomethodology*. New Jersey, Prentice Hall.

Giddens, A. (1984). *The Constitution of Society*. Cambridge, Polity Press.

Glaser, B.G. (1965). 'The constant comparative method of qualitative analysis'. *Social Problems* **12**(4): 436–445. https://doi.org/10.1525/sp.1965.12.4.03a00070

Glaser, B.G. and A.L. Strauss (1971). *Status Passage*. New Jersey, Aldine Transaction.

Glaser, B.G. and A.L. Strauss (2007). *Time for Dying*. New York, Aldine Transaction.

Hernes T. (2014). *A Process Theory of Organization*. Oxford, Oxford University Press.

Knorr Cetina, K. (1997). 'Sociality with objects; social relations in post social knowledge societies'. *Theory, Culture & Society* **14**(4): 1–30.

Latour, B. (2005). *Reassembling the Social: An Introduction to Actor-Network-Theory*. Oxford, Oxford University Press.

May, C. (2013a). 'Agency and implementation: understanding the embedding of healthcare innovations in practice'. *Social Science & Medicine* **78**: 26–33.

May, C. (2013b). 'Towards a general theory of implementation'. *Implementation Science* **8** (18): https://doi.org/10.1186/1748-5908-8-18

May, C. and T. Finch (2009). 'Implementing, embedding, and integrating practices: an outline of normalization process theory'. *Sociology* **43**: 535–554.

Mol, A.M. (2002). *The Body Multiple: Ontology in Medical Practice*. Durham, NC, Duke University Press.

Mol. A. M. (2008) *The Logic of Care: Health and the Problem of Patient Choice*. Oxford, Routledge.

NICE (2011). *Hip fracture: Management, Clinical Guideline CG124*. National Institute for Health and Care Excellence. https://www.nice.org.uk/guidance/cg124

Nicolini, D. (2012). *Practice Theory, Work and Organization: An Introduction*. Oxford, Oxford University Press.

Nugus, P., A. Holdgate, M. Fry, R. Forero, S. McCarthy, and J. Braithwaite (2011). 'Work pressure and patient flow management in the emergency department: findings

from an ethnographic study'. *Academic Emergency Medicine* **18**(10): 1045–1052. https://doi.org/10.1111/j.1553-2712.2011.01171.x
Pavalko, E.K. (1997). 'Beyond trajectories: Multiple concepts for analyzing long-term process'. *Studying Aging and Social Change: Conceptual and Methodological Issues*. M.A. Hardy. Thousand Oaks, CA, Sage Publications: 129–147.
Pescosolido, B.A. (2014). 'Patient trajectories'. *The Wiley Blackwell Encyclopaedia of Health, Illness, Behavior, and Society*. W.C. Cockerham, R. Dingwall, and S.R. Quah. Hoboken, New Jersey, John Wiley & Sons, Ltd. https://doi.org/10.1002/9781118410868.wbehibs282
Rheinberger, H.-J. (1997). *Towards a History of Epistemic Things: Synthesizing Proteins in the Test Tube*. Stanford, CA, Standford University Press.
Skovgaard, A.L., M.J. Jørgensen, T. Tjørnhøj-Thomsen, and M.T. Høybye (2022). 'Discharge readiness as an infrastructure: negotiating the transfer of care for elderly patients in medical wards'. *Social Science & Medicine* **312**: 11538 https://doi.org/10.1016/j.socscimed.2022.115388
Strathern, M. (1991). *Partial Connections*. Savage, MD, Rowman and Littlefield.
Strauss, A.L. (1978). 'A social world perspective'. *Studies in Symbolic Interaction* **1**: 119–128.
Strauss, A.L. (1982). 'Social worlds and legitimation processes'. *Studies in Symbolic Interaction* **4**: 171–190.
Strauss, A.L., S. Fagerhaugh, B. Suczet, and C. Wiener (1985). *Social Organization of Medical Work*. Chicago, IL, University of Chicago Press.
Strauss, A.L., Schatzman, L., Bucher, R., Ehrlich, D., and Sabshin, M. (1963). 'The hospital and its negotiated order'. *The Hospital in Modern Society*. E. Freidson. New York, Free Press: 147–169.
Strauss, A.L., Schatzman, L., Bucher, R., Ehrlich, D., and Sabshin, M. (1964). *Psychiatric Ideologies and Institutions*. London, The Free Press of Glencoe Collier-Macmillan.
Strong, P. and R. Dingwall (1979). *The Ceremonial Order of the Clinic: Parents, Doctors and Medical Bureaucracies*. London, Routledge.
Sutton E, M. Ibrahim, W. Plath, L. Booth, M. Sujan, P. McCulloch, and N. Mackintosh (2014). 'Understanding the enablers and barriers to implementing a patient-led escalation system: a qualitative study'. *BMJ Quality & Safety* **13**(1): 18–27. https://doi.org/10.1136/bmjqs-2024-017132
Taxis, K. and N. Barber (2003). 'Causes of intravenous medication errors: an ethnographic study'. *BMJ Quality & Safety* **12**: 343–347.
Timmermans, S. (1988). 'Mutual tuning of multiple trajectories'. *Symbolic Interaction* **21**(4): 425–440. https://doi.org/10.1525/si.1998.21.4.425.
Timmermans, S. and I. Tavory (2012). 'Theory construction in qualitative research: from grounded theory to abductive analysis'. *Sociological Theory* **30**(3): 167–186.
Tsoukas H. and R. Chia (2002). 'On organizational becoming: rethinking organizational change.' *Organization Science* **13**: 567–582.
Vindrola-Padros C, and B. Vindrola-Padros (2018) 'Quick and dirty? A systematic review of the use of rapid ethnographies in healthcare organisation and delivery'. *BMJ Quality & Safety* **27**(4): 321–330. https://doi.org/10.1136/bmjqs-2017-007226
Waring, J., F. Marshall, S. Bishop, O. Sahota, M. Walker, G. Currie, R. Fisher, and T. Avery (2014). 'An ethnographic study of knowledge sharing across the boundaries between care processes, services and organisations: the contributions to 'safe' hospital discharge'. *Health and Social Care Delivery Research* **2**(29). https://doi.org/10.3310/hsdr02290
Weick, K.E. (1995). *Sensemaking in Organizations*. CA, Sage, Thousand Oaks.
Zerubavel, E. (1979). *Patterns of Time in Hospital Life*. Chicago, University of Chicago Press.

PART 2

The Provisional Patient

The Unscheduled Care Assemblage

INTRODUCTION TO PART 2

Part 2 examines the unscheduled care assemblage, tracing the hip fracture trajectory from first contact with health services to referral to trauma and orthopaedic specialists. While unscheduled care spans multiple services, key providers in hip fracture include the Emergency Medical Response Services (EMS) Control Centre, typically the entry point to the formal care system, the EMS responders dispatched to the scene, and the hospital-based Emergency Department (ED). In this opening trajectory phase, the patient status is *provisional*, with object formation and coordination conditioned by triage, prioritisation, and mobilisation logics within fast-paced, resource-constrained environments.

Unscheduled care often serves as the default for urgent, unplanned needs, especially when other services are unavailable or uncertainty exists about where to seek help. Demand has long been a challenge. In Wales, ambulance calls have steadily risen, driven by factors such as population ageing, poverty, isolation, limited primary care access, and public confusion about service options (Mills and Whitehead, 2018). NHS data show that 44% of ED attendees are discharged without follow-up, and 16% are referred elsewhere, such as to GPs (Wales Audit, 2023). Meanwhile, discharge delays create 'exit blocks', limiting inpatient bed availability.

In Wales, national performance targets are in place for ambulance response times and ED assessment. These include an eight-minute response for 'Red' (life-threatening) ambulance calls – unmet since July 2020 – and a four-hour ED assessment target, achieved in only 58% of cases in February 2022. Cases, such as suspected hip fractures, classified as Amber 1 or 2, lack response time targets and are increasingly facing long waits.

DOI: 10.4324/9781003475019-7

The effectiveness of unscheduled care services is interdependent. Ambulances queueing outside EDs have become emblematic of wider NHS pressures. Strategies to address demand include hospital-based bed managers who expedite discharges and create surge beds to manage capacity and demand, and new models of care which enable EMS call resolution at the scene and expanded roles for advanced paramedics. Yet, services continue to struggle (National Audit Office, 2017; Welsh Ambulance Service NHS Trust, 2020; Welsh Government, 2023). At the time of writing, concerns were growing about 'corridor care' – patients treated in non-ward areas – and 'car park care,' where ED staff attend to patients in ambulances unable to offload due to full departments (Guardian, 2025; RCN, 2024).

*

The chapters in Part 2 draw on 18 hours of fieldwork with EMS Control Centre staff in one of three regional clinical contact centres in Wales, 37 hours with five emergency responders, 55 hours in a major ED, and analysis of key documents and artefacts. In the Control Centre, I shadowed three call handlers, two clinical support officers, and two dispatch operatives – sitting beside them at their workstations, listening to calls via a headset, observing their activities, and discussing their work between calls. I also conducted a recorded semi-structured interview with the centre manager to better understand the structures, technologies, organising logics, and interpretative repertoires shaping everyday practice.

I joined two ambulance crews and a paramedic in a rapid response vehicle (RRV) on 'ride-outs' and spent time with their colleagues at the ambulance station. Fieldwork with EMS responders presents unique challenges. While I avoided distracting drivers, many meaningful exchanges occurred in transit. I found note-taking feasible in moving vehicles, provided I paused occasionally to avoid travel sickness. I rode in the passenger seat with the RRV responder and alternated between the cab and the rear of the ambulance during crew ride-outs. Riding in the cab enabled close observation of dispatch communication, while travelling in the back during patient transfers offered insight into how responders gathered and documented information to enact the patient as an object of ED practice.

In the ED, patients were managed in different sections based on acuity. Hip fracture patients were typically cared for in Majors and the Assessment Unit. The former handled serious but not immediately life-threatening conditions, and the latter provided intermediate care for patients waiting for admission. Fieldwork focused on these areas. I shadowed two streaming nurses allocating patients to beds, three nurses and two healthcare support staff delivering care, and two ED doctors responsible for assessment and disposal decisions. My broader understanding of departmental operations was also informed by observing EMS crews and on-call trauma and orthopaedic doctors.

This part of the book is organised as follows. Chapter 3 explores the social world of the EMS Control Centre and the socio-material relationships through which patients were enacted for the purposes of prioritising care and allocating EMS sources. Chapter 4 centres on the work of EMS responders, focusing on the case study of Mary, who was later found to have fractured her hip. Chapter 5 describes and explains trajectory mobilisation in the ED, including front door triage and allocative processes, ongoing care, and disposal decisions. Chapter 6 analyses the relationships between services and the organisation of transitions.

References

Audit Wales (2023). *Annual Audit Report 2022 – Welsh Ambulance Service NHS Trust*. Auditor General for Wales. https://www.audit.wales/sites/default/files/publications/wast_aar_0.pdf (accessed 07/04/25).

Mills, S. and R. Whitehead (2018). *Amber Review – A Review of calls to the Welsh Ambulance Service Categorised as Amber*. https://easc.nhs.wales/publications/amber-review/. (accessed 07/04/25).

National Audit Office (2017). *NHS England NHS Ambulance Services HC972*. London, National Audit Office https://www.nao.org.uk/wp-content/uploads/2017/01/NHS-Ambulance-Services.pdf

RCN (2024). *Corridor Care: Unsafe, Undignified, Unacceptable*. London, RCN. https://www.rcn.org.uk/professional-development/publications/Corridor-care-unsafe-undignified-unacceptable-UK-pub-011-635

The Guardian (2025). 'England's NHS crews "watching patients die in back of ambulances" due to A&E delays', https://www.theguardian.com/society/2025/apr/06/englands-nhs-crews-watching-patients-die-in-back-of-ambulances-due-to-ae-delays (accessed 07/04/25).

Welsh Ambulance Services NHS Trust (2020). *Annual Report 2019–2020*. https://www.ambulance.wales.nhs.uk/Media/Documents/Annual%20report_ENG_v4.pdf

Welsh Government (2023). *Trends in NHS Urgent and Emergency Care Activity: As at March 2023*. https://www.gov.wales/trends-nhs-urgent-and-emergency-care-activity-march-2023-html

4

CALLS, CODES, DISPATCH

Emergency Medical Services Control Centre Work

This chapter examines the organisation of patients, care, and treatment in the Emergency Medical Services (EMS) Control Centre. Operating at the threshold of public need and formal care, the Centre received all '999' emergency medical calls. As hip fracture is an unscheduled event, the EMS Control Centre was typically the patient's first point of contact with the care system. The chapter begins by exploring the strategic action field, which conditioned hip fracture care within the social world of the Control Centre. It then traces how patients were enacted, and care was mobilised in real time, focusing on the practical and technological work through which urgency was assessed, resources allocated, and trajectories initiated.

The Social World of the Emergency Medical Services Control Centre

EMS Control Centre work entailed offering support and advice across a wide array of undifferentiated individual troubles, prioritising needs, and matching callers with the most appropriate service. This section explores the ecology of structures, organising logics, material arrangements, and interpretative repertoires that shaped how patients were enacted, urgency was categorised, and care was mobilised.

Structures

Service

The EMS Control Centre operated from a Clinical Contact Centre on an industrial estate outside a small Welsh town – one of three such centres in Wales. The facility also housed the Patient Care Service, which coordinated

DOI: 10.4324/9781003475019-8

transport for hospital appointments and day care; the Urgent Care Service, which dispatched non-emergency crews for patients needing basic care (e.g. pain relief); and the Community First Responders Service, which managed trained volunteers attending life-threatening emergencies until ambulance arrival. The Centre comprised a large open-plan space, typically staffed by around forty uniformed personnel at designated workstations, overseen by a duty control manager seated at a desk on an elevated, panoptical platform.

The EMS Control Centre Team

The Control Centre team comprised call handlers, who managed all incoming calls; dispatch operatives, who organised and allocated EMS resources; and clinical support officers, who staffed the Clinical Support Desk. Call handlers worked with the Advanced Medical Priority Dispatch System (AMPDS), a computer-supported triage tool that systematically prioritised cases and matched them to appropriate responses. EMS resources were coordinated by a two-person dispatch team: the 'allocator' managed demand, communicated with responders, and optimised resource use, while the 'assistant allocator' handled vehicle defects, staff absences, and crew breaks. The Clinical Support Desk, staffed by a nurse and a paramedic – the only clinically qualified team members – supported call handlers and dispatchers, reviewed all AMPDS-triaged calls, and identified cases needing further assessment to refine prioritisation.

Organising Logics

EMS Control Centre work was shaped by two interlinked administrative logics. The first, an allocative logic, focused on matching calls to the most appropriate service to preserve EMS resources for emergencies. Non-urgent calls could be redirected to a GP, pharmacy, out-of-hours service, or NHS Direct (a 24-hour nurse-led telemedicine service); referred directly to a specialist team; or assigned an EMS response. Available EMS resources included: emergency ambulance crews; rapid response vehicles (RRVs), operated by a single paramedic to provide timely care until ambulance arrival; advanced paramedic practitioners (APPs), intended to avoid unnecessary hospital transfers; emergency medical technicians (EMTs) and care assistants, trained in life support and typically involved in patient transport; bicycles, used in pedestrianised city centres; and an air ambulance.

The second, a triage logic, prioritised calls by urgency. At the time of the study, Wales used the Clinical Response Model, which categorised calls as: 'Red' (immediately life-threatening), 'Amber' (serious but not immediately life-threatening, requiring urgent care), and 'Green' (non-urgent, manageable through other services or self-care) (Mills & Whitehead, 2018).

Interpretative Repertoires

The AMPDS was central to the EMS Control Centre work. Introduced in the UK in 1997, formal prioritisation technologies like AMPDS are expert systems built on standardised rules and algorithms that encode the knowledge needed to manage emergency calls. Previously, call handlers asked whatever questions they deemed relevant.

> *Dispatch Operative:* 'A few years ago [...] all that they (EMS responders) needed to know was where they were going and why. Anything else was a bonus. Things have changed and now they are concerned with determining the most appropriate response. So, the information on what has happened needs to be more detailed'.

Call handlers entered information based on scripted questions, and AMPDS classified the patient's condition, generating a medical priority dispatch code used by dispatchers to allocate resources.

Clinical support officers used a second triage tool – the Manchester Triage System – a global clinical risk management tool for managing patient flow when demand exceeds capacity (Manchester Triage Group, 2013). It comprises 52 flowcharts based on primary symptoms (e.g. 'headache', 'shortness of breath', 'wounds'), each with ranked discriminators (e.g. 'airway compromise', 'severe pain', 'persistent vomiting'). Users select the relevant flowchart and work through discriminators top to bottom to assign clinical priority based on presenting symptoms, without assuming a diagnosis (Zachariasse et al., 2017).

Materials

Workstations

Call handlers, dispatch operatives, and clinical support staff each worked at dedicated stations equipped with monitors, keyboards, and headsets. All had access to the AMPDS-generated list of active calls, supplemented by role-specific tools and materials.

Call handlers used two monitors: one for AMPDS, the other for a dialling pad and crew location maps. They also kept a paper Kardex of AMPDS protocols as a backup and a notepad for information that couldn't be entered into the system. Clinical support officers used a similar dual-screen setup – one for AMPDS, the other displaying all open calls. They could re-categorise calls or add notes after triage. Dispatch operatives used the AMPDS and a GPS-enabled Computer-Aided Dispatch (CAD) system, which tracked EMS vehicles in real time to support efficient crew allocation.

Despite distinct roles, coordination was achieved through AMPDS, which provided shared access to all open calls – colloquially known as 'the stack' – serving as a common information space and coordination device.

The Patient Record

The AMPDS system generated the documentary record of the patient as a collective object of the EMS Control Centre practice. A composite triage, allocative, and transition object, it had the qualities of a technical object (Rheinberger, 1997) comprising a dispatch code, a reductionist case summary, and unstructured notes added by call handlers and clinical support staff. This enactment was deployed for multiple purposes and served as the formal record of Control Centre work.

The dispatch code translated the patient's undifferentiated bodily troubles into two interrelated objects of practice: a triage object (for prioritising the call) and an allocative object (for managing EMS resources). The code had four components:

1. A number (1–36) indicating the AMPDS protocol or complaint.
2. A letter or symbol denoting response severity, crew requirements, expertise needed, and urgency. An 'O' category indicated no ambulance was needed.
3. A number reflecting aspects of the patient's condition (e.g. alertness, suspected cardiac arrest).
4. An optional element capturing scene risks (e.g. combative bystanders, physical hazards, or unstable scenarios involving drugs, alcohol, or violence).

In addition to the code, AMPDS generated a structured, reductionist summary based on scripted questions and the assigned priority, which was shared with EMS crews when they were allocated a job. The following extract is illustrative.

> 46 male conscious
> Psych/abnormal behaviour/suicide
> Male suicidal thoughts
> Male
> Green 1

The final component was unstructured information, added by call handlers during the call, from multiple callers reporting the same incident, or by clinical support staff during secondary triage. This was selectively shared with EMS crews, for the purposes of transition with dispatch operatives mediating the flow of information (see Chapter 6).

EMS Control Centre Work

The Control Centre team managed a steady flow of calls. The workspace was filled with a shifting cacophony of one-sided conversations and clicking keyboards, rising and falling with the tempo of activity.

> The noise level is rising. One call handler is asking about bleeding – 'Is it soaking through a towel?' Nearby, another is guiding someone through chest compressions: 'Pump the chest and count out loud so I can count with you'. Next to us, a handler reassures a pregnant woman who is bleeding: 'Try not to panic… just lie in a comfortable position and wait for the ambulance crew'.

The ability to bracket off the background noise so as to concentrate on their respective work activities was a key skill for call centre staff.

> The nurse observed that call handlers got louder if they got more stressed in dealing with cases. It is very easy to get distracted by other conversations in the room. The nurse said that it took some skills to learn how to 'zone out' and concentrate on your own tasks.

Call handlers worked to performance targets, with compliance data displayed on overhead screens. They had 30 seconds to obtain the address and another 30 for case entry, with an overall call time target of two to four minutes – which was often difficult to meet. While targets did not visibly shape behaviour, they formed an important background feature of call handler work.

> *Call handler:* 'You ask what has happened? And when they start with 'Well what it is….', then you know that they are going to be an age. Some, even when you ask for an address they just go babbling on!'.

Even though calls came thick and fast, call handlers found time to chat to each other; sometimes in between cases, and sometimes if they were waiting on the telephone with a caller.

> As this call ends, call handler returns to the earlier conversation we had started about meningitis. I couldn't say how long has passed since we were having this conversation, it must have been 10–15 minutes and yet she picked up the thread as if it had been seconds. I was so engrossed in the scene I'd been observing I could barely remember that we had even had that conversation.

From their designated area, the officers on the clinical support desk reflexively monitored AMPDS information to identify those cases where a second level of triage was indicated. There were no formal standards for selecting cases; support staff were described as 'using their antennae' to determine whether a call required their attention.

Dispatch operatives used AMPDS codes to allocate resources, also working with performance targets: 95% of the calls had to be allocated within 30 seconds if a resource was available. Whilst the CAD system prompted the allocator to use the nearest vehicle, decision-making was mediated by other considerations, with allocators keen to stress that 'you use your head'. For example, once a resource had initially been allocated, in non-urgent cases, further consideration would be given to resource management.

> The best outcome for an allocator is not really thirty seconds of when they're allocated, it's about what they do after, in relation to re-mobilising a crew and standing a crew down and putting them onto another call.
>
> *(Control Centre Manager – Interview)*

> At this point he (allocator) is about to dispatch a crew [...] he then pauses, and says, 'But now I don't want to send this as I now have a UCS crew so I can send them and keep my emergency crew'.

Judicious use of emergency crews was key to allocators' work. In the following extract, the allocator explains why he is not deploying an RRV to respond to a possible hip fracture. RRVs are staffed by a single paramedic and reserved primarily for 'Red' calls.

> Another call comes through.
>
> *Allocator:* 'There you go. This example is a possible hip fracture – an elderly person has fallen off the toilet and cannot get up. This is coded Green One Bravo – so we don't send an RRV'.
>
> Allocator looks at the screen.
>
> *Allocator:* 'In fact, we can't send anyone for a minute. Which is rather a shame. OK. A crew has become available now and, in all fairness, they'd be better than an RRV. I don't have an issue with an RRV going out to a fall. But you can't have one person trying to get someone up, they end up hurting themselves and the patient. We've got twenty minutes running time. I could have sent an RRV but then they would have got stuck there as they need backup. Someone might ask why I haven't sent the RRV for reassurance, but I have to be cold and detached and there is nothing immediately wrong'.

Allocators were engaged in a continuous process of reflexively monitoring capacity and demand to dispatch the most appropriate resource within performance targets.

Making Patients and Mobilising Care

> It really starts with the call taker, cos if they don't get that right, then everything else has a domino effect, it all falls down [...] The call cycle really does start with them.
>
> *(Control Centre Manager – Interview)*

The organisation of care and treatment in the EMS Control Centre began with translating the person's undifferentiated troubles into the objects of EMS practice. Calls had to be triaged, categorised, and prioritised. Object formation was distributed across call handlers and the AMPDS, and in re-triaged cases, between clinical support staff and the Manchester Triage System. It was also shaped by informal, often invisible, practices of call handlers. This section examines these processes, how they shaped patient trajectories, and their implications for coordinating the emergency response.

Object Formation in Call Handler Work

All calls were initially managed by call handlers using the AMPDS. Expert systems, like AMPDS, are designed to limit user autonomy to ensure consistency and reduce risk. They are increasingly attractive in the context of rising costs and the need for fiscal constraint (Greatbatch et al., 2005). Call handlers, not clinically qualified, were typically employed on a comparable grade to healthcare support workers, often with backgrounds in customer services or telesales.

To translate caller troubles into dispatch priorities, AMPDS required call handlers to follow a standardised script in a fixed sequence. Progression through the system depended entirely on the caller's ability to answer key questions. Handlers could not proceed until each step was completed and data entered correctly. Compliance was routinely monitored. Unlike other research that has evidenced flexible user engagement with expert systems (Greatbatch et al., 2005; Pope et al., 2013), in this study user agency was more constrained. Call handlers were disinclined to operate outside the constraints of the technology, and consequently the AMPDS was a prominent actor in call interactions.

Call handler: 'We are concerned with basic questions relating to life and death and we can only ask the questions as set out. We can't elaborate [...] it's like a bible'.

Paramedic: 'The system is in its infancy and so we are adhering to it to the letter'.

A typical call began with the handler establishing the emergency location and a contact telephone number. Once it was entered into AMPDS, the call appeared on the 'stack', where it was visible to the dispatch team and the clinical desk. The handler then asked questions to identify life-threatening emergencies. If a 'Red' categorisation was ruled out, further questions determined the appropriate priority level. The following extract illustrates the typical sequencing of a call:

> *Call handler requests address and phone number.*
> *Once these details are verified call*
> *handler asks:* So, can you tell me what happened?
> *Caller:* My mother is ninety-two and she's had a fall. She's broken her finger, but I am more concerned about her back and ribs.
> *Call handler:* Is she awake?
> *Caller:* Yes.
> *Call handler:* Is she breathing?
> *Caller:* Yes.
> *Call handler:* When did this happen?
> *Caller:* About an hour and half ago.
> *Call handler:* How far did she fall?
> *Caller:* About four to five feet.
> *Call handler:* Off what?
> *Caller:* She stood on a chair and fell backwards and struck a radiator.
> *Call handler:* Is she alert?
> *Caller:* Yes, but she suffers with dementia.
> *Call handler:* Is she having any difficulty breathing?
> *Caller:* No.
> *Call handler:* Is she in pain?
> *Caller:* Yes.
> *Call handler:* OK well I have organised help, and I will tell you what to do. Don't move her. Help is on its way. Listen to the recorded advice. Call handler said that this generated a 30-minute response; it is not life threatening.

Once a call was prioritised, the call handler either ended the call – typically leaving a recorded message – or, if indicated (e.g. the patient was not alert), remained on the line until the ambulance arrived. AMPDS included scripted instructions for supporting callers while awaiting help, including life-saving interventions like CPR.

Efficient call management was essential to gather the information needed for AMPDS to generate a response priority within performance targets.

A major challenge for call handlers was maintaining an 'institutionally constrained focus to the talk' (Whalen and Zimmerman, 1987), guiding callers to respond precisely so the system could proceed. Handlers faced three types of interactional challenge in generating the required information: caller-derived, script-derived, and algorithm-derived.

Caller-Derived Challenges

Callers seeking emergency assistance varied widely in circumstances and emotional states. They might be very young or old, drowsy, intoxicated, physically injured, distressed, or have limited language or communication skills – all of which could affect their ability to provide the critical information call handlers needed (Cromdal et al., 2012).

In the following example, a caller is distraught over a malfunctioning stoma. She contacted EMS out of desperation, having waited anxiously for a delayed GP home visit. In everyday conversation, such distress would typically prompt a supportive response. But in the EMS Control Centre, call management took precedence. To process the call, the handler had to orient the caller towards the institutional and instrumental demands of the interaction.

> The next caller is very distressed. The call concerns a patient who has a colostomy 'which is pouring out'. She is apologetic for contacting the ambulance service, but she has called the GP and has been told that they are on their rounds, 'So who knows when they will get here'.
>
> *Call handler:* OK. I know this is very distressing, but I am just going to process the call.

This example shows how the call handler briefly acknowledges the caller's distress before reframing the interaction around the need to 'process the call'. She clearly signals a shift away from the supportive responses expected in everyday social contexts, towards an institutionally constrained format with different normative expectations.

Script-Derived Challenges

The AMPDS is founded on a script (Akrich, 1992) that assumes callers can provide the information needed to triage cases. In practice, this often was not the case. Callers were frequently not co-present with the patient, curtailing their ability to answer key questions. In such situations, handlers typically instructed the caller to move to a position where they could see the patient, or if that was not possible, ended the call to speak to the patient directly.

> This call is from a neighbour calling on behalf of a lady who has collapsed in the toilet. She is calling from her own home, and this makes it difficult for her to answer the call handler's questions. When the call handler asks whether she is conscious, the neighbour cannot answer, and the call handler asks if she can put the phone down and go and check for her. However, the caller hangs up and despite four attempts to call her back we fail in reconnecting.

Calls from personal alarm services were also challenging. These services support frail older people living alone, with pendant alarms linked to remote monitoring teams. When the monitoring team contacted EMS, they were not co-present with the patient, making it difficult for them to answer the handler's questions.

> Call handler said that one of the challenges they had was calls from organisations like 'Lifeline'. These are the organisations that respond to the community alarm system. The call handler said that very often they do not have the information the call handler needs. 'If they would only ask a few more questions because when we call the patient they often won't answer'.

The following example is illustrative:

> This is a call from someone who gives their first name and says they are from Lifeline. She reports that she has just taken a call from a confused patient, and she provides the telephone number and the address. Call handler asks what has happened.

Caller:	She's 82 and collapsed to the floor. She's not hit her head but is dizzy.
Call handler:	Is she awake?
Caller:	Yes.
Call handler:	Is she breathing?
Caller:	Yes.
Call handler:	When you say collapse what happened?
Caller:	That was their words; the call has just come through.
Call handler:	Do you know what the cause was?
Caller:	I don't know.
Call handler:	Is there serious bleeding?
Caller:	No.
Call handler:	Are they alert?
Caller:	I spoke to the husband and when I spoke to her, she was a bit confused.

> There is then a discussion about how to get entry to the home – which the caller is evidently reading from notes on her own system [...] Call handler terminates this call and rings the patient.

In this case the patient was contacted directly. Although the patient was slightly disoriented, and the call was cut off multiple times, the call handler managed to re-establish contact and confirm key details. The patient was identified as having diabetes, with the fall attributed to dizziness; she also noted that her breathing was 'heavy'. The call handler instructed the patient to 'stay on the line' to receive further information before ending the call, reassuring them that help was on the way and would arrive 'as quickly as possible'.

Algorithm-Derived Challenges

The final category of interactional challenge stemmed from the standardised format imposed by the AMPDS algorithm. As Berg (1997) notes, expert systems are inherently reductionist, seeking singular answers to complex, multifaceted issues. They impose a formally rational, individualist structure on work that is, in practice, social, affective, and interpretive (Greatbatch et al., 2005: 803). In Greatbatch et al.'s study of NHS Direct, nurses worked flexibly with the system, allowing it to recede into the background and enabling more conversational interactions. In contrast, call handlers in this study were reluctant to deviate from AMPDS, creating several interactional difficulties.

Storytelling is a common way people make sense of experience. A frequent issue arose from the tension between callers' desire to narrate their concerns and AMPDS's demand for decontextualised, specific information – often resulting in a struggle for control of the interaction.

> The next call comes from an anxious parent who is incredibly challenging to discipline and seems unable to recognise there is a process the call handler must work through. Call handler finds it difficult to get her to comply with the questions and their sequencing. The call relates to a child that has a gastroscopy tube which appears to have blocked off. The caller refers to the child gagging and blood coming from the tube as a result of the child straining. The AMPDS questions make it very difficult for the caller to give a full picture of what is happening and so she must disrupt the interaction in order to tell her story which is difficult to fit into the standard questions about breathing, alertness, awake etc.
>
> There is question about bleeding.
>
> *Call handler:* Which part of the body is the bleeding from?
> *Caller:* Where he is straining through the tube, it's not loads. He's been gagging.
>
> My notes indicate that call handler then asked something about whether the bleeding was serious, and the caller said it was 'where he has been straining' adding, 'He's normally got a PEG (a feeding tube placed through the abdominal wall and into the stomach) but this is a temporary wire. I've not put anything down it. I am too scared'.

Call handler says she is organising help.

Caller: He's been like this since I gave him his medicine.

Call handler then takes the caller's name and the name of the patient.

The system indicates that she should be referred to NHS Direct for a more detailed assessment. When call handler shares this news with the caller, she is clearly very unhappy.

Caller: Oh dear! Oh dear! I think you should just come and get him love.

Call handler instructs the caller to listen to the recorded message and then to clear the line so NHS Direct can call her back.

This reflects a well-documented issue: everyday talk must often be reshaped to fit formalised or specialised encounters (Atkinson, 1982). In loosely structured face-to-face settings like medical clerking, there is flexibility to adapt to narrative accounts. But AMPDS offered no such latitude – caller storytelling could not be accommodated within its rigid format.

Effects?

While call handlers worked diligently within AMPDS constraints, there was broad agreement within the EMS Control Centre that the technology was a 'blunt instrument'. The triage process often produced inappropriate response priorities, with consequences for EMS operations and care quality. A paramedic described the system as unfit for purpose, calling for a more robust alternative. Because AMPDS relied on keywords and required handlers to input caller responses without interpretation, mis-categorisation was common.

Clinical Support Officer: 'One challenge is that callers must use particular words—if they don't, you can end up with the wrong response category'.

In the first extract below, a clinical support officer outlines the range of priority codes AMPDS might generate for a suspected hip fracture. In the second, the control centre manager, explains how this variation can arise.

Clinical Support Officer: 'The call handlers are non-clinical, and the category codes depend on the answers to the questions the caller has been asked. So, a hip fracture could be a Red 2, Green 2 or it could come in as a Green 3'.

> I mean, all that they've got, actually, is if it's a dangerous or like a proximal area these are the questions that they ask from there … how far did she fall … how did she fall … what part of the body's injured? It depends, then, on what they say … where the pain is…. I mean a lot of the time I know that's all we have … the patient falls on the floor … very rarely do we have the patient … that the information says the patient's actually fractured their femur.
>
> *(Control Centre Manager – Interview)*

Object Formation in Clinical Support Officer Work

The limitations of AMPDS were widely acknowledged, prompting the establishment of the clinical support desk following the McClelland Review of the Welsh Ambulance Service (2013). Clinicians monitored triaged calls to identify candidates for reprioritisation. By embedding clinical expertise into triage and dispatch, the aim was to improve resource use and ease service pressures by downgrading calls. The desk covered all three regions served by the Welsh Ambulance Trust, though staff focused on the busiest region.

While clinical support staff used a formal triage tool, their socio-material practices differed markedly from those of call handlers. The Manchester Triage System allowed greater professional discretion, and interactions were not constrained by technology or scripts. Clinicians could explain questions, seek clarification, and apply interpersonal and interpretive skills to make more nuanced assessments.

> She pulled up the screen on the last case she was looking at. A 45-year-old who had removed some rungs from a ladder into his loft and forgot and has fallen […] The nurse said that after speaking to the patient they then decide on what card it is most appropriate to use. In the case in question, she has chosen limb problems rather than falls. Each card contained prompts, which the nurse explained must be explored in language which is tailored to the patient. She said her experience in working for NHS Direct was good preparation for this. She contrasted this practice with that of the call handlers who must stick more rigidly to a script. The nurse said that man she had just spoken to had assessed his pain as seven out of ten and moderate. But he also says he cannot move, so she has categorised it as severe. In this case, she has asked for a 20-minute response but has discussed with the patient whether he is happy for a non-qualified person to go. He has said he thinks he will be able to stand with gas and air to get into the ambulance. So, this allows her to use a cheaper resource or at least a less in demand resource.
>
> *Nurse:* I have not got rid of a Red Call, but I have freed up the qualified crew.

Object Formation Repair Work

Although AMPDS did not allow call handlers to formally apply their sensemaking skills in triaging calls, these insights still informed EMS object formation. In addition to the second-level triage provided by the clinical desk, call handlers could make a 'warm transfer' to speak with clinical staff or dispatch operatives if concerned about a call's categorisation. While the clinical desk focused on downgrading calls, call handlers were most attuned to cases that had been under-prioritised.

> Call handler said that sometimes a case which sounded like meningitis would be put through to NHS Direct but that before this was done, she would 'speak to the desk' and say, 'They're not saying, but they have all the symptoms'.
>
> Call handler said that she had had a case earlier this shift in which a woman had taken an overdose of DNP (a diet pill) and she was burning up inside. The system had suggested that she only required a 30-minute response, but she was clearly in a bad way, so she went over and spoke to the Dispatch Desk.

While this was a largely informal and invisible process, the sensemaking skills of call handlers in detecting inaccurate response categories was recognised by clinical desk staff.

> *Paramedic:* 'They are not clinical and so it is not fair to make judgement calls. But they are very good the call takers. They will come up and say, this has come out as a Green Three – no way! So, we had an example of an eight-year-old child who was having an allergic reaction, and the call handler came across to alert me to their concerns with the category. Otherwise, if its low on the stacks – say Green Three – then you may be three pages back and not necessarily triaged (by the clinical desk) [...] I had a code which was a child who was very short of breath and had pruritus – they were itching for Wales – and they could still feel the peanut in the back of their throat. There was an APP around the corner and the first thing they did was to bang them full of adrenalin. And in the words of the APP if the call handler hadn't looked at this then the child would have been dead. He owes his life to a proactive call handler. We all have to work together'.

*

Object formation in the EMS Control Centre was a layered process involving algorithmic logic embedded in the AMPDS, formal risk mitigation through the clinical support desk, and the informal, often tacit, interpretive interventions of call handlers. These elements worked in concert – though not always successfully – to shape how patients were enacted and trajectories set in motion (see Figure 4.1).

Trajectory Mobilisation

Whether formal or informal, there was a limit to what risk mitigation strategies could achieve in overcoming the limitations of the AMPDS. While under-prioritised cases could sometimes be flagged by call handlers, over-prioritised calls were harder to detect. For urgent 'Red' cases, an EMS resource was often dispatched before re-triage could occur, reducing capacity for Amber calls – a major source of frustration for EMS responders.

> *Paramedic:* 'What you will notice is that what comes through and what the patient says it is often way off the mark. I went in to a young man supposedly with chest pain, who said that he called about a headache, and he said, 'They asked me if I had chest pain and I did, two weeks ago'. Similarly, we went into a guy who had called NHS Direct about a tooth abscess, and they started questioning him and asking him if he had pain in his jaw. Which he did, but he stressed that he was not having a heart attack and did not need an ambulance, but because he said he had pain in his jaw he got a hot response'.

While prioritising life-threatening cases is essential, unnecessary escalations strain EMS resources. Complaints were more likely from lower-priority patients displaced by higher-priority calls than from those receiving urgent responses.

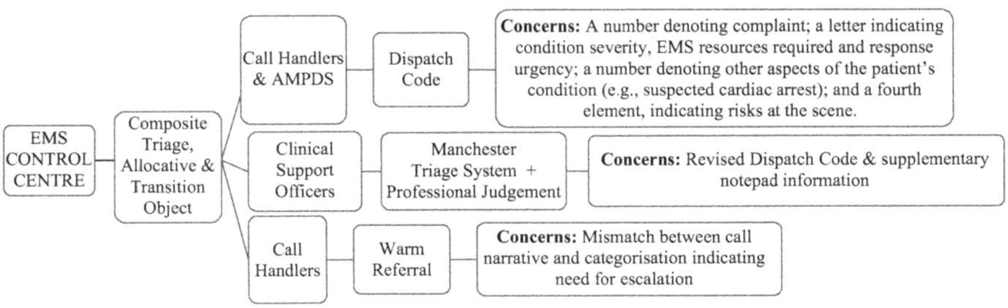

FIGURE 4.1 Object formation in EMS Control Centre work.

> It's ironic, really, because out of all the complaints generated from that, we would have probably more complaints from Green One calls than Red One or Red Two, because really speaking with a Red One or Red Two our resources usually ... not in every case, but our resources will be found for Red One or Red Two ... they have a pretty good service, really.
>
> *(Control Centre Manager – Interview)*

These contingencies in how patients are enacted as objects of practice by EMS staff can shape the initial hip fracture trajectory. The following comment, though reflecting a moral judgement about patient deservingness (Jeffrey, 1979), highlights the competing demands on the service and their implications for hip fracture care:

> There was an interesting comment made by a call handler over lunch when I said I was interested in hip fractures, which was that at the weekend crews are often called to people who are drunk and score higher than hip fracture patients and who then get left on the floor.

This final point underscores a recurring theme in the book, often overlooked in the pathways literature: individual care trajectories are ineluctably shaped by their intersections with others. While studies directly linking ambulance response times to hip fracture outcomes are limited, existing research shows that delays in the acute phase – from injury to surgery – adversely affect morbidity and mortality (Moja, et al., 2012).

Summary

This chapter examined the work of the EMS Control Centre – the first point of contact in the hip fracture trajectory. Here, a wide range of undifferentiated troubles were prioritised and matched to appropriate services. Care and treatment at this stage involved translating the patient into a two-part object of practice: a triage object for prioritising clinical care, and an allocative object for guiding EMS resource distribution. These were configured through a four-part dispatch code, with object formation distributed between call handlers using AMPDS and clinical staff using the Manchester Triage System. AMPDS-generated information was shared with EMS responders when they were allocated a call.

Expert systems like AMPDS are designed to limit user autonomy to ensure consistency and reduce risk, making them attractive for use by lower-skilled workers. This chapter highlighted the challenges call handlers faced in working with the system, the formal and informal strategies used to mitigate its limitations, and the potential impacts of these processes on the hip fracture trajectory.

References

Akrich, M. (1992). 'The de-scription of technical objects'. *Shaping Technology/Building Society: Studies in Sociotechnical Change*. W.E. Bijker and J. Law. Cambridge, MA, MIT Press: 205–224.

Atkinson, P. (1982). *Medical Talk and Medical Work*. London, Sage.

Berg, M. (1997). *Rationalizing Medical Work: Decision Support Techniques and Medical Practices*. Cambridge, MIT Press.

Cromdal, J., D. Persson-Thunqvist, and K. Osvaldsson (2012). '"SOS 112 what has occurred?" Managing openings in children's emergency calls' *Discourse, Context and Media* **1**: 183–202. https://doi.org/10.1016/j.dcm.2012.10.002

Greatbatch, D., G. Hanlon, J. Goode, A. O'Caithain, T. Strangleman, and D. Luff (2005). 'Telephone triage, expert systems and clinical expertise', *Sociology of Health & Illness* **27**(6): 802–830 https://doi.org/10.1111/j.1467-9566.2005.00475.x

Jeffrey, R. (1979). 'Normal rubbish: deviant patients in casualty departments', *Sociology of Health & Illness*, **1**(1): 90-1-7 https://doi.org/10.1111/1467-9566.ep11006793

Manchester Triage Group (2013). *Emergency Triage: Manchester Triage Group*, 3rd Edition Oxford, Wiley Blackwell.

McClelland, S. (2013). *A Strategic Review of Welsh Ambulance Services* available at: https://pgab.gig.cymru/cyhoeddiadau/adroddiad-mcclelland/ (accessed 08/04/25).

Mills, S. and R. Whitehead (2018). *Amber Review – A Review of calls to the Welsh Ambulance Service Categorised as Amber*. https://easc.nhs.wales/publications/amber-review/. (accessed 07/04/25).

Moja, L., Piatti, A., Pecoraro, V., Ricci, C., Virgili, G., Salanti, G., Germagnoli, L. (2012). 'Timing matters in hip fracture surgery: patients operated within 48 hours have better outcomes. A meta-analysis and meta-regression of over 190,000 patients'. *PLoS One* **7**(10): e46175. https://doi.org/10.1371/journal.pone.0046175

Pope, C., S. Halford, J. Turnball, J. Prichard, M. Calestani and C. May (2013). 'Using computer decision support systems in NHS emergency and urgent care: ethnographic study using normalisation process theory'. *BMC Health Services Research* **13**: 111. https://doi.org/10.1186/1472-6963-13-111

Rheinberger, H.-J. (1997). *Towards a History of Epistemic Things: Synthesizing Proteins in the Test Tube*. Stanford, CA, Standford University Press.

Whalen, M.R. and D.H. Zimmerman (1987). 'Sequential and institutional contexts in calls for help'. *Social Psychology Quarterly* **50**: 172–718 https://www.jstor.org/stable/2786750

Zachariasse, J.M., N. Seiger, P.P. Rood, C.F. Alves, P. Freitas, F.J. Smit, G.R. Roukema, and H.A. Moll (2017). 'Validity of the Manchester Triage System in emergency care: a prospective observational study'. *PLoS One* **12**(2): e0170811. https://doi.org/10.1371/journal.pone.0170811

5

BETWEEN CRISIS AND CARE

Emergency Medical Services Responder Work

This chapter examines how Emergency Medical Services (EMS) responders organise patients, care, and treatment. EMS personnel attend diverse emergency and urgent calls, deliver immediate on-scene care, determine appropriate action, and provide continuous support during transport. In cases like suspected hip fracture, decisions typically end with conveyance to the Emergency Department (ED).

The first part of the chapter outlines the social world of EMS responders and key features of the strategic action field that shaped their practice. Centred on the case of Mary, who fell at home, the second part analyses the enactment of patients as objects of practice to support disposal decisions and ensure safe, timely transfer to ED.

The Social World of EMS Responders

Never routine or fully planned, EMS work spans diverse scenarios – from road traffic accidents to incidents in homes, care facilities, streets, heritage parks, nightclubs, sports events, and rural areas. Offering unparalleled backstage access to people's lives (Palmer, 1983), the role is concrete and immediate (Metz, 1981). Responders must act swiftly to stabilise patients, make disposal decisions, and coordinate safe transfer to the next care stage. This section explores the ecology of EMS practice – the structures, organising logics, materials, and interpretative repertoires – through which patients were enacted, and care mobilised.

DOI: 10.4324/9781003475019-9

Structures

Service

At the time of the research, EMS in Wales operated across three regions. The study focused on the busiest, a mix of urban and rural areas serving a diverse population – from affluent suburbs to post-industrial communities. It included three Health Boards, eight EDs (three major), nine ambulance stations, and a wide range of EMS resources (see Chapter 4, p. 44).

To cover high-demand areas, responders were stationed at designated standpoints when not on calls. Health Boards monitored real-time ED capacity to prevent overcrowding; hospitals could go on 'divert' when full, rerouting patients to nearby facilities. Life-threatening cases or significant trauma were directed to major trauma centres. To ease ED pressure, alternative disposal options included referral to primary or community care, direct transfer to specialised services (e.g. maternity, mental health, alcohol treatment), or resolution at the scene via the 'See and Treat' model, where Advanced Paramedic Practitioners use guidelines to determine if on-site treatment is appropriate.

The EMS Responder Team

Over the past thirty years, EMS roles in the UK have evolved from manual, first-aid-based work (McCann, 2022) to a tiered system of practitioners. These include paramedics with graduate-level training; Emergency Medical Technicians (EMTs) with Level 4 apprenticeships; and Emergency Care Assistants (ECAs) with 6–9 weeks of basic training. More recently, Advanced Paramedic Practitioners (APPs), with postgraduate training in advanced clinical decision-making, have been introduced to resolve more calls on scene.

In addition to clinical expertise, EMS personnel are trained in emergency driving – a source of pride and enjoyment for many.

> I remarked that I would like to do the paramedic job, but I would not like the driving elements.
>
> *Paramedic:* That's the best bit!

The following extract is from my first day in the field.

> As soon as we logged in, a call appeared on the cab screen. EMT, in the back, asked, 'What's the job?' Paramedic, driving out of the station, read: 'Ninety-three-year-old female, bleeding with a cut arm'. The screen displayed: '93, female, haemorrhage, address, cut arm, won't stop bleeding,

pt on Warfarin, sore on arm, top came off and now arm bleeding'. A 'Green 1' call – not life-threatening but urgent – sent us speeding down River Road at 6 a.m. with blue lights flashing and sirens blaring.

Paramedic: What kind of passenger are you, Davina?
Me: 'Not great!'
Paramedic: We'll try not to throw you around too much!

My adrenaline was already high, as it often is at the start of fieldwork in unfamiliar settings. I was worried about interrupting the driver, getting travel sick, and whether I could take contemporaneous notes.

The crew knew it was my first ride-out, and in hindsight, the experience had a performative element. The quiet road didn't warrant the siren, and the passenger question was intended to showcase that EMS skills extend beyond clinical expertise.

Organising Logics

EMS response work was shaped by three organising logics. First, a clinical logic focused on addressing immediate medical needs (including reassurance, comfort, and potentially life-saving interventions), assessing the situation to inform disposal decisions, and managing the patient during transport. Second, mirroring the allocative logic of the EMS Control Centre, disposal decisions were guided by the imperative of prudent resource use. Responders were acutely aware of ED pressures and aimed to avoid hospital conveyance when alternatives were available. Third, a mobilisation logic underpinned the transition to the next care stage. Once a destination was identified, responders oriented to matters of concern to enact the patient as an object of practice for transfer.

These logics, closely interwoven in practice, were inscribed in the EMS Patient Care Record (PCR), which both accounted for EMS actions and translated the patient into a trajectory object to support onward mobilisation.

Materials

The Patient Record

The PCR was a central actor in the formal constitution of the patient. An A3 carbon paper form, the white original was retained by the ambulance service, microfiched, and served as the official record of EMS practice.

Paramedic: 'The paperwork is seen more as covering your arse rather than for patient continuity. We're constantly being warned, "It's not just what you do but what you do not do that will hang you out to dry". It doesn't matter if I kill someone as long as I document it'.

A yellow copy accompanied the patient and became part of the accumulative acute care medical record.

A highly structured document, the PCR included information on basic patient details, involvement of other agencies, medications administered at the scene, and electrocardiogram results. Reflecting the breadth of EMS work, there were specialist sections for obstetric cases, mental capacity assessments, airway and breathing, cannulation, burns, trauma, stroke, road traffic accidents, spinal injuries, safeguarding, and non-conveyance decisions. The form was predicated on a script which assumed patients would remain emergency responders' responsibility for only a limited period, with space for documenting ongoing care restricted to three fields for recording physiological parameters. Most entries were numerical or tick-box and had a technical quality; a small free-text section captured call context, medical history, and other relevant information considered pertinent to the patient's subsequent trajectory in narrative format.

Documentation occurred alongside care. In dual crews, the non-driver might begin the PCR en route. RRV paramedics sometimes made entries while awaiting ambulance crews. During transport, the responder travelling in the back of the ambulance with the patient typically completed the form, though fast-moving events often meant finalising it in the ED post-handover.

Equipment

EMS responders used a wide array of materials and technologies – from everyday items like bandages, splints, IV supplies, medications, and airway devices to advanced tools such as cardiac monitors, defibrillators, and pulse oximeters. Each shift began with vehicle checks to ensure all necessary equipment was present.

> When I arrived at the station the night shift was going off duty and Paramedic was checking the ambulance before the day shift. He informed me that all crews are required to do this. He asked his colleague from the night shift whether there was anything she was aware of that needed to be restocked.

There was also an informal practice of replenishing supplies from EDs. Though unofficial – since services operated separate budgets – it avoided unnecessary returns to base, preserving EMS availability.

Communication Technologies

Beyond clinical care, communication devices were central to the work. Responders received case information from the Control Centre via handheld radios and mobile data terminals. AMPDS-generated data appeared on in-vehicle screens.

Radios enabled real-time communication with Dispatch for support, and a dedicated phone line allowed responders to pre-alert EDs when transporting patients needing immediate care.

Interpretative Repertoires

Like other healthcare professions, responders' work was mediated by formal protocols. These included not only guidelines for clinical management but also protocols governing disposal decisions and referral mechanisms. In practice, however, these were rarely visible. Decision-making largely relied on internalised knowledge and professional judgement, tailored to the specific demands of each call.

EMS Responder Work

EMS crews typically worked 12-hour shifts. After preparing vehicles and restocking supplies, they logged into the system to indicate availability. Across all fieldwork episodes, we were allocated jobs straight away and rarely returned to designated standpoints. Except for brief lunch breaks, shifts involved a near-continuous stream of calls.

> As soon as we are back in the ambulance, we get another job. This patient is just around the corner. It is 0908.
>
> EMT said that the crews worked under immense pressures. In the past it wasn't uncommon for crews to only get a handful of calls per shift. Now the pressure is constant with teams moving from one call to the next, little time for meals, breaks being missed, and teams routinely working overtime.

Each clinical encounter was time-limited. The aim was to address any immediate patient needs, decide on disposition, and ensure safe transfer of care. Crews discouraged prolonged on-scene intervention, emphasising rapid assessment and escalation.

> *Paramedic:* 'An important rule is "Don't stay and play". The most important quality of a paramedic is to be able to look at someone and say, "They are ill and need secondary care"'.

In the same way that hospital work requires staff to have the ability to function in conditions of organisational turbulence (Melia, 1979; Allen, 2015), crews were required to work in chaotic environments, and management of the scene was often a prerequisite for management of the patient. In one case we were called to on a Friday evening, a man had been hit by a car on a busy street in the heart of the night-time economy, and the work of assessing the patient had to be undertaken amid a melee of inebriated friends and onlookers. In another, responders calmly managed three young children while attending to their father for a suspected heart attack.

Operating in moving vehicles was another challenge. Over the course of the fieldwork, I marvelled at responders' ability to function in circumstances that left me overwhelmed by nausea.

> The journey to the hospital is horrendous. I am travelling backwards, seated behind the patient stretcher. The vehicle bumps around constantly, and I have very real concerns I am going to be sick.
>
> At one point the IV Paracetamol falls on the floor. Paramedic seems to move around the truck with ease – and maintains her balance adopting a wide leg stance across the centre of the vehicle [...] Paramedic is adding more details to the Patient Care Record. How she manages this is beyond me.

Between jobs, crews cleaned vehicles and replenished supplies. Occasionally, they snatched a drink from the ED, but hydration and caffeine requirements had to be balanced with toilet access – especially difficult for RRV paramedics, who rarely took cases to the hospital.

> I commented on the lack of downtime. Paramedic said crews used to have only a few jobs per shift. 'If you're in a car (RRV), you can go from job to job – and they forget about your needs'. She sometimes uses patients' homes or calls Control to request a toilet break.

Over the fieldwork, several respondents referred to the poor morale amongst the crews, attributing it to the intensity of front-line work and a lack of understanding of its psychological demands from the wider service.

> She said many of the crews were on antidepressants. Paramedic: 'You get so little joy in this job and all it needs is for a little chink and the job gets under your skin'.

One RRV paramedic reflected on a particularly difficult period.

> The RRV driver was clearly struggling with the work. He made reference to a period of time in which he dealt with a number of cases in close succession: 'A woman who'd thrown herself in front of a train and was dead obviously; a ninety-seven-year-old who'd been hit by a taxi and had a fractured femur stuck out here (indicates site of fracture) – she did really well actually I checked; and a ten year old who died in Glebe Road, hit and run. It's too much. You can't do a genuine job all the time. You'd go mad'.

The reference in this second extract to 'genuine jobs' is insightful. EMS personnel often expressed frustration at the volume of calls they saw as inappropriate, echoing Hughes' (1971) concept of 'dirty work' and ethnographic accounts characterising crews as 'trauma junkies' (Palmer, 1983) who reject 'puke' or 'bullshit' jobs (Seim, 2017; Corman, 2018). While such calls may conflict with professional identity, they may also help mitigate the psychological toll of managing high volumes of legitimate emergencies. This raises questions about the impact of service intensification on responder well-being, especially if efforts to reduce inappropriate calls succeed.

Notwithstanding the recurrent discussions about morale, crews consistently displayed outward cheerfulness, often using humour to reassure patients – a quality frequently praised by families and patients.

Making Patients and Mobilising Care

EMS work involved rapid assessment and decisions about treatment and conveyance, often under conditions of limited information, unstable environments, and constrained resources. This section explores how patients, care, and treatment were organised at this phase of the trajectory, focusing on the case of Mary – the only call I attended where it transpired the patient had sustained a hip fracture.

Object Formation in EMS Responder Work

In EMS practice, patients were enacted as two closely coupled objects: a professional object to support clinical assessment and disposal decisions, and a trajectory object aligned with ED diagnostic and administrative needs, facilitating onward care. Object formation involved assessing visible clinical signs through standard tests, while also reconstructing the circumstances of the injury. Information was gathered from the patient, bystanders, or – on occasion – drawn from prior knowledge of the individual.

Scene interpretation was also central to sensemaking, offering insights into the patient's condition and history.

> *Paramedic:* 'Observation is key. While someone is looking at the patient, the other can be scanning the room, looking at pills, potions, nursing notes, GP letters. All that kind of detritus tends to get left lying about. This lady must be OK. Her bedroom is still upstairs, so she's still managing to navigate up and down and she lives alone. The nursing notes look quite new'.

This extract echoes Goodwin's (1994) concept of professional vision and how seeing is shaped by professional objectives. The reference to 'detritus' highlights responder expertise in discerning and interpreting environmental cues that might seem trivial to others.

Enacting a Professional Object of Practice

I was riding in the back of the ambulance when the dispatch call for Mary came in and struggled to see the screen. Notably, there was no reference to a potential hip injury in the information received.

> After restocking at ED, the crew calls Control to confirm availability. We are immediately allocated a job: an 85-year-old woman who has fallen and cut her head.

EMS responders received AMPDS-generated information on the call, but owing to their distrust in the system's accuracy, they approached each case as a tabula rasa, relying on their own experience and judgment to guide their decisions.

> *Paramedic:* 'You learn not to go in with preconceived ideas. Otherwise, you can end up going down the wrong path and it is hard to get back from that. So, you have to go in to assess what you are dealing with. It doesn't take long to do the basic tests'.

Sensemaking began on arrival.

> A man, with blood all over his sweater, lets us in. It is Mary's husband. Mary is seated on a chair with a nasty gash on the right side of her forehead and connected to an oxygen cylinder.
>
> Paramedic greets the patient and asks what has happened.
>
> *Mary:* I was out there (in the kitchen) and I don't know what happened, but I ended up on the concrete.
>
> As she is talking Paramedic is examining the wound using her pen torch. The EMT, who is scanning the room, notices some empty wine bottles and asked:
>
> *EMT:* What have you been doing this evening? Have you had a little tipple?
> *Mary:* A small glass of fortified wine. Only this much.
> *Paramedic:* Enough to send you flying?
> *Mary:* Oh no!

The presence of a significant head wound, quickly assessed as requiring closing, meant the decision to take Mary to hospital was straightforward.

Paramedic: That is going to need closing, either glue or stitches, so we're going to have to take you to A&E.
Mary: Oh no!
Paramedic: Sorry. It's too big to leave.

Enacting a Trajectory Object of Practice

Once a disposal decision was made, EMS responders engaged in further sensemaking to enact the patient as a trajectory object for ED. This involved constructing a coherent account of the incident, detailing injuries and symptoms, establishing relevant medical history, and gathering any additional information pertinent to the case. Depending on the circumstances, this distributed activity took place at the scene, in the ambulance, or during the journey to hospital.

Sensemaking unfolded in multiple forms. It included tailored inquiries that addressed specific aspects of the clinical situation and evolved in response to the emerging understanding of the case. It also involved standardised questions aligned with the institutional requirements of the PCR and the administrative needs of ED. In addition, it was embedded in the small talk used to manage social interaction and reassure patients. These seemingly casual conversations, often centred on the body and health, provided opportunities to collect relevant information while maintaining rapport.

In Mary's case, although the head wound prompted an immediate disposal decision, it was through this broader sensemaking process that additional information suggestive of a hip fracture emerged. After confirming the need for hospital transfer, the responder asked further questions about the incident and whether Mary had sustained any other injuries beyond the visible wound.

Paramedic: Did you lose consciousness at all?
Mary: No.
Paramedic: Have you got any other injuries?
Mary: Yes, my shoulder is stiff.
Paramedic: Any neck pain?
Mary: My neck is always stiff as I broke it.
Paramedic: Any new pain?
Mary: No.
Paramedic: How about your back? Any new pain?
Mary: My hip.
Paramedic: Did you hit your hip?

Husband: When I went out, she was on her front.
Paramedic: She didn't lose consciousness?
Husband: No.
Paramedic: Did she call out?
Husband: No.
Paramedic: Did you trip over the cable (oxygen tubing)?
Mary: No. I'm used to it.
Paramedic: Why are you on the Oxygen?
Mary: Because my lungs are useless.

[…]

Paramedic: About your lungs, which you say are knackered?
Husband: Knackered – that's one way of describing it!
Mary: Did they give you any words to describe what was wrong?
Mary: I had TB.
Paramedic: Was it COPD? Bronchiolitis?
Mary: That's it.
Paramedic: Bronchiolitis?
Neighbour: She was covered in blood.
Paramedic: Are you on any blood thinning medications?
Mary: No.
Paramedic: Are you on any other tablets?
Mary: Yes.

While hip pain is mentioned, the history taking focuses primarily on Mary's underlying medical problems. Her husband's comment – 'she was on her front' – implies he does not associate the accident with a hip injury. The hip only becomes a focus when Mary tries to stand to get into the wheelchair to be taken to the ambulance.

Arrangements are made to assist Mary into a wheelchair. As she is transferring, she complains of pain in her hip. She tells Paramedic she broke her hip several years ago.

Paramedic: How does this pain compare to when you broke it before?
Mary: I think I have just jarred it.

Once she is in the wheelchair Paramedic and EMT prepare to take Mary to the toilet, but she struggles to stand.

A neighbour who has come over to assist the couple asks if she can help but her offer is declined.

Paramedic: Are you sure you want to do this (go to the toilet)?
Mary: Maybe not.
Paramedic: Why don't we wait until you are in ED.

Mary agrees to this.

Mary was transferred to the ambulance, where her head wound was dressed and pain medication administered. Before departure, further sensemaking took place. With hip pain now a concern, the paramedic examined her hip and revisited the circumstances of the fall. A cardiac monitor revealed irregularities, prompting additional questions about her medical history.

Once Mary is settled on the trolley, Paramedic says: I am going to be a pain and ask if I can take your shoes off. I am looking to see if one leg is shorter or rotated (this would be indicative of a fracture).

Paramedic: What's causing more pain: your head or your hip?
Mary: My hip.
Paramedic: Have you had any painkillers today?
Mary: I had some Paracetamol this morning.
Paramedic: Would you like some more?
Mary: I think I can ride it out.
Paramedic: Are you sure?
Mary: OK then it might be better.
Paramedic: Would you like a tablet or a needle?
Mary: I can manage a tablet.

[…]

Paramedic: Are you normally steady on your feet?
Mary: Yes. I walk with a stick when I go out.
Paramedic: Did you have your shoes on when you fell?
Mary: My slippers.
Paramedic: Did you have them on properly?
Mary: Yes.
Paramedic: And there was nothing on the floor?
Mary: Not until I spilt the water.
Paramedic: So, you spilt the water and slipped on it?
Mary: Yeah.

Paramedic is looking at the monitor.

Paramedic: Have you got any heart problems?
Mary: Yes, an aneurysm.

Paramedic: An aortic aneurysm?
Mary: Yes – they're not worried about it though.
Paramedic: (studying the heart reading) Has anyone told you that you have got an irregular heartbeat?
Mary: Yes.

[…]

Paramedic: Right, you said you had an irregular heartbeat. Atrial fibrillation?
Mary: What's that?
Paramedic: If you don't know what it is then you don't have it! Can I put some stickers on so we can check out your heart? It's a bit irregular at the moment, which is why I am asking. What are your normal SATS? (measurement of blood oxygen saturation).
Mary: The doctor did them in the week and they were eighty-eight.
Paramedic: Is that normal for you as it wouldn't be for me?
Mary: That's what he said: good for you but not for me.

[…]

The husband has now locked up the house and joins us in the ambulance.

Paramedic: A couple more tests and then we can get going.

Once Mary was stabilised and her immediate needs addressed, she was transported to hospital, with object formation continuing en route. As Hughes (1980) notes, the ambulance journey is a key site for generating information for ED staff – a finding echoed in my observations. It also provided an opportunity for crews to begin completing the EMS PCR, even while in motion.

During the journey, the paramedic resumed history taking. In the following extract, we see a shift from a tailored inquiry into Mary's specific troubles to the standardised data collection required by the PCR, marked by the phrase: 'I'm just going to jot a few things down'. I observed this transition frequently, as EMS responders moved from relational engagement with patients and supporters to a more formal orientation towards documentation. At this point, the form becomes a visible actor in the interaction, having previously remained backstage. When focused on the patient, crews often deferred formal documentation, recording clinical observations on gloves or the ambulance whiteboard rather than directly into the PCR.

Paramedic: The pain in your hip. How would you describe it? Does this feel numb? Can you wriggle your toes?
Mary: It's just jarred.

Paramedic: Is it worse when you move and weight bear?
Mary: Oh Yes!
Paramedic: Any pain in your head?
Mary: No.
Paramedic: I am just going to jot a few things down. How's your breathing been the last few days?
Mary: Normal.
Paramedic: No coughs, colds?
Mary: No.

Paramedic pauses for a minute and studies the ECG.

Paramedic: OK I need some information. Is […] your official name?
Mary: Yes.
Paramedic: Can you tell me your date of birth please?
Mary: […]
Paramedic: And this is your home address?

[…]

Paramedic: You say you were in the kitchen, and you fell through the back door to outside. Were you going out or in?
Mary: Out.
Paramedic: And you say there was water on the floor, and you slipped?
Mary: Yes.
Paramedic: Do you think you landed on your right side?
Mary: Yes, I did.
Husband: But I found you on your front.
Paramedic: Did you roll onto your front?
Mary: Yes – I fell on my right and rolled onto my front.
Paramedic: And was it the patio?
Mary: I just fell outside.
Paramedic: But was it onto grass or pavers?
Mary: It was concrete.
Paramedic: So, you've got an aortic aneurysm, irregular heartbeat, you've had a hip replacement. When?
Mary: Just over a year ago.
Paramedic: Any high blood pressure?
Mary: No.
Paramedic: You said you had bronchiolitis following TB and I can see steroids here. Is there anything else I've missed off?
Mary: I have arthritis in my hands but that is normal. I broke my neck.
Husband: You broke your shoulder and neck.
Paramedic: Which bones?

Mary:	C2 I think?
Paramedic:	Did you do this when you broke your hip?
Mary:	No, that was two and half years ago.
Paramedic:	How did you do that?
Mary:	The phone went in the night, and I got up and tripped over.

[...]

We arrive at the hospital and Paramedic says, 'I haven't finished my writing yet'.

Paramedic:	Why are you on water tablets?
Mary:	No idea!
Paramedic:	Have you had swollen ankles?
Mary:	Yes.
Paramedic:	Do you have any allergies?
Mary:	No.
Paramedic:	Right. I am going to book you in.

Prior to ED arrival, EMS responders enacted the patient as a dual object of practice, shaped through distinct constellations of concern. First, as a professional object, the patient was constituted through immediate clinical and logistical imperatives – those necessary for on-scene intervention and disposal decisions. Second, as a trajectory object, she was configured in relation to the broader temporal and biographical context of the call, oriented towards the work purposes of ED. These enactments were materially mediated through the PCR: the (technical) professional object was inscribed in its structured, reductionist fields, while the trajectory object was constituted through narrative entries. Object formation processes in EMS responder work are summarised in Figure 5.1.

Despite the sensemaking invested in generating the trajectory object – often involving extensive history taking and interpretive work – this effort was constrained by the documentation infrastructure. Several respondents noted that the PCR format was insufficient to accommodate the complexity and volume of information generated, revealing a misalignment between the work of object formation and the representational capacities of the form.

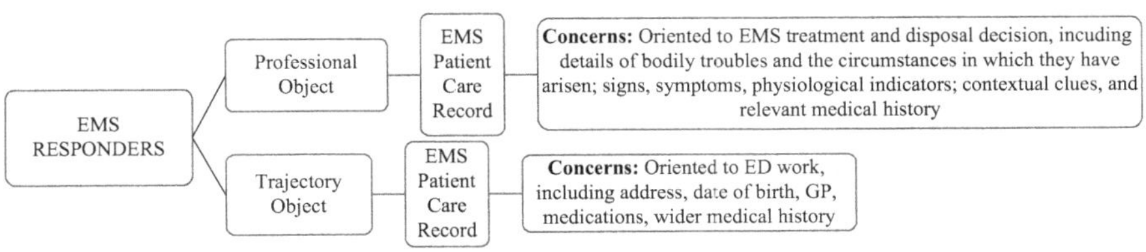

FIGURE 5.1 Object formation in EMS responder work.

> Paramedic is an experienced clinician and expressed the view that the documentation has changed very little over the years, although they now write a more comprehensive narrative than they once did. Paramedic: 'We're expected to put more stuff in it, but the actual size has remained the same. There is a more fulsome narrative, in previous sheets the narrative section was about a third of the size it is today. It's still far too small'.

This enactment of the patient was central to managing transition with ED staff and will be explored in more detail in Chapter 6.

When we left Mary and her husband at the ED, her diagnosis remained undetermined. EMS responders typically do not learn the outcomes of the cases they attend. However, later that day, while returning to the same hospital with another patient, we encountered Mary's husband, who confirmed that she had sustained a hip fracture.

> I notice the husband of our earlier patient waiting outside. It looks as if he is waiting for a cab, and I surmise that his wife is to be admitted. I pointed him out to Paramedic, when she returned to the ambulance, and she informed me that the lady had been confirmed to have a hip fracture. Paramedic: But the doctor said that the type of fracture would not have caused any shortening or rotation.

Summary

This chapter has shown how EMS responders mobilise care by enacting patients as two closely coupled objects of practice: a professional object to support clinical disposal decisions, and a trajectory object to facilitate ED transfer. With little reliance on AMPDS-generated information, each case was approached as a tabula rasa. Despite limited time on scene, responders constructed a more expansive patient object than the reductionist version produced through control centre work. This included clinical signs of bodily trouble, the circumstances of the event, environmental cues informing disposal, and aspects of medical history and social context relevant to ED sense-making. Conveyance of an undifferentiated EMS call to ED marks a significant status passage in the hip fracture trajectory – closing the episode for EMS and initiating a new phase for ED.

References

Allen, D. (2015). *The Invisible Work of Nurses: Hospitals, Organisation and Healthcare.* London, Routledge.

Corman, M.K. (2018). 'Street medicine: assessment work strategies of paramedics on the front lines of emergency health services'. *Journal of Contemporary Ethnography* **46**(5): 600–623.

Goodwin, C. (1994). 'Professional vision'. *American Anthropologist* **96**(3): 606–633.

Hughes, D. (1980). 'The ambulance journey as an information generating process'. *Sociology of Health & Illness* **2**(2): 115–132.
Hughes, E.C. (1971) *The Sociological Eye*. New Brunswick and London, Transaction Books.
McCann, L. (2022). *The Paramedic at Work: A Sociology of a New Profession*. Oxford, Oxford University Press.
Melia, K.M. (1979). 'A sociological approach to the analysis of nursing work'. *Journal of Advanced Nursing* **4**: 57–67.
Metz, L.D. (1981). *Running Hot: Structure and Stress in Ambulance Work*. Cambridge, MA, Abt Books.
Palmer, C.E. (1983). '"Trauma junkies" and street work: occupational behavior of Paramedic and Emergency Medical Technicians'. *Urban Life* **12**(2): 162–183. https://doi.org/10.1177/0098303983012002003
Seim, J. (2017). 'The ambulance: toward a labor theory of poverty governance'. *American Sociological Review* **82**(3): 451–475.

6

FROM ARRIVAL TO ADMISSION

Emergency Department Work

> In the Emergency Department people are at an early stage of their entry into the healthcare system; staff are still trying to assemble a picture of what has happened and reach a diagnosis from a host of signs, symptoms, histories and investigations. As collective objects of practice, patients are working scenarios – provisional understandings – in an evolving clinical scene of information seeking, sensemaking, synthesis, and tests of various kinds.
>
> (Fieldnote Memo)

This chapter focuses on the organisation of patients, care, and treatment in the Emergency Department (ED). The ED specialises in the urgent and acute care of individuals who present without prior appointment, either independently or by ambulance. Alongside initial treatment for a wide range of conditions – some requiring immediate attention – the ED acts as an organisational gatekeeper. Once life-saving interventions are ruled out, the key task is to determine whether the patient can be treated and discharged or requires referral and admission to hospital. Hip fracture always necessitates inpatient care.

The chapter begins with an overview of the social world of ED work, then explores how patients with hip fracture are enacted through ED practices, culminating in diagnosis and referral to the orthogeriatric team.

The Social World of the Emergency Department

This section explores the structures, logics, resources, and interpretative repertoires that shape how patients, care, and treatment are organised within the

DOI: 10.4324/9781003475019-10

social world of the ED. EDs are fast-paced, unpredictable environments where a highly differentiated patient population must be managed efficiently within externally imposed time constraints.

Structures

The Department

The ED at the study site was among the busiest in the UK. As a major trauma centre, it received around 140,000 patients annually, including 33,000 children. Like the EMS Control Centre (see Chapter 4), the ED was subject to national performance targets: a 15-minute window for EMS handover, with crews recording arrival, handover initiation, and completion; and a four-hour target for reaching a disposal decision – either discharge or referral for inpatient care.

The ED was divided into distinct sections, each with specific resources (beds, staff, equipment, expertise). Patients needing life-saving interventions were allocated to one of three Resus beds, with EMS crews using a dedicated 'red phone' to alert ED staff. These calls were triaged by an ED nurse who coordinated preparations and, if needed, alerted specialist teams. Non-life-threatening cases unlikely to require admission were managed in 'Minors', typically involving treatment and discharge with follow-up arranged. People requiring a thoroughgoing medical assessment, like suspected hip fractures, were assessed in 'Majors', which included two trolley bay areas, with capacity for 12 patients, and an Ambulatory Care Unit for those not requiring a bed.

The ED also housed a 12-bed Assessment Unit (AU), designed to free up ED capacity. Patients successfully referred to inpatient services were cared for in AU until a hospital bed became available. Those not requiring admission but unfit for immediate discharge were cared for in the Clinical Decision Unit (CDU). All children were treated in a separate paediatric area.

The ED Team

Nurses, doctors, healthcare support staff, and receptionists formed the ED's front-line workforce. Receptionists booked patients into the department and served as the first point of contact. The nursing team included registered nurses and healthcare support workers responsible for clinical care, alongside senior nurses managing patient flow. ED and AU had separate nursing teams with distinct management structures. The medical team comprised rotating resident doctors at various training stages, overseen by consultants. Together, nurses, support staff, and doctors mobilised patients through the department, addressed immediate needs, synthesised diverse information sources to reach disposal decisions, and facilitated onward trajectories.

Beyond the core ED team, many others circulated through the department: EMS responders bringing new patients; specialist teams supporting specific cases (e.g. stroke, trauma, mental health); service managers monitoring performance, bed availability, and flow; patients' relatives and supporters; occasional police officers and security staff; and a range of clinical specialists reviewing referred patients.

Organising Logics

ED work was driven by clinical, administrative, and mobilisation logics, which shaped both the organisation of care and the matters of concern through which patients were enacted as objects of practice. Clinical logics underpinned nurses' attention to immediate care needs and doctors' efforts to reach a diagnosis and disposal decision. These were interwoven with administrative and mobilisation logics aimed at prioritising cases, managing resources, and coordinating patient trajectories.

Administrative logics reflected ED's role as one of the most open points in the healthcare system (Hillman, 2014), receiving patients with conditions ranging from minor to life-threatening. A central organising principle was the need to interpret and act on undifferentiated troubles according to clinical urgency, with nurses responsible for triaging all arrivals. Alongside this imperative was an allocative logic focused on resource use – evident in efforts to avoid unnecessary admissions, manage bed availability, and maintain patient flow. A third, closely aligned logic centred on mobilisation. Clinical staff engaged in continuous reflexive monitoring of activity to track patient trajectories, ensure timely case closure, and support comprehensive handover to the next point of care.

Interpretative Repertoires

Nurses triaged all patients on arrival using the Manchester Triage System (see Chapter 4, p. 45), categorising individuals on a 5-point scale from most (1) to least (5) urgent. Experienced nurses had internalised the system, and the process appeared routinised; I saw no visible use of the material tool. However, participants noted that junior nurses, more sensitive to the responsibility of triage, were more likely to consult the formal protocol.

ED Nurse: 'We work quite autonomously down here, you are making decisions and caring for patients before they have been seen by the doctor. When I first started, I would categorise all patients as two when maybe they didn't need that. There's a book somewhere, but we've all been here for so long we just do it. Sometimes you see the new nurses with the book'.

In enacting patients as triage objects of practice, nurses produced a summary of the patient's history using the SBAR (Situation, Background, Assessment, Recommendation) format – a communication tool introduced by Kaiser Permanente in the early 2000s and now widely adopted to support patient safety and reduce errors.

ED nursing care was mediated by standardised risk assessments (e.g. falls, skin integrity, pressure ulcers, manual handling, nutrition), each with visual or pictorial scales to guide interpretation. Nurses used clinical judgment to determine which assessments were appropriate, documenting these decisions explicitly to distinguish them from omissions.

Materials

The Patient Record

Patient care in ED was recorded in two documents: the Clinical Assessment Services (CAS) Card and the Adult Patient Assessment Booklet. The CAS Card – a four-page A4 booklet – served as the formal multidisciplinary record, with designated fields for documenting the patient's trajectory through the department. It functioned both as an accumulating and coordinating device (Berg, 1999), bringing together diverse matters of concern as ED doctors made sense of the case, and as an accounting tool, formally recording care delivered.

Nursing care was documented in the 16-page Adult Patient Assessment Booklet, or 'nursing notes'. It included risk assessment tools and sections for monitoring physiological indicators (e.g. temperature, blood pressure, pulse, respirations, oxygen saturation, neurological status, fluid balance, and bowel movements). Two pages were allocated for free-text entries on nursing interventions. The form also captured additional patient information – accommodation, religion, language, caring responsibilities, safeguarding concerns, and community support – much of which was not directly relevant to ED care but reflected the mobilisation logic of nursing practice, anticipating needs for inpatient care or discharge planning.

Clinical Information Technologies

ED work was supported by priority imaging and laboratory services. Digital systems enabled access to laboratory results, imaging data, comprehensive patient histories, and electronic patient discharge and communications with primary care physicians via the Welsh Clinical Portal (https://dhcw.nhs.wales/product-directory/our-digital-services/welsh-clinical-portal/).

Coordination Technologies

ED work was supported by a range of coordination technologies. Staff accessed EMS flow data to track incoming ambulances, including estimated arrival times and patient details, as well as information on self-presenting patients. ED coordinators used a management system to monitor hospital bed occupancy and patient flow, with real-time access to performance indicators such as patients at risk of breaching the four-hour disposal target and ambulance handovers exceeding 15 minutes. Whiteboards in each ED section provided a visual overview of patient trajectories through the department.

ED Work

Fieldwork took place during the summer, a period many respondents described as less busy than winter. Nonetheless, during my time in ED, there was a steady stream of new cases, with periodic surges triggered by serious illnesses or injuries.

Unlike EMS responders, who moved sequentially from case to case, ED staff managed multiple patients simultaneously, each at a different trajectory stage. The rhythm of ED work reflected the need to balance clinical urgency with caseload management under time and resource constraints. Nurses were assigned dedicated roles to oversee departmental activity: a streaming nurse liaised with EMS crews to allocate patients, while senior nurses in 'controller' roles managed patient flow.

> *Unit Manager:* 'They challenge flow, chase things up, trouble shoot and escalate, liaising with bed management'.

> The controller described her role as 'operational' and she worked to develop a 'helicopter view of both ED and AU'.

Care and treatment were primarily delivered by doctors and nurses. Doctors worked with a case-based model, prioritising patients, initiating investigations, and awaiting results – often managing several cases at once. They could be called away to attend front-door emergencies, during which hours might pass before they could return to earlier cases. The pace of work could shift rapidly, from intense activity to relative calm.

Nurses, by contrast, were assigned to specific areas. Their work was shaped not only by the fluctuating clinical needs of their patients but also by the need to coordinate with multiple doctors and manage the movement and handover of patients through the department. Both nurses and doctors worked in shifts, with continuity maintained through brief handovers focused on the current caseload within each team.

Making Patients and Mobilising Care

As patients progressed through ED, they were enacted as multiple objects of practice. Initial object formation centred on matters of concern related to bed allocation and the prioritisation of care, and thereafter, for the purposes of diagnosis, ongoing care and treatment, and trajectory mobilisation. In the four-hour performance target for reaching a disposal decision, collective understanding of the patient evolved into a stabilised narrative object of practice focused on diagnosis, overall trajectory, and future plan.

In the following section, I examine these processes, highlighting the matters of concern that informed care and treatment, the sensemaking strategies deployed by ED staff, and the conditions influencing patient-making. The analysis attends to both visible and invisible processes of object formation.

Initial Object Formation

Enacting the Patient as an Allocative Object

All suspected hip fracture patients were admitted to Majors, where the streaming nurse allocated them to one of several areas: a trolley space, a seat in the Ambulatory Care Unit (ACU), or, occasionally, re-routing to Minors, where patients were shuffled between the waiting area and examination cubicles. Within Majors, further distinctions existed – with specific beds equipped for cardiac monitoring.

Nurses play a central role in bed management across healthcare systems, making situated 'match-making' decisions to align patient needs with available resources (Allen, 2015a, 2015b). In ED, the streaming nurse engaged in continuous reflexive monitoring to maintain awareness of capacity and anticipated demand. This was essential for managing patient flow and ensuring space for incoming cases. The streaming nurse had access to EMS Control Centre data, displayed on a screen, and regularly appraised this to anticipate arrivals.

> She said that this information was useful as it 'shows demand on the system and in the community, what level the calls are and the location of crews. There are eight outstanding and most look like they are coming in. You can see, if they're eighty-eight with falls they are likely to come in and need a trolley space'.

Nevertheless, this was noisy information. Not all EMS cases came to Majors – some went directly to Resus or, in the case of primary care referrals, to the AU. Part of the streaming nurse's work in maintaining awareness of capacity and demand was reconciling the information on the screen with observed activity on the ground in and around the ED.

> Streaming Nurse is back at the screen. She has a problem: one EMS crew hasn't notified their arrival. Suddenly, we hear the air ambulance. I ask if it was expected.
>
> *Streaming Nurse:* 'They're not, but sometimes they use the service to drop someone off. I'm going to put my head in Majors to see what's going on'.
>
> She disappears. According to the screen, the second trauma case – 9824 – has arrived. I wonder if it's linked to the helicopter. I realise I'm engaged in the same kind of sensemaking as the streaming nurse – matching screen data with unfolding events.
>
> *Streaming Nurse returns:* 'The crew has gone. That's annoying'.
> *DA:* '9824 has arrived. Was that the helicopter?'
> *Streaming Nurse:* 'No. I'll go over to Resus and see if she's there. I don't know where 9824 is. Could be the Assessment Unit'.

Another source of noise in the EMS system was the quality of case descriptions generated by the Advanced Medical Prioritisation Dispatch System (AMPDS) (see Chapters 4 and 5). Like EMS responders, ED nurses treated these cautiously, as they often misaligned with the actual patient presentation.

> I explained that I had spent some time in the EMS Control Centre and unprompted she observed, 'Well its very interesting how the information you get from there is very different from what is actually found'.

In enacting patients for allocative purposes, the streaming nurse did not assess patients directly. Bed placement decisions were based on brief discussions with EMS responders while the patient remained in the ambulance. If no suitable bed was available, the patient remained under EMS care. Beds were only allocated when need was unequivocal, as patients could not be moved once placed. No structured proforma guided this process; decisions were based on professional judgement and proxy indicators negotiated with EMS crews. These discussions were typically brief, with both parties oriented to their circumscribed purpose. This is illustrated in the following extract, where the streaming nurse and EMS crew reach consensus to allocate a male patient to a trolley space in Majors with cardiac monitoring. The decision is not clear-cut: the patient is young, and most physiological indicators are within normal limits, but the streaming nurse concludes that, as the case 'sounds a bit cardiac', monitoring is warranted.

Streaming Nurse:	Who have you got?
EMS Responder:	A forty-year-old male with left sided chest pain. Sounds cardiac; it is going down his left arm. Obs are OK, but BP is high. Not known to have cardiac problems, (sotto voce) but he is a really big guy. He had a similar episode in 2009 – and had a range of tests but they found nothing. He's had aspirin and GTN (glyceryl trinitrate, Medication used for chest pain) and says that he feels a bit better.
Streaming Nurse:	What's his ECG? (electrocardiograph).
EMS Responder:	(hands over ECG print out) ECG is normal.
Streaming Nurse:	Because it sounds a bit cardiac, he'd better go into six for monitoring.

Age was a key factor in allocation decisions. In the first example, as soon as the streaming nurse learns that the patient is a 22-year-old and before she has been informed of the presenting problem, she asks whether they are suitable for Minors. This contrasts with the second extract, where the responder assumes a 72-year-old 'young lady' will be allocated a bed in Majors.

Streaming Nurse:	Who have you got?
EMS Responder:	A twenty-two-year-old.
Streaming Nurse:	Is he suitable for Minors?
EMS Responder:	No, a big metal sheet has gone down his leg and it has gone like this (mimics a slicing motion).
Streaming Nurse:	Ouch!
EMS Responder:	I have a young lady for you; she is seventy-two years young. Jarred her knee stepping up. She's got arthritis but now cannot weight bear, but she's American and here on holiday. Her husband is a physician. Is she going to come in here?
Streaming Nurse:	Let me see how many spaces on each side. Bear with me a second.

These interactions were highly routinised. EMS responders had a good social world's understanding of the service and were oriented to the criteria likely to influence allocation decisions. EMS Responders and ED staff were often well-known to each other, and nurses trusted their assessments. Most decisions were based on the oral handover, with follow-up questions as needed. The EMS Patient Care Record (PCR) was occasionally consulted, but this was the exception.

I asked whether she looked at the EMS PCR as part of the handover.

Streaming Nurse: It depends. If I know the crew and I know that what they say is going to be correct, then I'll take their handover. But if I don't know the crew or have doubts, then I will check the PCR. It's a bit like nursing – if you know someone you will go with their handover; but if not, you might dig around a bit more and check the obs [...] If I am sending someone to ACU I would check the PCR and to see whether the obs (physiological observations) are saying what they (the crew) say they are?'

The understanding of the patient as an allocative object of practice centred on a delimited number of situated concerns consequential for their placement in the department. Object formation was not formally documented; instead, the streaming nurse indicated the patient's location by circling the relevant option on the CAS Card. This served as the official record of where care was delivered and enabled doctors to locate their assigned patients. However, the concerns and sensemaking processes underpinning the allocation decision remained undocumented.

Enacting the Patient as a Triage Object

Once a bed was allocated, EMS responders formally transferred the patient to ED (see Chapter 7 for a discussion of transitions), and a copy of the EMS PCR was incorporated into the hospital record. Under the care of the ED nurse, the patient was constituted as a triage object to determine their priority for medical review. This process was typically interwoven with relationship-building and attention to comfort needs.

In the following extract, two nurses attend to a patient brought in after an epileptic seizure. One inserts a cannula and takes blood, while the other conducts assessments and history-taking to inform triage. As with EMS responders (see Chapter 5, p. 68), social talk is interspersed with formal clinical tasks.

ED Nurse 1: Have you got any pain?
Patient: Yes definitely, I have pain here where I hit my head and here where I slid down the ridge.
ED Nurse 1 takes his blood pressure: I am going to pop a line in and take some bloods.

[...]

ED Nurse 2: How are you feeling hon (honey, a local term of endearment)?

Patient: I feel drunk, very dizzy, and have a headache like you wouldn't believe.
ED Nurse 2: Did you have any warning?
Patient: No warning, unfortunately, I do not get any warning.

[…]

ED Nurse 2: Why were you in town?
Patient: I was just having a look around and getting a birthday present. But I didn't get very far.

While she is asking these questions, ED Nurse 1 is completing the CAS Card – this, I discover, is the triage process.

ED Nurse 1 (who is taking blood): Do you take Warfarin?
Patient: No.

ED Nurse 2 is writing down the patient observations – looking backwards and forwards between the monitor and her paperwork. At one point she moves closer to the monitor and scrutinises it.

The patient asks what time they are working until, and the nurses inform him it is until 1930.

ED Nurse 2 inquires as to his work and the patient explains that he takes calls for a transport company.

ED Nurse 2: Do you know where you are?
Patient: Yes. I am in Royal, no in [correct name of hospital].

[…]

We are interrupted by one of the EMS responders who is completing the PCR, a copy of which is subsequently left with the patient.

ED Nurse 2: Who's your next of kin?

[…]

ED Nurse 2: Do you live alone?
Patient: No; we live together.
ED Nurse 2: Any past medical history?
Patient: Yes, appendicitis and I had it out, twenty years ago.
ED Nurse 2: And you are confirmed epileptic?
Patient: Yes in 2004 by Dr […].

> As she is having this conversation, ED Nurse 2 is also reading from the PCR and appears to be copying information from here at the same time as she is asking the patient questions. The questioning stops and she is now clearly copying information from the PCR onto the CAS Card. It read:

S:	Tonic Clonic Fit
B:	Known epileptic, felt dizzy and remembers falling against a wall and sliding down.
She pauses and asks:	They don't know how long it lasted?
Patient:	No, they said fifteen seconds or something, but I don't know.

> ED Nurse 2 returns to the task of completing the form and makes the following entry: 'Not sure how long lasted. Also fit in ambulance lasted a few seconds'.
>
> This patient was assessed as a '3' on the triage system.

ED Nurse 2:	He will probably end up with a CT (scan) but then because he is a known epileptic maybe not.

In contrast to triage in the EMS Control Centre, the Manchester Triage System was not a prominent actor in ED work, having been largely internalised by experienced nurses. Similarly, while the Situation and Background components of the SBAR tool structured a brief clinical summary – typically based on the EMS PCR – the Assessment and Recommendation elements were less relevant, as triage had already occurred.

> Back at the central desk, I ask if this is the triage process. She confirms it is, but only a 'brief triage', noting 'there isn't very much space on the form'. She explains she's using SBAR: 'S is subject [sic], B is background'. When I ask about Assessment and Recommendation, she points to the observations section marked 'A' and says her recommendation is 'ref to dr'.

Through this process, the patient was enacted as a technical object for the purposes of triage: clinical urgency was assigned a numerical category, accompanied by a brief SBAR-structured summary. These data were recorded on the CAS Card and placed in a carousel used to manage medical workload.

Initial object formation for allocative and triage purposes was, respectively, locally situated and highly reductionist – rapidly assembled, narrowly focused, and designed to support immediate decision-making. In contrast, enacting patients for care and treatment was a more extended, distributed process. Sensemaking was shared between the ED nurse and doctor, and understanding evolved incrementally towards a disposal decision. Object formation at this stage encompassed a broader range of concerns than in EMS work – some highly standardised and inscribed in organisational artefacts, others more individualised, shaped by the singularities of the case. What counted as relevant emerged dynamically within the evolving clinical scenario.

Object Formation in Medical Practice

ED doctors were responsible for reaching a provisional diagnosis and determining a disposal decision within the four-hour performance target. These decisions were binary: they either resulted in discharge or referral to an inpatient specialist service. Medical object formation entailed enacting the patient as a professional object of practice oriented to matters of concern for reaching a diagnosis. Depending on the outcome, the patient was subsequently enacted either as a referral object to facilitate specialist in-patient care, or as a transition object, to support discharge to primary care.

Enacting a Professional Object of Practice

Doctors picked up new cases from the ED triage carousel, following an unwritten rule to see patients in order – no cherry-picking of interesting cases. As a site of medical education, sensemaking was mediated through the medical hierarchy: resident doctors' enactments of the patient required senior review before a decision was finalised.

Patients were enacted as professional objects of practice through the clinical clerking process, which involved taking a history, performing a physical examination, and initiating and interpreting tests. The CAS Card included an open-text section for documenting this process, reflecting the diversity of presentations in ED. While clerking styles varied, all doctors followed a broadly similar format, adapting their questions to the unfolding narrative of symptoms and signs to progressively focus on the main concern.

The following extract illustrates key features of ED medical sensemaking and object formation. It begins with the doctor consulting the clinical portal for prior hospital admissions – a common practice, as professionals routinely review existing records before seeing the patient. The in-person assessment opens with an invitation for the patient to tell their story, with further details elicited as the narrative unfolds. In this case, the patient, who has a longstanding cancer diagnosis, provides a clear history. This was not always possible, and family members or supporters often played a crucial role in sensemaking.

> ED doctor's next patient has been admitted with haematuria (blood in the urine). Doctor looks him up on the clinical portal. He reads for a little while and observes, 'He's quite a poorly chap'. I can see that the patient has a diagnosis of metastatic pancreatic cancer. Doctor expresses surprise that there is so little information on the clinical portal for a patient with this kind of medical history – only three referral letters – 'there are not many letters for someone with this history'.

[...]

We go to see the patient. The nurse has just finished taking an ECG. She remains in the cubicle while the following conversation takes place.

ED Doctor: So, tell me your story.

The patient explains that he had an operation a couple of weeks ago to address a 'blockage on both sides'. He said he had just come back from [another country] where they had concluded that he had some fibrosis.

ED Doctor: What was the cause of this?
Patient: They said it was fibrosis, and I had metastatic cancer some years ago, so whether it is that? Either way, they have put in a stent, they called it a stent, but it is in fact pig tails, I think.
ED Doctor: That just describes the shape of the end.
Patient: Anyway, they were both fine and it went well, that was last Friday.
ED Doctor: Are you feeling unwell?
Patient: Yes. It is painful across there (indicates area on lower abdomen) and I feel very tired and that has got worse and worse since I got home. My last blood test was 8.9 and my doctor was sufficiently concerned to contact my oncologist to organise a blood transfusion.

[...]

ED Doctor: So, the cancer originated where?
Patient: Pancreas.
ED Doctor: You've done very well.
Patient: I've had treatment in [another country] and some treatment here.
ED Doctor: Were they attempting a cure or getting your symptoms under control?
Patient: My impression was that it would delay things.

[...]

ED Doctor: So, when you are peeing is it red? There are no clots?
Patient: My wife has some samples.

At this point the wife produces some jars containing pink coloured urine.

ED Doctor: No pain?
Patient: I have some pain urinating.
ED Doctor: Back pain?
Wife: He has pain in his back.
Patient: I have back pain from an old injury.
ED Doctor: Is it any worse?
Patient: It varies so much it is hard to answer that question. The only pain I have is just across there (indicates lower abdomen) when I am urinating and this morning when I was urinating, which made me wonder whether something had gone wrong.
ED Doctor: Yeah, it could be a bit of an infection.

ED Doctor then examines the patient. He starts with his back and asks the patient to indicate whether any of his actions produce pain. He then asks the patient to lie flat and examines the patient's abdomen – asking the patient to drop his hands by his sides to make the abdomen as soft as possible. As he is carrying out the physical examination he asks about allergies and medications: 'Meds-wise, you're on chemo, but you're not receiving chemo now?'. He then asks: Is there anything I can hurt?

The patient indicates an area on his right lower abdomen.

Patient: Also, my right testicle has swollen up, but they didn't think it was anything significant.
ED Doctor: I see that they have put an ultrasound on it.
Patient: It hasn't healed itself – it's twice the size it should be.
ED Doctor: OK. Well, it seems more likely to be an infection. We'll get some bloods off, and I'll talk to the urology team. Are you on any medications other than painkillers?

His wife produces a packet of tablets from her bag: sleeping pills and 'one other tablet'.

ED Doctor asks how many sleeping pills he takes and the reason for the other medications.

Patient: Something I had from the chemotherapy – the tips of my fingers and toes went numb.

ED Doctor asks whether he will take blood should he need it.

ED Doctor: OK. We'll do bloods, urine and I'll talk to the urology team.

Several features stand out in this extract. First, the patient is a longstanding cancer patient with detailed knowledge of his condition, care, and healthcare processes. He actively contributes to sensemaking – for example, clarifying that his back pain is pre-existing and unrelated to his current presentation. Second, the couple arrive prepared, bringing a urine sample and the patient's medication. Third, the extract illustrates how the archival patient record is used as a sensemaking resource in new presentations. Beyond its content, the record's materiality – its size and scale – signals the complexity of the patient's medical history. In this case, the ED doctor is puzzled by the record's lack of detail, which is later explained by the patient's treatment history outside the UK.

The complexity of object formation in ED medical work varies. In some cases, doctors reached decisions based on the concerns elicited during clerking. Such as the young mother presenting with pain after an accident, where the doctor ordered a precautionary spinal X-ray but immediately prepared the discharge letter in the expectation that this would not reveal anything of concern. Or the referral to the medical team of a high school student admitted after a collapse, when it emerged that this was one incident in a wider pattern of unexplained collapses, the reasons for which had not been formally investigated.

Disposal decisions for suspected hip fracture were typically straightforward. In the absence of other injuries or urgent medical issues patients were sent straight to X-ray and if the injury was confirmed, they were referred to the Trauma and Orthopaedic Service. In many other cases, however, reaching a disposal decision was more protracted, requiring consideration of a wider range of concerns. Further tests and investigations could be required, and the results interpreted by appropriately qualified specialists. In such cases, reaching a disposal decision within performance targets was challenging.

> Doctor has a look at the CT scan results. We have now received the report on the sternum and L4 (fourth lumbar vertebrae) but still await the report on cervical spine – this must be done by another specialist radiologist. So, there are multi specialists reporting on the same scan.

> Today, one of the ED consultants, having asked me about my project, questioned why I was focused on hip fracture patients. I tried to explain that my interest was in processes, and I had taken the hip fracture pathway as a tracer condition through which to explore the relevant parts of the healthcare system. He continued to press the point about which patients I was interested in. He then offered the view that with hip fracture patients doctors at least had a diagnosis, but for other kinds of patient this was less clear-cut, and that staff were working with an uncertain and dynamic picture. He said that when he was a young doctor the juniors would clerk the patients, assemble all the relevant information to inform the diagnostic process, and then this would be followed by a senior review. In the current climate, patient flows are such that consultants are required to undertake a senior review much earlier in the information gathering process and as such the clinical picture can continue to evolve. It is also the case, that often they simply do not have the information

> required in order to reach a diagnosis. The senior review is a prerequisite for requesting a bed, however. So theoretically, the senior medical staff are being required to request a bed for patients on very provisional grounds. This issue is particularly challenging with patients with co-morbidities.

This extract highlights the tensions between clinical and administrative logics in the ED. The consultant's reflection reveals how time pressures and throughput targets have reshaped diagnostic practices, requiring senior reviews to occur earlier in the patient journey – often before sufficient clinical information is available. This shift not only challenges traditional models of medical decision-making but also introduces risks associated with premature diagnosis, particularly for patients with complex or comorbid conditions. The requirement to request a bed based on provisional assessments underscores how administrative logics – driven by capacity management and flow imperatives – can condition clinical practice, potentially leading to misallocation of inpatient resources and further straining bed capacity.

Enacting a Transition Object of Practice

Once a disposal decision was made, new enactments of the patient were needed to support their onward trajectory. For discharged patients, ED doctors had to create a transition object to transfer care to the GP. This was relatively straightforward. A digital discharge system, shaped by primary care information needs, standardised most concerns. The patient was enacted for transfer via drop-down menus prompting input (e.g. investigation results) and a free-text clinical summary.

ED doctors often batched discharge tasks during quieter periods, though this carried risks related to performance targets. Regardless of the patient's actual journey, the disposal decision had to be recorded 'on time'. Without a completed discharge, the target could be breached despite the material reality. In the first extract, a patient has left, but the system still shows them in ED because the GP letter is not done. In the second, the time taken to complete the letter causes a missed target, ironically adding to clinicians' workload.

> The coordinator approaches the ED doctor: Did you see the TIA (transient ischaemic attack) who was discharged? Can you do a discharge letter, as I can't get them off the system!

> *ED Nurse:* Have you seen [name]'s bloods are back? They are normal – can he go?
> *ED Doctor:* Yes. But I am happy to have a chat with him if he is concerned.
> *ED Nurse:* I am being nagged by the Controller as he is about to breach!

ED doctor goes into the digital system and makes an entry for this patient. He enters the clinical summary for the purposes of the GP letter entirely from memory.

> Despite the doctor's efforts to discharge the man with abdominal pain, he has breached by three minutes. He is now required to enter a reason for this. He ponders for a bit and then adds 'waiting for investigations and for me to look at that'.

Enacting a Referral Object of Practice

If hospital admission was needed, more extensive object formation was required to enact the patient as a referral object. This involved aligning histories, signs, and symptoms with the professional objects of the relevant specialty – to 'sell patients' (Hilligoss, 2014; Nugus et al., 2009). Medical interlocutors described this as time-consuming and frustrating. Enacting a referral patient entailed emphasising salient case features and sometimes ordering additional investigations – not for their own decision-making, but to meet specialist expectations. For hip fracture patients, referral was straightforward; a broken bone was unequivocally the responsibility of the trauma and orthopaedics team, and the radiological image performed the translational work necessary to accomplish a referral.

All referrals, other than medical referrals, were made in a telephone conversation with a doctor on the specialist team. ED doctors typically took time to assemble the case and mentally rehearse the history to justify the referral. The version of the patient that emerged was specifically tailored to this goal. For less experienced doctors, creating a referral object could be difficult, in part because of the power imbalances within the medical hierarchy, but also because they were less aware of referral norms or how to enact a referrable case.

> The doctor returns to the desk again. She still cannot achieve a referral for her 'Triple A' patient.
>
> *ED Doctor 1:* The medics don't want him either without a scan. No one will accept him. It's my fault, before I saw the patient I looked at the ECG with [ED consultant] and he said that the patient must go to the medics. The surgeon's won't see him until he has had a CTA, radiologists will not do the CTA until creats (blood test which measures creatinine levels in the blood to assess kidney function, which is required before a CTA scan).
>
> *ED Doctor 2:* You've not done creats?
>
> *ED Doctor 1:* No.
>
> *ED Doctor 2:* You should do.
>
> *ED Doctor 1:* I really should speak to [ED consultant]. Please someone take him!

If further investigation was needed and no other specialty was appropriate, Medicine became the default referral. The on-call medical team worked from the ED and reviewed patients in the AU. In these cases, referrals were made by adding the patient's name to a whiteboard in the Doctors' Office. The patient was still enacted as a referral object, oriented to the work of medical colleagues, but the process didn't involve formal negotiation with the team.

> ED doctor returns to completing his notes on the elderly lady. He pauses, 'I am trying to phrase something useful for the medical team'.
>
> We then walk round to the little office the medical doctors use, and ED doctor enters the details of the patient onto the white board. He adds her name and then hesitates in making the entry about the presenting complaint. He has written, 'collapse query cause', but then pauses and ponders out loud, 'How can I convey my concerns here?', he then adds to the entry 'previous collapse during sports'.

In the absence of having to negotiate directly with a gatekeeper, making medical referrals was less onerous than specialist referrals and senior colleagues cautioned juniors against settling prematurely on a medical referral as this was an easier option.

> 1515 and the consultant starting the evening shift arrives. There is a discussion about a recent near miss in which 'a fractured cervical vertebra was overlooked in the rush to bounce to medicine'

Making a successful specialist referral represented closure for the ED. The patient record was finalised, and the CAS Card was placed in the 'referred' section of the carousel where it could be retrieved by the specialist team.

Object Formation in ED Nursing Practice

Patients were cared for by nurses in Majors until a medical disposal decision was made, and then in AU until an inpatient bed became available. Nursing work involved addressing immediate needs and mobilising patient trajectories. Object formation generated two overlapping objects of practice: a professional object focused on clinical care, and a trajectory object focused on patient flow.

Enacting Professional Objects of Practice

Nurses in Majors were responsible for formally enacting the patient as a professional object of practice. Central to this was the Adult Patient Assessment Booklet (APAB), which brought together several mandatory risk assessment proformas – manual handling, tissue viability, falls, and nutrition. While these assessments supported the identification of immediate nursing care needs, their completion also served as an important organisational quality indicator, subject to audit in the event of a complaint.

Nurses drew on diverse sources to enact patients as professional objects: bedside assessments, conversations with patients or families, listening to medical clerking, reviewing documents like the EMS PCR and CAS Card, searching the clinical portal, and seeking additional information as needed. In the following extract, I join a nurse completing the documentation.

> ED nurse was doing a patient admission when I arrived. She had the EMS PCR and the APAB in front of her. I asked whether they used the PCR for the purposes of their information gathering.
>
> *ED Nurse:* I do; you can pick up the past medical history – so here it is dementia and hypertension.
>
> In the narrative section in the APAB, she wrote: 'Admitted to ED after being found on floor by carer'. She then completed the Waterlow Score (a widely used risk assessment tool for pressure ulcer development) and the Pat-A-Bac tool (a manual handling assessment). She commented: 'I've got to do an ECG and check to see whether she is on the falls list' (a reference to a community care initiative designed to support people at risk of falls).
>
> *DA:* How will you do that?
> *ED Nurse:* Her daughter.
>
> She goes to the trolley bay where the patient is located accompanied by her daughter.
>
> *ED Nurse:* Has she any history of falls?
> *Daughter:* No. Oh yes. A couple of nights ago she had a stumble.
> *ED Nurse:* Is she continent?
> *Daughter:* Yes.
> *ED Nurse:* Sorry to ask these questions. Is she steady on her feet?
> *Daughter:* She's a little unsteady.
>
> (As she asks these questions, ED Nurse makes entries into the APAB).

In this example, the nurse draws on multiple sources. She begins with the EMS PCR, then seeks further information from the patient's daughter. Some interactions are clearly shaped by institutional requirements – for example, 'Is she continent?' – driven by the need to complete documentation. Others are more relational, such as the apologetic repair: 'Sorry to ask these questions'. This case was straightforward, as the relative could provide the necessary information, but that was not always the case. Creating nursing objects of practice could involve more extensive, time-consuming efforts – contacting distant relatives, care homes, or GPs.

> ED nurse greeted me warmly. ED Nurse: I have just triaged this lady, and my main job is finding out the contact number for her next of kin. She is confused and neither of the numbers I have are long enough. This is what it is like, particularly with elderly patients.
>
> She tries one of the phone numbers, but it is not a legitimate number.

There was a normative expectation that enacting and documenting the patient as a professional object of nursing practice should be completed by the nurse responsible for the admission. This was not always possible because of wider work demands – nurses worked with multiple patients – and the speed with which patients were mobilised through the department. Failure to complete object formation challenged professional relationships across section interfaces in the ED.

> On the way back from AU to Majors ED Nurse observed: Some of them over there (AU) will rip you apart with the handover.

DA:	In what sense?
ED Nurse:	Oh 'why haven't you done this and why haven't you done that?' But when they say we have to move them round then we have to go.
DA:	So, it's more about the stuff they think you should have done than the quality of the information?
ED Nurse:	Yeah.

Enacting Trajectory Objects of Practice

Beyond attending to individual care needs, nurses played a vital but largely invisible role in trajectory management (Allen, 2015a). In ED, this involved attention to factors affecting patient flow: test results, doctors' disposal decisions, discharges, referrals, and future care plans. While professional objects were formally constituted in nursing documentation, trajectory objects were generated informally – yet remained resource-intensive.

Amid organisational pressures and national performance targets, there was a shared imperative to maintain awareness of patients awaiting disposal decisions. ED doctors, managing multiple cases simultaneously, reflexively monitored test result progress.

> After the handover, ED doctor seeks out the notes of the road traffic accident patient, who is now in AU. He is trying to establish what the Cardiologists have said about the results of the Echo (Echocardiogram). He has some difficulty finding the information – mainly because the report has mistakenly been entered into the nursing notes rather than the patient's medical record. The entry is difficult to read. ED doctor says, 'It's difficult to read and interpret, but as far as I can see there is nothing obvious there'.
>
> The anaesthetists spend time intubating the patient, who is then taken for a scan. Meanwhile the Registrar leaves the bedside and starts checking up on the formal reports on another patient with the fractured sternum.

Maintaining real-time trajectory awareness in all patients was not easy, however. Doctors could initiate investigations and then become enrolled in other activities in the department. To a considerable extent, then, they relied on ED nurses for this purpose.

> I asked whether he actively chased up results or whether he relied on the nurses to tell him. ED Resident Doctor: 'We do rely on the nurses to chase us; as you have seen, you get pulled into other things'.

ED nurses proactively monitored patients, informed doctors of test results, and prompted action when targets risked being breached.

Beyond managing patient flows, nurses' maintained trajectory awareness for transition management. Patients were mobilised through the department at short-notice and nurses needed a comprehensive understanding of the evolving trajectory for the purposes of handover, whether from ED to AU, or AU to the wards.

Nurses enacted patients as trajectory objects through care trajectory narratives – informal artefacts that encapsulate a 'working knowledge' (Ellingsen & Monteiro, 2003) of care (Allen, 2015a). These narratives had a retrospective-prospective structure: summarising the trajectory to date and orienting to future care. Though absent from formal communication systems, they were key to cooperative action.

In Majors, these narratives were largely mental models – working understandings stabilised for AU transfer. In AU, maintaining trajectory awareness was more demanding. Whereas patients remained in Majors for about four hours, length of stay in AU was variable. Some patients could move through the department quickly, if a bed was available, but many others remained for several days, and care could evolve quite rapidly during this time. In addition, while the nurses in Majors worked with known ED doctors, AU nurses interacted with a broader range of specialist teams. A core component of AU nursing work was maintaining awareness of trajectory awareness under conditions in which patients could be transferred at short notice and medical-nurse communication was exacting.

To manage these challenges, AU nurses deployed an informal structured proforma, colloquially known as 'the handover form', which functioned as a coordinating and accumulating device (Berg, 1999). It was inscribed with the concerns that constituted the patient as a trajectory object: presenting problem, past medical history, diagnosis, and plan, with a structured section focused on the patient's nursing care needs. Nurses used the proforma to maintain a rolling summary of each patient's evolving care trajectory. While some entries were contemporaneous, I often observed nurses stepping away from clinical work to review and update the form.

> AU nurse is updating a handover form. I watched her as she looked through the notes and then periodically added new information to the form – sometimes double-checking her sources. She also ticked a few boxes to show certain things had been completed.
>
> *DA:* Are you updating the form?
>
> *AU Nurse:* It makes handover easier, and this chap is complicated, and I wanted to make sure I've got everything.
>
> *DA:* Does this ensure you have everything to hand if you need to transfer someone? You don't get much notice, do you?
>
> *AU Nurse:* No. You can be with a patient five minutes and then be expected to handover.
>
> Updating the handover forms often involved nurses periodically reviewing patient notes to identify and distil key developments. This could mean flipping back and forth through narrative-style entries. The form consolidated all information needed for handover in one place – a systematic process of updating the care trajectory narrative in a context where multiple medical teams might briefly engage with the patient and leave isolated entries.
>
> In AU, where trajectories evolved rapidly, nurses needed a ready overview in case of sudden transfers. The handover form helped stabilise this. Today, I observed one nurse rewriting a form to reflect changes in a patient's condition, and another updating and adding to it. A senior nurse noted their usefulness but stressed the importance of keeping them current. She pointed to a form from a patient admitted the previous day, noting that much could have changed since. Completed documentation alone was no guarantee of up-to-date information.
>
> *(Fieldnote Memo)*

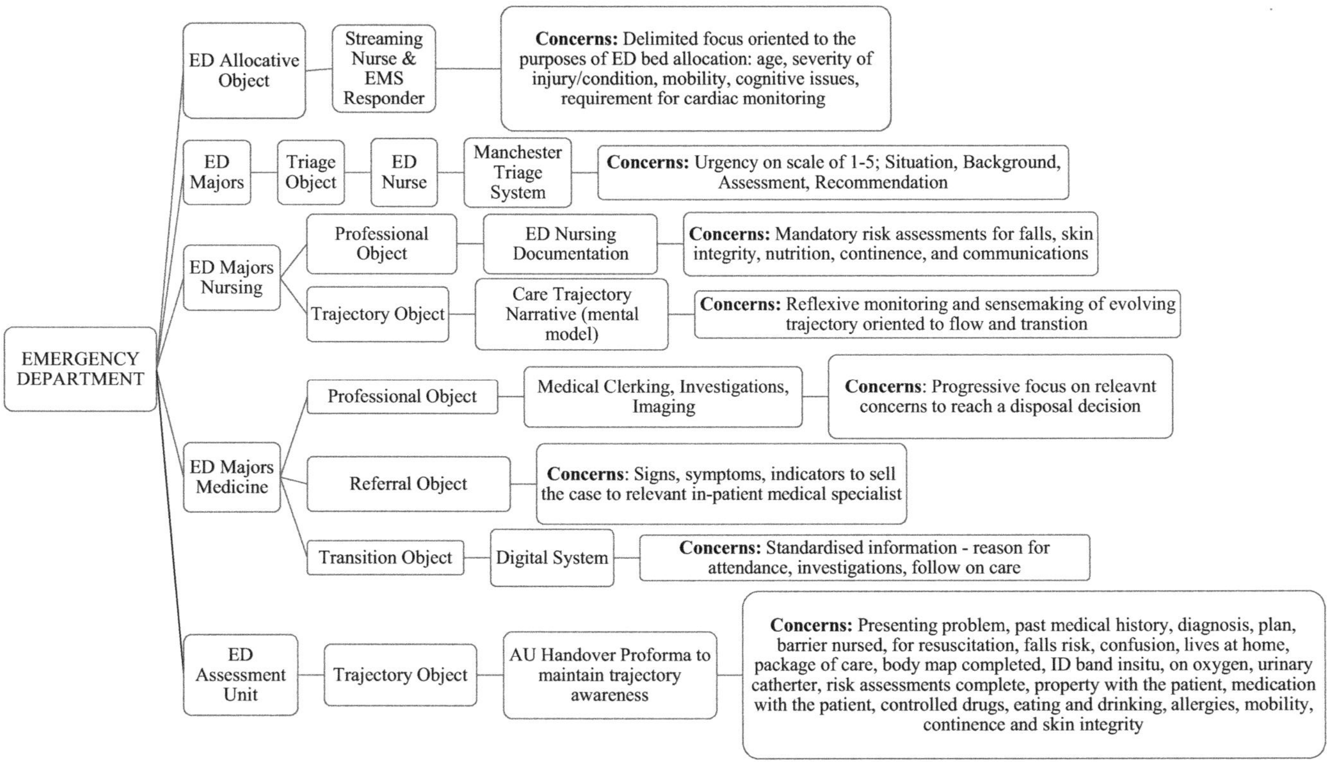

FIGURE 6.1 Object formation in ED work.

DA:	Are you updating the form?
AU Nurse:	It makes handover easier, and this chap is complicated, and I wanted to make sure I've got everything.
DA:	Does this ensure you have everything to hand if you need to transfer someone? You don't get much notice, do you?
AU Nurse:	No. You can be with a patient five minutes and then be expected to handover.

Updating the handover forms often involved nurses periodically reviewing patient notes to identify and distil key developments. This could mean flipping back and forth through narrative-style entries. The form consolidated all information needed for handover in one place – a systematic process of updating the care trajectory narrative in a context where multiple medical teams might briefly engage with the patient and leave isolated entries.

In AU, where trajectories evolved rapidly, nurses needed a ready overview in case of sudden transfers. The handover form helped stabilise this. Today, I observed one nurse rewriting a form to reflect changes in a patient's condition, and another updating and adding to it. A senior nurse noted their usefulness but stressed the importance of keeping them current. She pointed to a form from a patient admitted the previous day, noting that much could have changed since. Completed documentation alone was no guarantee of up-to-date information.

(Fieldnote Memo)

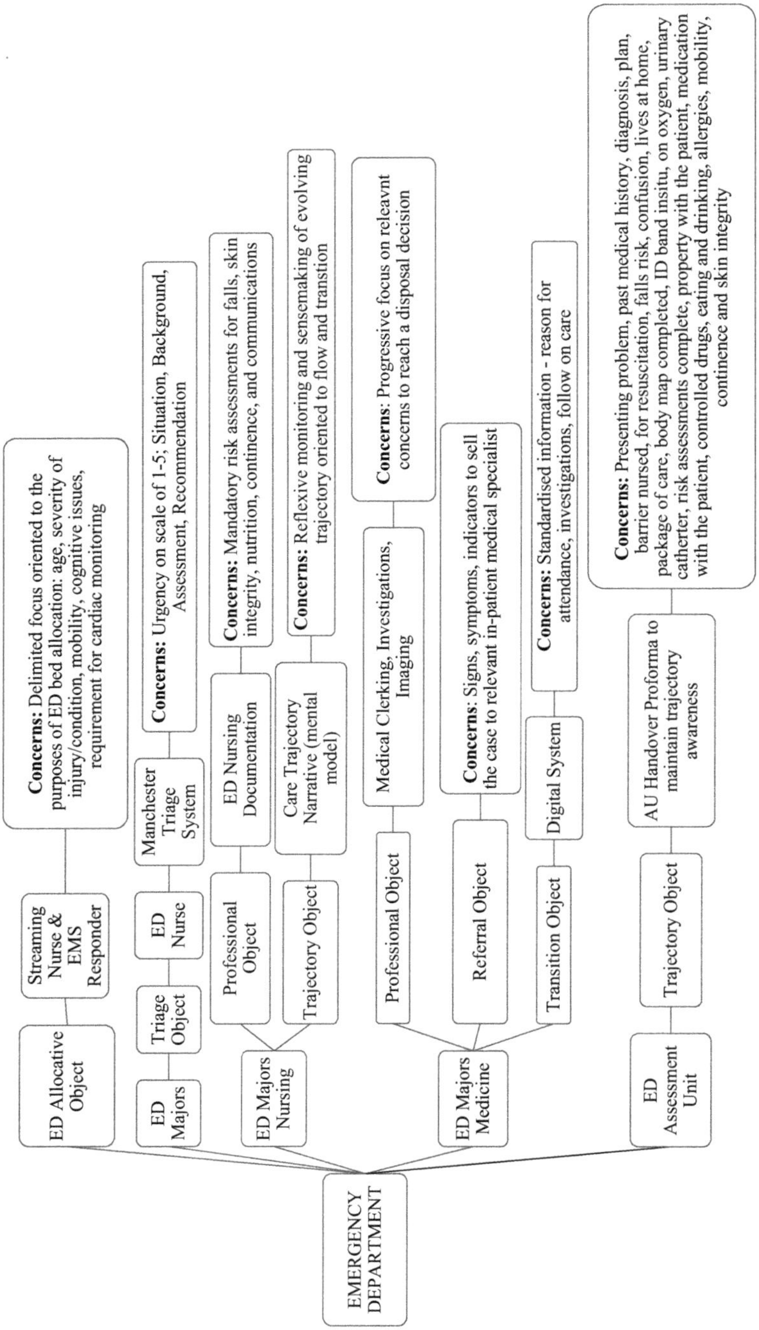

FIGURE 6.1 Object formation in ED work.

While the handover form was integral to nursing practice in AU and, as I will describe in the next chapter, it played a central role in managing transitions, it was primarily a working record (Fitzpatrick, 2004) – a documentary counterpart to nurses' working knowledge. It was not retained in the formal medical record and was discarded after the patient had been transferred to the ward.

Summary

This chapter has examined how patients were enacted as multiple objects of practice to mobilise care and treatment through the ED. Activity was shaped by tightly coupled clinical, administrative, and mobilisation logics, aimed at prioritising care within externally imposed time constraints. Initially focused on narrow concerns for bed allocation and care prioritisation, more expansive versions of the patient were incrementally constructed by nursing and medical staff as professional objects for ongoing care and disposal decisions. Nurses reflexively monitored trajectories, enacting patients as trajectory objects. Though largely informal, these enactments played a crucial role in sustaining patient flow at this stage. Figure 6.1 illustrates these logics and the layered enactments of the patient across the ED trajectory.

References

Allen, D. (2015a). *The Invisible Work of Nurses: Hospitals, Organisation and Healthcare*. New York, Routledge.

Allen, D. (2015b).'Inside "bed management": ethnographic insights from the vantage point of UK hospital nurses'. *Sociology of Health & Illness* **37**(3): 370–384. https://doi.org/10.1111/1467-9566.12195

Berg, M. (1999). 'Accumulating and coordinating occasions for information technologies in medical work'. *Computer Supported Cooperative Work* **8**: 373–401

Ellingsen, G. and E. Monteiro (2003). 'Mechanisms for producing a working knowledge: enacting, orchestrating and organizing'. *Information and Organization* **13**(3), 203–229. https://doi.org/10.1016/s1471-7727(03)00011-3

Fitzpatrick, G. (2004). 'Integrated care and the working record'. *Health Informatics Journal* **10**: 291.

Hilligoss, B. (2014). 'Selling patients and other metaphors: a discourse analysis of the interpretive frames that shape emergency department admission handoffs'. *Social Science & Medicine.* **102**:119–128. https://doi.org/10.1016/j.socscimed.2013.11.034

Hillman, A. (2014). '"Why must I wait?" The performance of legitimacy in a hospital emergency department'. *Sociology of Health & Illness* **36**(4): 485–499.

Nugus, P., Bridges, J., and Braithwaite, J. (2009). 'Selling patients'. *BMJ* **339**: b5201. https://doi.org/10.1136/bmj.b5201

7

EVOLVING OBJECTS

Unscheduled Care Transitions

Building on the preceding analysis of the organisation of patients, care, and treatment within individual unscheduled care services, this chapter examines their interrelationships and the management of transitions. It considers two distinct transition processes: the technologically mediated interface between the EMS Control Centre and responders, and the relational narrative-based arrangements utilised across all other unscheduled care interfaces. The chapter begins by describing the transitional arrangements in unscheduled care and then brings these processes into view through empirical illustration.

Transition Arrangements

This section outlines the transitional arrangements through which patients were moved across service boundaries within unscheduled care. First, it explores the *transition interfaces* between services, highlighting the shared organising logics and mutual awareness of interdependence that shaped their interrelations. Second, it considers the socio-material *infrastructure* that mediated transitions. Finally, it examines how patients were enacted as *transition objects* to facilitate their transfer across organisational settings.

Transition Interfaces

A distinguishing feature of transition interfaces in the unscheduled care assemblage was the shared orientation of constituent services to prioritisation and mobilisation logics. As outlined in earlier chapters, care and treatment within each service were shaped by national performance targets and constrained by limited resources. EMS call handlers managed cases within a strict

DOI: 10.4324/9781003475019-11

two-to-four-minute window; dispatch operatives worked to time targets; EMS responders focused on rapid assessment, stabilisation, and timely conveyance; and in ED, the goal was to reach a disposal decision and initiate action within four hours.

Unscheduled care services faced significant demand pressures. Each had distinct functions and challenges, but there was strong mutual awareness of their interdependence. EMS responders sought to avoid unnecessary ED transfers when alternatives were available, and ED staff – via EMS Control Centre data – could monitor community demand and the impact of ED delays on ambulance availability.

Streaming Nurse: In the winter, you could be sat here with a list of incoming jobs and a list of jobs that you have sat outside in the ambulances thinking about who you need to prioritise to offload [...] If we are holding crews outside, you can see the effects of this on the community in terms of the reduced availability of crews.

Shared organising logics and mutual understanding of service interdependencies created a practical alignment of interests across the unscheduled care assemblage, shaping transition management.

Transition Infrastructure

Technology was a significant actor in the coordination of activity at the interface between the Control Centre and front-line EMS crews. The AMPDS (Advanced Medical Priority Dispatch System) structured information flow from the initial call, shaping the categorisation of urgency. Dispatch operatives used APMDS codes to allocate resources, and crews received AMPDS-generated summary data on screens within their vehicles.

By contrast, transitions across the rest of the unscheduled care assemblage relied mainly on human actors. EMS responders and ED nurses acted as representatives of their respective social worlds, mobilising patients across service boundaries. In addition to shared organising logics and mutual interdependence, they held reciprocal understandings of each other's work. EMS responders made frequent ED transfers and often had established relationships with staff. Within ED, transitions between Majors and AU were similarly underpinned by familiarity. Majors nurses typically understood AU workflows, with many having worked in both settings. AU nurses were also familiar with ward routines, having previously worked or trained there.

This cross-boundary familiarity enabled what Boland and Tensaki (2001) describe as 'perspective-taking', which facilitated handover alignment with the concerns and practices of the receiving service. As described in previous chapters, transition management was deeply embedded in the everyday work of EMS responders and ED nurses, with trajectory object formation closely interwoven with the enactment of patients as professional objects of practice.

Transition Objects

The AMPDS was the principal actor in constituting the patient as a transition object at the Control Centre-EMS responder interface. Mediated by call handlers' interactional skills, it translated callers' narrative accounts into a codified object, through structured triage and classification (see Chapter 4). The understanding of the patient produced by this process was inscribed in a standardised call summary. At dispatch operatives' discretion, additional information from call handlers or clinical support staff was sometimes relayed to responders, supplementing the AMPDS output. This is reflected in the capitalised sentence at the end of the following extract, which is a fieldnote of the screen display in the ambulance.

> **32-year-old female conscious breathing
> Preg/childbirth/miscarriage
> High risk complications
> Miscarriage
>
> 1 1st trimester
> 2 This is not a reported miscarriage
> 3 There is a serious bleed
> 4 She has HIGH RISK complications.
>
> BEEN IN HOSPITAL OVERNIGHT WITH LOSSING (sic) BLOOD FOR FEW WEEKS.**

As this extract illustrates, the patient is enacted as a technical object. The complex processes that have gone into the constitution of the case in the control centre work are largely invisible to the end user, and as an object of practice, the patient is fixed, stable and immediately available.

At all other interfaces within the unscheduled care assemblage, transition objects had a narrative quality. Nurses were the primary actors in managing transitions and, as described in Chapter 6, routinely deployed care trajectory narratives in their work (Allen, 2015). Their flexibility supported recipient design (Heritage, 1984) and allowed for revision as care evolved, or new understandings emerged. Unlike the fixed immutable forms generated in EMS Control Centre Work, narrative objects enacted patients as mutable mobiles (Allen, 2015; Rolland et al., 2006) – adaptable across contexts and responsive to trajectory dynamics. Constructing an adequate narrative was a collaborative sensemaking activity, typically developed in dialogue between service representatives at the transition interface. Though relatively unstructured, this work was a visible and significant marker of professional competence.

Transition Processes

This section examines how transition was practised across the four unscheduled care interfaces, focusing on object formation and the mobilisation of the patient trajectory across organisational and professional boundaries. Drawing on empirical materials, including the case of Mary introduced in Chapter 4, it illustrates both the processes through which transitions were accomplished and the conditions which mediated their timing, form, and content.

EMS Control Centre–EMS Responder Transition Interface

When EMS responders were allocated a job, they received an AMPDS-generated enactment of the patient via the in-cab display. This included automated call summary data and, occasionally, free-text notes from control centre staff. While these entries formed part of the wider sensemaking practices of call handlers and clinical support officers, their quality varied, reflecting the circumstances of their production.

> Call handlers could only view a small text box, typing while multitasking and switching between screens. Once submitted, entries disappeared, leaving no chance for review. Today, one typed 'flow' instead of 'fall' and didn't notice. Other examples I have observed include 'Melina' for 'Melaena' and 'kndd' for 'knee'. In fact, when I was with the dispatch operative, he actually had a look at the adjacent letters on the keyboard to try and decipher the intended word in the note pad.
>
> *(Fieldnote Memo)*

In enacting patients as transition objects, dispatch operatives acted as intermediaries, filtering out and interpreting this information. In practice, then, not all notepad data reached crews. As one dispatch operative explained:

> We only send what's obviously relevant. We don't want to prompt too many questions, but we don't want to withhold information either. Sometimes we talk on the radio or ask the clinical desk to follow up. The system shows who took the call, and not all call handlers are as good [...] I wouldn't want that job – it's not easy, and many are quite young. It must be daunting.

Once an address was confirmed, the case appeared on the AMPDS and could be dispatched. It was not uncommon for crews to be allocated a job without any initial information.

> 0939 – We get our first call out to Summerfields. We do not know the details of the case.
>
> *Paramedic:* It's a nice long drive so hopefully we will know more when we get there.
> *DA:* Do you ever get to a job and not know the case?
> *Paramedic:* If we get close and there's still no information we can radio through or someone from control will call.
>
> (Control comes through on the radio).
>
> *Paramedic:* There you go.

Crews also had to interpret information that was unclear, misleading, or incorrect. In the following fieldnote, the clinically significant difference between vomiting and coughing blood had not been resolved in the transmitted information.

> I remarked on the quality of the information we were given for the last case, i.e. there is a big difference between vomiting and coughing blood. When I made this observation Paramedic said: 'That's right because the crew asked whether he was vomiting. I'd forgotten that that was what it had said'.

EMS responders were widely sceptical about AMPDS reliability. While screen data offered age, gender, and some clues as to the equipment to be taken from the vehicle into the location, as described in Chapter 5, EMS responders treated each call de novo, warning of the dangers of preconceived ideas.

> *Paramedic 1:* 'One of the things I learnt when I was newly qualified, was not to be blinkered by the screen. You need to keep an open mind. I learnt that lesson. I was called to a fella who was scruffy and had fallen off his bike. It was boiling hot. He was unconscious, had pinpoint pupils and was sweating. I assumed he was on heroin – but I just did a blood glucose reading as you do routinely, and he was hypo (hypoglycaemic, i.e. low blood glucose levels). I could have Narcaned (Narcan is a medication administered to block the effects of opioids) him and missed the hypo!'.
> *Paramedic 2:* 'To be honest you learn to take the information you are given with a pinch of salt. The only thing I do believe is if they say that there is a cardiac arrest, and CPR is being performed at the scene'.

Thus, while AMPDS-generated patient enactments were designed as immutable mobiles (Latour, 1987) – standardised representations meant to travel across sites (see Chapter 3) – they did not circulate as intended. They remained largely immutable in form, but they were not mobile in practice, because crews distrusted and discounted them. Although dispatch operatives oriented to AMPDS enactments as transition objects, responders treated them less as sensemaking resources and more as mechanisms of allocation. At this interface, the object of practice did not travel; only the job did.

EMS–ED Transition Interface

On arrival at ED, the patient remained in the ambulance under EMS care. The second crew member entered the department to book the patient in at Reception and liaise with the streaming nurse to secure a bed (see Chapter 6). Only once a space was allocated could the patient be transferred and formally handed over to the responsible nurse.

To trace this transition in detail, we return to Mary's case at the EMS–streaming nurse interface. In this initial interaction, object formation focused on concerns relevant to determining Mary's placement in ED. Though not a formal transfer of care, it played a key role in shaping subsequent object formation for transition, where professional identities were at stake. The EMS responder begins with a concise narrative: what happened, what injuries are evident or suspected, and relevant aspects of Mary's medical history that are salient for the streaming nurse's purposes.

EMS Responder:	I have got [Mary] an eighty-five-year-old lady who lives with her husband. She was trying to go out the door and she slipped on some water, and she fell out onto the patio. She has a 'lac' (laceration) to her head and right hip pain. She can't weight bear because of the pain, but there is no shortening, no rotation (reference to indicators of hip fracture). She has chronic bronchitis and is on permanent oxygen. ECG's (electrocardiogram) a bit irregular (shows the ED nurse the printout). It's nice and regular and then she throws an ectopic and it looks like a bundle there. So, she's irregularly irregular. Says she's got an aortic aneurysm.
Streaming Nurse:	Did you do bilateral BP?
EMS Responder:	No. No loss of consciousness, GCS (Glasgow Coma Scale) is fine.
Streaming Nurse:	What's her NEWS (National Early Warning Score) score?

EMS Responder hasn't done this either.

EMS Responder:	I've got it (NEWS scoring system) on the phone.
Streaming Nurse:	Haven't you got the table?

The EMS responder and ED nurse consult the NEWS chart on the wall. There is some debate about what to do about the SATS (blood oxygen saturation levels) which are normal for Mary but also a trigger for NEWS. They decide that these should be included and generate a score of five.

Streaming Nurse:	Fine. I've got a trolley in Majors. I'll make sure there's a cardiac monitor.

Not all ED beds had cardiac monitors, and at this stage of Mary's trajectory, it was cardiac risk – not the head wound or hip pain – that shaped the allocation decision. The streaming nurse asked probing questions to determine bed placement, with priorities differing from those of EMS responders. Bilateral blood pressure was not routinely measured, but a different reading on each arm can indicate a bleeding aortic aneurysm – a possible cause of Mary's fall. However, in Mary's case, the EMS disposal decision focused on the visible need to suture the head wound, with the aneurysm only emerging in the ambulance, though the medical history.

In accounting for this omission, the EMS responder appealed to standard neurological criteria 'no loss of consciousness and a satisfactory GCS' to justify the absence of a detailed cardiac assessment. The reference to the NEWS score, used to identify acutely ill patients, similarly, reflected the streaming nurses' orientation to the cardiac history. Crews did not routinely calculate NEWS scores, but this was a significant concern for the streaming nurse. Back in the ambulance, the EMS responder performed a bilateral blood pressure reading – an action I interpreted as prompted by the streaming nurse's earlier question. These new data, along with the recently calculated NEWS score, subsequently became part of the handover.

The formal transfer of care involved a more detailed narrative than that used for bed allocation. It had a retrospective focus on the incident and EMS disposal decision, but also included medical history relevant to ED diagnostic work. Sometimes the EMS narrative sufficed, but more often nurses contributed to sensemaking, surfacing aspects of the case for their own purposes. In Mary's handover, the nurse clarified that the fall was a 'slip not a trip' – a distinction important for diagnosis, as slips tend to cause more serious injuries. This reframed the hip pain as a more prominent concern.

We 'off-load' Mary from the ambulance and take her into the designated cubicle. I offer my arm as support to the husband who is a bit unsteady.

EMS Responder:	Who's looking after Mrs [name]?

ED Nurse comes forward.

EMS Responder: [Mary] is an eighty-five-year-old lady who was at home and slipped. She landed on her right side and has lacerated her head. A neighbour helped her get up. She can't weight bear. There is no obvious shortening, no rotation (reference to indicators of hip fracture). I've given her Paracetamol. She's OK when she is still. She has told me she has not got heart disease, but the 3-lead (ECG) shows a left bundle and ectopic [...] She's got an aortic aneurysm which they are keeping an eye on. Her bilateral BP (blood pressure) is fine. She's broken her back in the past but has no new pain. No pain in her head. She's on constant oxygen. Her SATS are ninety-one but that's normal for her. She has a NEWS score of five, but this is because of her SATS. She's got bronchitis associated with TB, which is why she's on Oxygen. She didn't trip over the tube.

ED Nurse: So, a slip not a trip?

EMS Responder: Yes. She's had half a glass of wine. The wound had stopped bleeding when I got there.

We leave the patient with the nurse and EMS responder finds a surface to lean on and completes the PCR.

EMS Responder: I'll just finish writing. I've been too busy talking.

[...]

EMS Responder checks through the notes, and the patient observes: There is so much writing!

EMS Responder: It's our saving grace!

As well as illustrating the extended narrative used for transfer of care, this extract also reveals that professional identities are implicated in handover processes. New information – the bilateral blood pressure and NEWS score – arising from the earlier interaction with the streaming nurse, are incorporated into the narrative. The EMS responder also notes the absence of shortening and rotation in their account of Mary's hip pain. While hip fracture is not explicitly mentioned, this utterance signals attentiveness to a potential injury and does performative work in the public display of competent professional practice.

EMS responders often completed patient records after handover. In Mary's case, this included the bilateral blood pressure readings and the NEWS score. Back in the ambulance, having handed over Mary's care, I asked the paramedic about the bilateral BP.

EMS Responder: 'It's because of her aneurysm. If there's a difference of twenty it suggests its bleeding. It didn't occur to me actually. There was so much going on and we were chatting away and the way it was presented it was not looking like a collapse'.

Majors– Assessment Unit Interface

Patients remained in Majors until the ED doctor reached a disposal decision. If ED was operating within national performance targets, this phase lasted up to four hours. During this time, they were cared for by an ED nurse and a healthcare support worker, who were responsible for a trolley bay area. With a capacity for six patients, they triaged all new admissions, conducted formal assessments to enact the patient as a nursing object, addressed ongoing care needs and managed transitions to the AU. As outlined in Chapter 6, a central element of nursing work in Majors was reflexive monitoring of cases to maintain awareness of evolving trajectories. This included checking the status of investigations, interacting with ED doctors, and reviewing CAS Card entries. Patients were transferred to AU once admission was deemed necessary.

Nurses managed transitions from Majors to AU. Compared with the EMS–ED interface, these transition narratives were wider in scope, reflecting the evolving trajectory. While traces of the EMS handover remained, they were brief, and the focus centred on nursing care needs, and future plans. The following extract is typical. It relates to an elderly female patient who, like Mary, has had a fall but has not sustained a hip fracture and has been referred to the specialist frailty team. Here both nurses are oriented to the formal nursing documentation, and the narrative enactment of the patient as a transition object emerges through joint sensemaking.

Majors Nurse: [Name] likes to be known as Grace, ninety.

Both nurses are attending to the patient record, and AU Nurse points to snowflake symbol which is a signifier of cognitive impairment.

Majors Nurse: I don't think she is. It says query on the form. She's completely deaf that's all. She was found on the floor by the carers, it's known that falls are a bit of an issue, she has visual impairment.

AU Nurse: Continent?
Majors Nurse: She wears pads and was dry when I last checked.
AU Nurse: Has she been seen by a medic?
Majors Nurse: Yeah, but not senior.
AU Nurse: And the plan?
Majors Nurse: 'FOPAL (Frail Older People's Assessment and Liaison Service).

Knowing the patient is a central to nursing practice (Allen, 2015) and delivering a comprehensive handover is a key marker of professional competence. ED nurses used mental models of patient trajectories through reflexively monitoring activity, but at transition points, they typically undertook further sense-making and translational work to stabilise case details for handover.

> After the call ended, the ED nurse updated the lady's notes [...] I realised she was transcribing details from the medical clerking on the CAS Card into the nursing assessment booklet. It became clear the patient was being moved to AU, and the nurse was finalising notes to ensure everything was in order before transfer.

Owing to front-door demands, patients were often moved from Majors to AU while the ED nurse was still making sense of the evolving trajectory. In such cases – when there was insufficient time to develop an understanding and construct a trajectory narrative – handover faltered, and nurses relied more heavily on the documented record.

> *ED Nurse:* 'This is [name], eighty-one. Came in with (urinary) retention. There was only five hundred and sixty-one mils residual, but they still catheterised him. He's a known COPD (chronic obstructive pulmonary disease), he's on fluids, and I've done his NEWS. I don't know anything else. He only came in at ten past ten.
>
> She pauses and reads from the medical clerking notes on the CAS Card.
>
> *ED Nurse:* Oh, he was very agitated when he came in and had some abdo (abdominal) pain. He's had bloods and ECG and has now been referred to urology.

In accounting for her incomplete knowledge of the patient by referencing the patient's brief time in Majors – 'he only came in at ten past ten' – the ED nurse is oriented to normative expectations about an adequate handover. In other scenarios I observed, the nurse had developed a mental model of the trajectory but had not had time to complete the formal documentation. In the following example, the handover has taken place to the satisfaction of the AU nurse, but the process of finalising the documentation, surfaces a detail that has been omitted.

> After the handover has finished the ED Nurse remains on the unit adding information to the notes. The process prompts her to provide more information.
>
> *ED Nurse:* She's got some old bruises on her head, and she's got this money (shows AU Nurse the notes).

Beyond its role in professional identity, the nurse's decision to re-engage with the AU nurse to share overlooked details highlights the value of care trajectory narratives as working knowledge in nursing. AU nurses rarely had time to reconstruct cases from notes alone; instead, they relied on the patient enactment conveyed at handover to organise care.

Assessment Unit–Ward Interface

Patients with hip fractures remained in AU until an inpatient bed became available. The hospital had several trauma and orthopaedic wards – spinal, trauma, and orthogeriatric. The goal was to admit hip fracture patients to Jenolan, the orthogeriatric ward, within 12 hours of referral. A dedicated Trauma and Orthopaedics Coordinator matched patients to appropriate beds. While patients were in AU, significant organisational activity supported admission, including moving patients within Jenolan, transferring trauma patients elsewhere, and/or expediting discharges.

Once a bed had been identified, the AU received little notice of the need to organise the transfer of care. The transition between AU and in-patient wards was managed by nurses and took place over the telephone. As described in Chapter 6 (p.97), to mitigate the challenges of maintaining trajectory awareness in conditions of high patient throughput and complex inter-professional communication mechanisms, AU nurses had developed a handover proforma. This served as a coordination tool and reference point for narrative construction. Without it, handovers could be hesitant, with nurses leafing through records to gather key details.

> AU Nurse is preparing to handover a second patient. She has the patient notes open in front of her and is reading from the medical admission proforma.
>
> *AU Nurse:* This one I will have to think through. I can't read a lot of it. I'm not saying my writing would be any better if I was writing in a hurry but....

AU Nurse 2: It's difficult, isn't it?
AU Nurse: (to person on the phone) Hi ya. Are you expecting [name]? Ok thanks.

She pauses; I notice that she has her fingers marking different sections in the notes to enable her to readily access key information. There is no handover form in this case.

At one level, the nurse's difficulty reflects the lack of consolidated information. At another, completing the handover form appeared to help nurses make sense of the patient's trajectory. The form acted as more than a checklist – it scaffolded the narrative, aiding recall and strengthening the nurse's grasp of what to communicate. This aligns with research on distributed cognition (Hutchins, 1995), which highlights how artefacts support memory and reasoning, and with psychological work on the 'generation effect', whereby generating information oneself leads to improved recall (Slamecka and Graf, 1978).

Sometimes, patients were moved before the AU nurse had handed over. As the handover sheet was not part of the formal record, it did not accompany the patient, making it a valuable resource for AU nurses to sense-check their mental model.

AU Nurse is still waiting for the ward nurse to come to the phone so that she can handover.

AU Nurse: When they are busy and they need to move someone out, and they see us waiting like this, they just take the notes and go. It's not ideal, but then if you had a relative on an ambulance wanting to come in then.

Summary

Trajectory mobilisation in the unscheduled care assemblage involved discrete services aligned through shared organising logics. The APMDS was a central yet problematic actor in managing transitions between the EMS Control Centre and front-line crews. While EMS infrastructure aimed to enact patients as stable, transferable objects, in practice, these enactments lacked mobility due to widespread distrust of technology-generated information. Crews treated them as allocative objects rather than sensemaking resources.

Elsewhere in the assemblage, transition relied entirely on the dynamic, mutable sensemaking of human actors. Rather than linear information transfer, it was a collaborative process of object formation grounded in shared social understandings. Despite – or perhaps because of – their unstructured nature, jointly enacted care trajectory narratives served as temporary stabilisations, enabling coordination and mobilisation of diverse patient populations

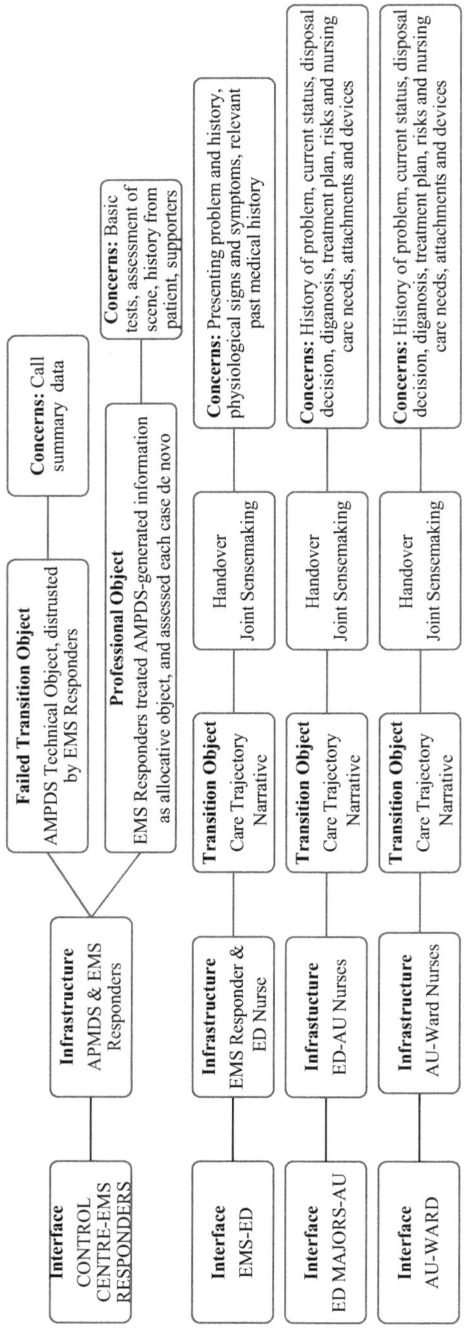

FIGURE 7.1 Transition arrangements in the unscheduled care assemblage.

as evolving objects of practice across service interfaces in a fast-paced, high-throughput environment. Figure 7.1 illustrates transitional arrangements in unscheduled care assemblage.

References

Allen, D. (2015). *The Invisible Work of Nurses: Hospitals, Organisation and Healthcare.* London and New York, Routledge.

Boland, R.J. and R.V. Tensaki (2001). 'Communication and collaboration in distributed cognition'. *Coordination Theory and Collaborative Technology*. G.M. Olson, T.W. Malone and J.B. Smith. New Jersey, Lawrence Erlbaum Associates: 51–66.

Heritage, J. (1984). *Garfinkel and Ethnomethodology*. Cambridge, Polity Press.

Hutchins, E. (1995). *Cognition in the Wild*. Cambridge, MA, Bradford Books.

Latour, B. (1987). *Science in Action: How to Follow Scientists and Engineers through Society*. Cambridge, Harvard University Press.

Rheinberger, H.-J. (1997). *Towards a History of Epistemic Things: Synthesizing Proteins in the Test Tube*. Stanford, CA, Standford University Press.

Rolland, K., H.V. Hepsø, and E. Monteiro (2006). Conceptualising common information spaces across heterogeneous contexts: mutable mobiles and side-effects of integration. *Proceedings of the 2006 20th Anniversary conference on Computer Supported Collaborative Work*, ACM.

Slamecka, N.J. and P. Graf (1978). 'The generation effect: delineation of a phenomenon'. *Journal of Experimental Psychology: Human Learning and Memory* **4**(6): 592.

SUMMARY OF PART 2

The chapters in Part 2 examined the making and mobilisation of the provisional patient in the unscheduled care assemblage, detailing the socio-material arrangements through which patients, care, and treatment were coordinated across the EMS Control Centre, EMS crews, and the ED. Operating under high demand, unscheduled care managed diverse conditions within strict timeframes and national targets. Despite distinct institutional roles, services were functionally interdependent, oriented to shared logics prioritising and mobilising patient care.

The AMPDS played a central but contested role in organising EMS work. Widely viewed as unreliable, it undermined coordination. Clinical staff and call handlers developed formal and informal risk-mitigation strategies, while EMS responders treated AMPDS outputs as allocative rather than transitional objects, approaching each case anew. Elsewhere in the assemblage, trajectory mobilisation relied entirely on human actors. Activity was grounded in professional judgment and reciprocal understandings, especially among EMS responders and ED nurses, where clinical and trajectory objects were tightly integrated in everyday practice.

As care progressed, patients were enacted in different ways. Early object formation reflected administrative logics, producing stabilised technical objects shaped by triage algorithms and operational needs. In contrast, treatment and disposal decisions emerged through incremental sensemaking. EMS responders and ED doctors synthesised diverse information sources to build evolving objects of practice, with clinical significance emerging dynamically through formal assessments and professional judgment. ED nurses played a central role in monitoring and supporting these processes, facilitating flow and ensuring

DOI: 10.4324/9781003475019-12

effective handover. They did so by constructing and circulating trajectory narratives, which were progressively revised as understanding deepened and earlier concerns gave way to new priorities.

AMPDS outputs were designed as immutable, transportable representations of the patient, but their perceived unreliability limited their mobility and effectiveness as transition objects. In contrast, trajectory narratives mediating EMS, ED, and ward interfaces functioned as dynamic, additive coordination tools. As transition objects, they enacted patients as mutable mobiles, enabling the mobilisation of diverse, emergent trajectories in a fast-paced care environment.

Part 3 shifts focus to the acute care assemblage and the organisation of patients, care, and treatment between the orthogeriatric team and the operating department. As the trajectory moved from diagnosis to surgery and immediate post-operative recovery, object formation centred on immediate care needs and surgical preparation.

PART 3

The Definitive Patient

The Acute Care Assemblage

INTRODUCTION TO PART 3

Part 3 of this book focuses on the *acute care assemblage*. It explores the social worlds of the orthogeriatric ward and Operating Department (OD), analysing the socio-material relations that mobilised the hip fracture trajectory from hospital admission, through surgery, and back to the ward. In this phase, the patient is reconfigured as a *definitive* patient – a clinically recognised object of practice, diagnosed and classified according to formal criteria and embedded within a highly structured and protocolised ecology of care. Non-human actors – technologies, tools, and protocols – take on a heightened role in shaping object formation, trajectory mobilisation, and coordination.

Hip fracture management in the UK is guided by clinical standards from the National Institute for Clinical Excellence (NICE, 2011), which emphasise early surgery and prompt treatment of correctable conditions to avoid delays. They also provide recommendations on pain relief, anaesthesia, and surgical procedures. While not mandatory, these guidelines inform practice and are supported by the National Hip Fracture Database – a nationwide audit of indicators which enable services to benchmark performance.

ODs are specialist infrastructures and critical healthcare resources. In the UK NHS, surgery accounts for over five million admissions annually (Fowler et al., 2021), with about a quarter being emergencies like hip fractures (Royal College of Surgeons, 2015). Given its high-risk nature, surgery is subject to extensive safety protocols, including WHO guidance (WHO, n.d.).

As high-volume, high-cost, high-risk services, OD efficiency affects hospital finances, clinical outcomes, and patient safety (Meredith et al., 2011). Their management is a national concern (Wales Audit Office, 2016). Initiatives like The Productive Operating Theatre (NHSI, 2011) aimed to improve scheduling,

DOI: 10.4324/9781003475019-14

standardisation, and patient flow. However, at the time of the study, the Wales Audit Office noted waning focus on OD efficiency, as attention shifted to unscheduled care pressures. OD productivity was also constrained by system-wide issues such as bed availability and preoperative preparation.

*

The chapters in Part 3 draw on observations of orthogeriatric and OD work, document analysis and staff interviews. Data from the orthogeriatric ward included 106 hours of fieldwork and interviews with two consultant orthogeriatricians, two frailty nurses, an associate specialist surgeon, and the ward manager. I shadowed an on-call registrar, two junior doctors, two frailty nurses, senior nurses; attended trauma and orthopaedic team meetings, medical handover, nursing handover, medical clerking, ward rounds, nursing admission process, trauma, and orthopaedic service seminars; joined staff for coffee, and conducted fly-on-the-wall observations of ward work.

Data on the OD comprised 12-hours of fieldwork, including observation of the full OD trajectory of Megan, a female hip fracture patient. I studied the receptionist managing patient throughput, shadowed the porters and healthcare support workers collecting patients from the wards and observed the anaesthetists and assistants in the anaesthetic room. I attended several operations, including hip fracture surgery; observing from various vantage points: sitting alongside the anaesthetist; watching the surgery, and noting the work of the wider team: the scrub practitioner supporting the surgery, the intermittent contributions of the radiographer in providing images, and the activities of circulators – OD staff who worked on the periphery of the operating table aiding the surgical team and anaesthetist. I also observed transfers to the Post Anaesthetics Care Unit (PACU) and shadowed the work of nurses as they supported patients' immediate post-anaesthetic recovery and returned them to the care of the ward. My observations were supplemented with interviews with five senior OD staff and a trauma and orthopaedic surgeon.

Part 3 is organised as follows. Chapter 7 examines the acute care trajectory on the orthogeriatric ward, focusing on how nurses and doctors enact patients for preoperative care. Chapter 8 explores the OD, tracing the patient trajectory from entry to the service, anaesthetic administration, surgery, and post-operative recovery. Chapter 9 analyses the management of transitions on entry into and out of the OD.

References

Auditor General for Wales (2016). *Operating Theatres: A Summary of Local Audit Findings*. Cardiff, Wales Audit Office. https://www.audit.wales/sites/default/files/operating-theatres-2016-eng_7.pdf (accessed: 14/04/25).

Fowler, A.J., T.D. Dobbs, and Y.I. Wan (2021). 'Estimated surgical requirements in England after COVID-19: a modelling study using hospital episode statistics'. *British Journal of Surgery* **108**: 97–103. https://doi.org/10.1093/bjs/znaa012

Meredith, J.O., A.L. Grove, P. Walley, F. Young, and M.B. Macintyre (2011). 'Are we operating effectively? A lean analysis of operating theatre changeovers.' *Operations Management Research* **4**: 89–98. https://doi.org/10.1007/s12063-011-0054-6

NHSI (2011). *The Productive Operating Theatre: Building Teams for Safer Care*. Coventry, NHS Institute for Innovation and Improvement. https://www.england.nhs.uk/improvement-hub/wp-content/uploads/sites/44/2017/11/The-Productive-Series-generic-flyer.pdf (accessed: 14/04/25).

NICE (2011). *Hip Fracture: Management, Clinical Guideline CG124*. National Institute for Health and Care Excellence. https://www.nice.org.uk/guidance/cg124

Royal College of Surgeons (2015). *The State of Surgery in Wales*. https://www.rcseng.ac.uk/-/media/Files/RCS/Library-and-publications/Non-journal-publications/RCS-State-of-Surgery-in-Wales-2015.pdf (accessed: 14/04/25).

WHO (n.d.). *Safe Surgery: Tools and Resources*. https://www.who.int/teams/integrated-health-services/patient-safety/research/safe-surgery/tool-and-resources (accessed: 14/04/25).

8

ASSESSMENT AND ALIGNMENT

Preoperative Orthogeriatric Work

> They bring you to ED. You're assessed by a nurse, triaged [...] if they think you're fractured, they send you for an X-ray, which will confirm, and then they send for a trauma doctor [...] to clerk you and consent you, and take bloods and ECG and any other investigations that may need to be done, and then they request a bed. And hopefully you get a bed allocated to you on Jenolan, you will be seen [...] by the team that are on call, plus the orthogeriatrician who comes down to have a look at your medical problems and make sure you're fit for surgery. And hopefully, you'll be put on the theatre list and have your operation, that day. The complication is age, co-morbidities, and medication and, a lot of the elderly are on a lot of medication.
>
> (Frailty Nurse – Interview)

People with hip fractures were typically admitted to Jenolan, a 38-bed specialist orthogeriatric ward providing care from admission to discharge for older patients with trauma and bone injuries. Hip fracture treatment is time-critical; NICE guidelines recommend surgery within 48 hours (NICE, 2011). This requires early preoperative preparation, prompt assessment and management of pre-existing conditions, and support for ongoing care needs. This chapter focuses on the preoperative phase of the hip fracture trajectory. It begins by describing the social world of orthogeriatric services and the strategic action field shaping practice. It then examines the enactment of patients for care, treatment, and surgical preparation through the nursing and medical admissions processes.

DOI: 10.4324/9781003475019-15

The Social World of Preoperative Orthogeriatric Care

Preoperative orthogeriatric care is oriented towards enacting the patient as a definitive patient. This involves rapid stabilisation of medical conditions, surgical planning, identification of nursing needs, and alignment of clinical priorities across geriatric, anaesthetic, orthopaedic, and nursing domains. This section explores the structures, organising logics, resources, and interpretative repertoires that conditioned orthogeriatric work during this phase of the trajectory.

Structures

Services

Preoperative care was shared between Trauma & Orthopaedics (T&O) and Gerontology. Collaborative models are recommended in hip fracture because of the prevalence of the injury in older people, and the effect of co-existing health and frailty issues that impact the patient trajectory (Middleton, 2018). Despite collaboration, the services operated with distinct clinical logics. Gerontology addressed a broad spectrum of medical, psychological, and social concerns across the trajectory, while T&O focused narrowly on injury and surgical intervention.

> At some point when we were discussing the quality of care, the T&O registrar remarked: ‘My bit is easy and constrained. Orthogeriatrician’s is much more complex, dealing with relatives and all that’.
> I was introduced to the trauma and orthopaedic consultant who I have not previously met. He asked about the project and when I explained its purpose he remarked: ‘Hmm we don’t normally think about those kinds of things’.

Orthogeriatrician:	‘Surgeons are only interested in fixing bones and not people’.
Senior House Officer:	‘Well people think they have sorted out the problem and then they don’t look any further. T&O are notoriously bad at this. They are just concerned with the bones!’.

Beyond the collaborative care team, anaesthetics was a key actor. Hip fracture surgery requires either general or regional anaesthesia, and anaesthetic risk is a key concern (Fox, 1994). With the power to cancel operations because of safety considerations, anaesthetists exercised considerable influence over surgical planning.

The Preoperative Orthogeriatric Team

Nurses and resident doctors were primarily responsible for patient care during the preoperative phase. A 24-hour nursing service was delivered by a team comprising a ward manager, a deputy, nurses, healthcare support workers, and two specialist frailty nurses. Ward nurses and support workers addressed daily care needs, while frailty nurses monitored surgical preparations and led discharge planning. Combining advanced clinical and trajectory management skills, frailty nurses typified the coordinator roles that have emerged in recent years in response to the challenges of increasing patient complexity and service use intensification (Allen, 2015). Ward nurses worked 12-hour shifts, coordinated through formal handovers at 7 am and 7 pm. The ward manager and frailty nurses worked weekdays, 8 am–4 pm. Nurse staffing levels were considered inadequate, with many newly appointed and recently qualified staff.

During core hours, resident doctors – overseen by consultant orthogeriatricians – provided daily medical care. The team included F1 doctors in their first clinical post (rotating every four months) and senior house officers on GP training programmes (rotating every six months). They covered all ward patients and the on-call rota, attending to ED and Fracture Clinic cases. An on-call team handled urgent issues overnight and at weekends. T&O comprised four consultant-led teams, including registrars, senior house officers, and a specialist associate doctor in hip fracture. Due to unfilled training posts, locum doctors were regularly employed. Consultant led teams covered a surgical on-call rota and were responsible for managing emergency admissions and acute cases during their designated day, night or weekend.

Beyond nursing and medical teams, Jenolan had a dedicated occupational therapist and pharmacist, and access to physiotherapists, though they typically only became involved postoperatively (see Chapter 11).

Organising Logics

Clinical and mobilisation logics conditioned orthogeriatric work in the preoperative phase. Activity focused on ongoing care and surgical preparation aligned with national standards (NICE, 2011). Institutional priorities also required early consideration of discharge planning, reflecting pressures to minimise length of stay. These logics were embedded in formal interpretative repertoires coordinating the work of resident doctors and ward nurses and provided the rationale for investment in the frailty nursing role.

Interpretative Repertoires

Several formal tools were enrolled in preoperative activity. The Hip Fracture Proforma was a central actor in mediating medical work. It had been developed by the orthogeriatric consultants and frailty nurses to coordinate the activity of transient resident doctors.

> Usually, the very first patient contact with our team is with the most junior doctor, the F1 doctor um who is on call dealing with hip fractures. As you know, the F1 doctors change every four months [...] they'll be trying to juggle that patient with the two drunks in casualty with a broken arm and the motor accident that's coming in. So, they're juggling things ... they're putting hip fracture into their priorities.
>
> *(Orthogeriatrician – Interview)*

The Hip Fracture Proforma was an eight-page A4 booklet comprising a Clerking Template and an Initial Treatment Regime. The Initial Treatment Regime provided clinical guidance and decision support for preoperative medical management (see Chapter 11). The Clerking Template enacted the patient into a technical object (Rheinberger, 1997) aligned with the professional objects of T&O, Orthogeriatric, and Anaesthetic Services. It addressed anaesthetic risk, underlying health conditions, and the patient's usual activity, function, and independence. This information informed surgical planning and preoperative preparation and was used to anticipate the recovery trajectory.

> It's largely a process of the house officers learning about what the anaesthetist needs to know and that's most of the contents of it ... but it also has the information that I need to know if I'm going to work out whether I need to get engaged with somebody. "Lives alone is fully mobile, does own shopping and has no aids". This tells you a lot about the patient. I know that she has cognitive functioning because she can manage her finances, write a shopping list, do her shopping. And this is confirmed by her mini mental (short assessment of cognitive capacity) which is ten.
>
> *(Orthogeriatrician – Interview)*

A range of formal artefacts supported the organisation of nursing work. Central to the admissions process was the Adult Generic Patient Assessment Booklet, used across all adult-inpatient wards, and colloquially referred to as the 'yellow booklet'. It contained a bundle of risk assessment tools (falls, skin integrity and pressure ulcers, manual handling, nutrition, continence, stool chart, and intravenous infusion site assessment), scoring guides, and decision algorithms to prompt appropriate actions and inform care planning. Though duplicating ED risk assessments (see Chapter 6), policy required repetition upon each ward transfer, reflecting their dual role: informing nursing care and managing unit accountability for adverse events. In addition, standardised nursing care plans addressed specific needs – for example, medication dependence, catheter use, hygiene assistance, immobility, confusion, and anxiety. Each pre-printed plan outlined required interventions and featured tick-box options for tailoring to individual patients.

Ward nurses also completed the Jenolan Admission Proforma, which included a Unified Baseline Assessment tool designed to enact the patient as a trajectory object for discharge planning. Based on national policy promoting health-social care collaboration in the community, it translated individual needs into matters of concern for social care work. While used selectively elsewhere, Jenolan had adopted it as the standard admission form for all patients.

Materials

The Patient Record

In the unscheduled care assemblage, documentation was confined to a limited number of artefacts – EMS PCR, CAS Card, and the nursing care record. In contrast, the acute care assemblage featured a more complex and expanded patient record, shaped by the progression of the patient's care and treatment, their movement across different settings, and involvement of multiple providers.

All patients had a set of 'medical' notes, the primary accumulative record, housed in an A4 ring binder organised by dividers. Sections included test results (blood gases, electrocardiographs, radiography reports, blood tests, microbiology tests), ED documentation (copies of the EMS PCR, ED CAS Card, and nursing record), and 'surgical notes' (consent forms, anaesthetic chart, OD patient care record, operating notes). A key component was the running record – a narrative account of medical work, maintained by junior doctors, often summarising the evolving trajectory. Other actors (nurses, physiotherapists, occupational therapists, social workers, pharmacists, dieticians) contributed to the running record, but for communication purposes. Each profession also maintained separate records, but with the exception of nursing, these were not retained on the ward.

The other ward-based record was the Nursing Evaluation of Care document. This 34-page A4 booklet, was kept at the bedside, and comprised free text fields for documenting nursing interventions in real time. The aim was to capture individual nursing interventions as they happened, improve visibility and pattern recognition in patient needs, rather than the nurse making a summative entry at the end of the shift. Owing to workload pressures, however, entries were often retrospective.

> I observed one of the nurses completing her real time nursing notes at the nurses' station. She is making a series of individual entries, each of which is given a time, which extend from 1500. It is now 1700.
>
> *DA:* So much for 'real time' nursing notes. Are you writing those in retrospect?

Nurse: I know. I should really write 'written in retrospect'. I like this though as I don't miss anything. On some wards, like where my friend works, what they write is really broad, and I wonder how that would stand up in a Court of Law.

Nurse is complaining that she has not had time to write her 'real time' nursing notes and is trying to catch up now.

Nurse (to physiotherapist): What time did you get [name] up? Help me out with my real time notes!
Physiotherapist: Umm?
Nurse: Nine thirty? Does that sound OK? (writes an entry in the notes).

In addition to the medical and nursing records, patients had bedside charts for monitoring bodily functions. Some were universal (e.g. vital signs, medication), others reflected individual care requirements (e.g. fluid balance, nutrition). They were maintained by nurses and healthcare support workers and later filed in the accumulative medical record.

Clinical Information Systems

Like ED, the Jenolan team used various digital technologies to support clinical activity, including access to laboratory results and imaging data and comprehensive patient histories via the Welsh Clinical Portal. Nurses also entered data into a clinical workstation that captured high-level information about the status of individual patient trajectories. The system was accessible to senior nurses and hospital bed managers to support the coordination of patient flow across the organisation. At the ward level, it generated handover sheets that nurses used to organise their work. Nurses carried these sheets in their pockets and updated them in response to patients' evolving trajectories of care. Like the proforma used in the Assessment Unit (Chapter 6), the handover sheet functioned as a highly portable coordination device that supported nurses in maintaining trajectory awareness.

The Trauma and Orthopaedic Service also used a dedicated digital case management system, which included summaries of all T&O patients, including operating notes and theatre lists. Resident doctors were responsible for adding new cases to the system. Although designed for team-wide remote access, respondents observed that information was often out of date, and Jenolan doctors expressed a preference for the ward-based clinical workstation maintained by nurses to monitor patient's ongoing management.

Preoperative Orthogeriatric Work

The orthogeriatric patient population encompassed older adults with a broad spectrum of injuries at different trajectory stages. Ward activity encompassed preoperative care, postoperative recovery, rehabilitation, and discharge planning. The orthogeriatric consultant attended the ward daily and led a weekly ward round. Patients were also under the care of one of the four trauma and orthopaedics teams, whose involvement beyond the surgery was limited to a weekly ward round.

Resident doctors clerked new patients, managed preoperative preparations, addressed acute medical issues, wrote discharge summaries, prescribed medications, and handled routine ward work, such as documentation and organising investigations. Their work was fragmented, involving frequent task switching and interruptions for urgent issues, ward rounds and ED admissions. Twice-daily handovers coordinated activity with the out-of-hours team but focused selectively on cases likely to require medical intervention.

Most patients required high levels of direct nursing care, and in addition to mobility issues, many had cognitive impairment.

> Throughout the nursing handover, a female patient is calling out from the ward corridor. She is well known to the nurses and has been on the ward for 140 days. In addition, a male patient in the cubicle is shouting obscenities. At one point Senior Nurse looked to me and said something to the effect of 'welcome to the mad house' and it is true; the environment is chaos. It raises some very interesting questions about how the nurses can filter out this background noise to do their work. Throughout the handover, different nurses were conversing at intervals with the two confused patients in the central ward area, reminding a man that breakfast would be available soon, informing a woman that a toilet was occupied, and she would need to use an alternative.
>
> *Frailty Nurse:* 'The patients here are very physically and emotionally demanding, and staffing is not great. They all need a standing hoist or a Stedy (a standing frame). The nurses can struggle, and the geography doesn't help as if you're in the end bay you need to stay there for safety reasons [...] They're having to do the washes and everything, whereas I'm free to chase up the other things. If they've got ten or nine patients to look after, how do you do the physical work that needs doing and then all the management?'.

As discussed in Chapter 5, nurses play a key role in trajectory management (Allen, 2015). Yet, given Jenolan's patient population and staffing levels, combining clinical care with trajectory mobilisation was challenging. Frailty and ward nurses shared this work. Frailty nurses focused on preoperative trajectory management aligned with hip fracture standards, monitored resident doctors' enactments, collected audit data for the National Hip Fracture Database, and led discharge planning (see Chapter 11). Ward nurses managed admissions, coordinated daily care, responded to emergent needs, and created information flows around the patient – joining ward rounds, liaising with doctors and the multidisciplinary team, and interacting with families and other visitors.

Thus, whereas frailty nurses' care trajectory management was proactive and oriented to care standards, ward nurses' care was responsive and embedded in ongoing clinical care. This division of labour reflects Strauss' (Strauss, et al. 1985, Strauss, 1988) distinction between coordination –mobilising planned and formal processes – and articulation – responsive interventions oriented to the management of contingencies (see Chapter 2).

Making Patients and Mobilising Care

This section examines how medical and nursing staff enacted patients for preoperative care and treatment, focusing on the matters of concern foregrounded at this trajectory stage, the information sources used, and the role of formal tools in mediating these processes. It also highlights mechanisms of object formation that remained invisible to the formal record.

Object Formation in Preoperative Medical Practice

Preoperative orthogeriatric medical care was interdisciplinary and required the generation of multiple specialist professional objects. Initial object formation was undertaken by resident doctors using the Clerking Template to enact the patient around the concerns of gerontological, T&O and anaesthetic work. This interdisciplinary understanding informed surgical planning, medical care, and recovery trajectory projections.

Enacting Professional Objects of Practice

Medical object formation began with clinical clerking, typically conducted in ED. This was a structured sensemaking process in which different types and sources of information were consulted to enact the patient as a technical object aligned with the information requirements of the Clerking Template. As with ED doctors (see Chapter 6), it involved assembling background information before seeing the patient in person.

> We find a seat at the workstation where the requisite paperwork is already laid out: ED CAS Card, EMS PCR, the Hip Fracture Proforma, drug chart.

> Doctor scrutinises the ED CAS card observing: It sounds mechanical, laceration to the head and hand, pain score OK. He's 81 was brought in by ambulance.
>
> Doctor looks at the yellow ambulance PCR chart and reads: Lives with wife, occasional alcohol, non-smoker.

As described in Chapter 5, EMS responders gathered detailed medical information to inform ED work, but for enacting a definitive hip fracture inpatient this was largely disregarded. Having established the circumstances leading to the injury, the doctor used the clinical portal to assemble a medical history. These data related to the individual's previous healthcare interactions, including letters between specialists and the patient's GP. These letters often contained valuable contextual data beyond their primary focus.

> Doctor opens the patient's file on the clinical portal and groans at the long list of out-patient letters. She begins scanning the letters, extracting information on past medical history as she does so. She notes that the patient has type 2 diabetes – this information is found in a letter from Memory Clinic. There are many letters from the Memory Clinic which she moves through very quickly and does not extract further information. In one letter there is a reference to thrombocytosis, and she says: 'That's why she's on [medication]. That's good'. She writes 'thrombocytosis' under the Past Medical History section on the Clerking Template. A subsequent letter evidently offers extra details as she adds in brackets 'essential thrombocythemia' and observes, 'Ok things are quite static'.
>
> *Doctor:* So, she has assorted complications and cataracts and macular degeneration. She has carers in to assist with medications and that was in January.

As this extract indicates, doctors typically moved swiftly through what could often be a large volume of data, extracting what was relevant for clerking. This entailed a sensitivity to information relevance and trustworthiness. Sensemaking was hermeneutic – fragments were interpreted through their logical relationships, the circumstances of their production, and the evolving understanding of the case.

Once the preparatory work was complete, the doctor progressed to the in-person clerking. Unequivocally an institutional encounter, the interaction followed the structure of the Clerking Template, with the doctor controlling the agenda, asking questions, and adjudicating on the relevance of information. When the patient, or more typically, family members, threatened to derail the conversation, disciplining strategies were deployed to retain a focus on medical concerns. If the patient was unable to answer questions, the doctor relied on family or friends to supply the necessary information.

Typically clerking began with a question inviting an account of the injury. The following fieldnote relates to a male patient who has fallen in the park; he is accompanied by his wife and niece.

We go to see the patient. Doctor asks what has happened.

Patient: I was walking the dog, and I was going up an incline into the park and I staggered backwards.
Wife: He's had a terrible chest infection. He's just started on antibiotics, and I was surprised he wanted to go out. I was in the hairdressers.
Doctor: Did you have any light-headedness?
Patient: No.
Doctor: Did you have any chest pain?
Patient: No.
Doctor: Shortness of breath?
Patient: No.
Wife: He's not that steady because he's not been eating. [name] (nodding towards the niece) saw him yesterday and said he looked washed out.

[…]

Patient says he banged his head on the gate.

Doctor: Have you fallen before?
Patient: I tripped up a step.
Wife: Yes, but that was ages ago. You've not fallen for a long time.

In this extract, the doctor's questions are oriented to the tick boxes on the Clerking Template used to categorise the history of the fall: 'trip, slip or accident'; 'palpitations, chest pain, shortness of breath'; 'aura, fit, tongue biting, incontinence'; 'dizzy, lightheaded, pale, sweaty'; 'unexplained loss of consciousness'. The patient's account identifies the fall as an accident, excluding a fit or loss of consciousness as predisposing factors, but the doctor asks further questions to establish whether he has experienced chest-pain, shortness of breath or light-headedness. The history of a chest infection and unsteadiness caused by not eating, introduced by the patient's wife, furnishes relevant background information, but these are not listed as concerns in the Clerking Template, and the doctor does not invite elaboration.

Inquiries designed to establish the circumstances of the fall were typically followed by questions about medical history. This section of the proforma included both a free-text area for detailed notes and tick boxes to highlight 14 specific concerns related to anaesthetic risk and surgical planning, such as heart conditions, hypertension, diabetes, respiratory issues, deep vein thrombosis, anticoagulation, jaundice, neurological issues, smoking, alcohol or addiction, and previous cancer. Relevant information for the purposes of completing this section was normally assembled from the clinical portal as part of the initial preparatory work, and this part of the in-person clerking typically had a broader orientation. The following extract relates to a female patient, accompanied by her son and daughter. The patient is drowsy, and in contrast to the previous example, the doctor elicits the required information from the son and daughter.

Doctor: Is she falling regularly?
Daughter: She has tinnitus, and they gave her medication for that. The last few nights she's had problems with her breathing.

[…]

Doctor: So, you don't think she's falling regularly?
Son: We're not aware but then she hides things from us.
Daughter: But we've been shopping today, and she was fine.
Doctor: So, nothing out of the ordinary?
Daughter: No.

[…]

Doctor: Any other problems?
Daughter: I know her balance was going which is why she's taking these tinnitus tablets.
Doctor: Do you have them?
Daughter: No.
Doctor: Do you know what they are?
Daughter: Sorry, no.
Doctor: Can you bring them in? Has she had any previous surgery?
Daughter: She had a hernia but other than that, just teeth work.

Having established any additional relevant medical history, the clerking typically turned to the individual's social circumstances. This section of the template was organised under four headings with associated tick box categories: home (house, bungalow, downstairs flat, upstairs flat, residential home, nursing home, hospital); home support (living alone, living with someone, living with carer, home care package, institutional care); usual mobility (able to do own shopping, able to get out of the home, unable to shop, and home bound); and usual walking aids (none, one aid [stick, crutch] two aids, frame, wheelchair/bed bound).

Doctor: So, what is the situation at home? Is it a house or bungalow?
Wife: Bungalow.
Doctor: Is it just the two of you?
Wife: Yes.
Doctor: Any adaptations?
Wife: We had the bath taken out and a large shower put in.
Doctor: Is it a wet room?
Wife: It's not a wet room but it's very big.
Doctor: Anything else?
Wife: We have rails down to the garden.
Doctor: Who does your shopping?
Wife: We do it together. I do the gardening.
Doctor: Do you have a stick?
Wife: I've got it here.
Doctor: Any stairs to the house?
Wife: No.
Doctor: Wheelchair?
Wife: No.

[…]

Doctor: Are you OK with cleaning and washing and dressing?
Wife: Yes, I help him with his socks.

One of my medical respondents, a General Practitioner in training, noted that the social circumstances section of the Clerking Template was more circumscribed than their usual clerking process. However, its primary purpose was to prefigure matters of concern relevant to the surgical plan and trajectory prediction, rather than for organising discharge. As I will describe below, the 'Nursing and Multidisciplinary Assessment', within the Jenolan Admission Proforma, was designed to assemble more detailed information for this purpose.

Although the clerking process closely followed the structure of the proforma – and its mediating effects on the work of resident doctors was evident to an observer familiar with the artefact – unlike the Advanced Medical Priority Dispatch System (AMPDS) described in Chapter 3, the Clerking Template was not an obvious actor in the doctor-patient interaction. The one exception was the formal cognitive assessment. This section included a short mental state assessment scored out of ten, and a clock face drawing task. The latter prompted doctors to ask the patient to 'fill in the numbers of this clock face and draw in the hands of the clock pointing to three o'clock'. Completing the task required following instructions, language comprehension, visualising object orientation, and motor coordination – functions often impaired in dementia.

At one level, the prominence of the Clerking Template at this point in the interaction reflected the need for patients to complete the clock face test on the form. At another, it was clear that while cognitive impairment is a legitimate preoperative concern and predictor of recovery, doctors felt discomfort administering the test on all patients. In the following example, the doctor's explicit orientation to the institutional requirement to undertake the test, and reassurance that the questions 'might seem silly', distances the interaction from any implied judgement about the individual's cognitive capacity.

Doctor: I am going to ask some questions which are the same questions we ask anyone who comes in with a hip fracture. They might seem silly, and I don't want you to be offended.

The final phase of clerking took place away from the bedside and involved completing the relevant sections of the template and initiating tasks prescribed in the Initial Treatment Regime. This included reviewing medications (typically abstracted from the ED CAS Card), prescribing analgesia, aperients, and IV fluids, assessing alcohol withdrawal risk, and ordering standard preoperative tests and any other indicated investigations.

The medical clerking process is a systematic methodology for producing a differential diagnosis and an investigation and management plan. It is a core clinical skill, formally assessed during medical education, and individual doctors develop their own routines aligned with professional standards. Several respondents acknowledged that working with the Clerking Template impacted their normal clerking practices.

Resident doctor: I find that it does constrain the history taking and makes it less free flowing.

Moreover, in hip fracture, the diagnosis had been reached before the patient was accepted into the team's care. Thus, clerking served not to generate a differential diagnosis but to assemble matters of concern relevant to the management of the case. Some resident doctors described this as 'rubbish work' that simply involved 'paperwork'.

Resident Doctor: 'This is an odd process in terms of information flow as the registrar has already made the decision to do an operation, so this is just a formality. When you do a clerking in trauma you make no decisions, even in ED when you clerk the hip fractures, the fracture has already been confirmed. So, you don't have many responsibilities'.

Nonetheless, the quality of clerking was crucial for surgical planning, and arranging any necessary tests was essential to ensure timely surgery.

Once clerking was complete, the registrar provided a 'senior review'. The understanding of the patient that emerged from this process encompassed a wide range of concerns, aligned with the discrete professional objects of practice of T&O, orthogeriatric and anaesthetic work.

Enacting Interdisciplinary Objects of Practice

Patients were enacted as interdisciplinary objects of practice for surgical planning during the trauma and orthopaedic team morning meeting, also attended by the orthogeriatric consultant. At this stage, patients had the qualities of epistemic objects (Knorr Cetina, 1997), not fully known. Held in an office away from the ward, hip fracture patients were reviewed alongside other trauma admissions. Each presentation typically began with the radiographic image displayed on a large screen, with consultants seated at the front.

Consultant 1:	Next! (image appears on the screen)
Registrar:	It's a simple hip [...] it looks like an intracapsular fracture from where I'm standing but it is hard to see because of his girth!
Consultant 2:	If you make it one screen then you can invert the image (the image is changed). Hmmm? Clear as mud!'

The registrar, using the completed Clerking Template, gave a brief oral summary, highlighting key concerns for determining surgical strategy. Options included the use of various fixation devices (screws and nails) or a full or partial joint replacement. Choice of surgery depended in part on the location of the fracture, but age was also an important consideration.

Registrar:	Hemi (hemiarthroplasty, partial hip replacement) would be my first choice because of what she's had done before.
Consultant 1:	How old is she?
Registrar:	Eighty-seven but she's very good.
Consultant 1:	I'm not being ageist, but she's probably got two years of being morbidity free.
Consultant 3:	Sometimes you need to decide standing in front of the bed.
Registrar:	She's saying that she's happy with a matching pair!
Consultant 3:	I think I'll do that then.

Chronological age is a poor proxy for health status, and this extract illustrates the fragmented versions of the patient generated in the preoperative period. Resident doctors undertook the clerking in direct interaction with the patient, but rarely consulted the X-ray, and consultants, who had never seen the patient made the final decision on the most appropriate surgery. In this context, the

T&O registrar – who had accepted the ED referral and conducted a senior review – played an important boundary spanning role in translating the patient for the purposes of surgical planning.

While T&O surgeons and orthogeriatricians shared a commitment to operate on all hip fractures, anaesthetic risk could cause disagreements (Fox, 1994). Anaesthetists did not attend the planning meeting, but the Clerking Template was designed to enact the patient as a prospective anaesthetic object of practice, alerting the consultant orthogeriatrician to cases requiring a pre-emptive discussion to allay anaesthetist concerns.

> They need to know that we know about the patient's problems and the decision to take somebody to theatre has been made with our eyes open [...] so from my point of view, if you don't have hip fracture surgery [...] you die. You might end up in a nursing home, if you don't die, but you don't go home again. So, nobody goes home without the hip being fixed. It's a death sentence not to have surgery ... it's a death sentence largely applied to people who were going to die anyway but, in terms of palliative care, it's pretty ghastly to be nursed in bed unable to get onto a bed pan. So, essentially, we operate on pretty much everybody who's not just about to expire in front of us and that needs to be documented. But the anaesthetist, if you ask them to do this palliative care procedure on this patient, which involves putting them to sleep while we do an operation, they will generally say yes, but that involves having labelled this as palliative care. So, they need to know we understand the risk ... they need to know we've addressed the things that might be treatable ... and they also need to know that actually, when it goes wrong, I'll put my hand up and say it was the right thing to do, I'll talk to the coroner, which is where I was last week, so that they don't feel responsible.
>
> *(Orthogeriatrician – Interview)*

Object Formation in Preoperative Nursing Practice

This section explores how patients were enacted in preoperative orthogeriatric nursing practice. As with resident doctors, clinical and mobilisation logics were closely coupled in nurses' work. Object formation involved generating professional objects focused on nursing care needs, and trajectory objects oriented to ongoing coordination and discharge planning. The nursing admission process involved substantial paperwork – respondents estimated up to 45 minutes – which ward nurses rarely had time to complete in one sitting. As a result, the work was often distributed among staff or interspersed with other tasks.

While formal artefacts played a central role in mediating nurses' enactment of patients as technical objects aligned with care standards and accountability, object formation in nursing practice was also embodied, situated, and emergent – largely invisible to the formal record.

Enacting Professional Objects of Practice

On admission, initial nursing object formation involved completing risk assessments, determining care plans, and selecting bedside charts. Some hospital wards used standard admission packs, but on Jenolan, documentation was assembled de novo for each patient. After reviewing any accompanying records, nurses selected the necessary forms from the pigeonholes lining the wall behind the nurses' station. The following extract captures a newly appointed staff member preparing documentation for an incoming patient.

> The new patient's ED notes are at the nurses' station, retrieved by the ward manager. The staff nurse is preparing for admission, standing in front of the pigeonholes behind the desk. I watch with interest, trying to anticipate which forms she'll select based on my earlier review of patient records. She retrieves the following, in order:
>
> - Behaviour chart – for documenting problematic behaviours, antecedents, and consequences
> - DNAR chart – Do Not Attempt Resuscitation
> - Jenolan Admission Proforma – she takes time locating this
> - Adult Generic Patient Assessment Booklet
> - ID bracelets
> - Real-time nursing documentation– also takes time to locate

The Adult Generic Patient Assessment Booklet (AGPAB) was a central actor in the formal constitution of the patient as a professional object of nursing practice. It had to be completed within six hours of admission to demonstrate that all areas of risk had been assessed. Skin integrity was routinely checked on arrival. As the following extract suggests, this practice reflected concerns with unit accountability as much as risk assessment. Pressure ulcers were an organisational quality indicator, and any occurrence was reported as an adverse event.

> *Nurse:* 'We check them when they come up from the ED, and we see them into bed, we normally roll them and check what their pressure areas are like when they come in, so then you can fill in your Waterlow (pressure ulcer risk) score from that, because I've said if anybody's seen a patient into bed, one quick glance you can see if they've got any sores or not. Because obviously if they've come in with a sore, then it's important that we document that, so that we know that it hasn't developed while they were on our ward'.

Beyond checking for skin integrity, other risk assessments were undertaken away from the bedside. Nurses had latitude in determining if a risk assessment was applicable in individual cases but were required to formally record this as an active clinical decision.

The admission process also involved assembling the nursing care plan. Care plans emerged in the UK in the 1970s as part of the nursing process, a systematic and patient centred framework for delivering care which was part of a wider effort to professionalise nursing. It represented a shift from task-based care to a more deliberative individualised model (Walton, 1986). The methodology involves assessment, developing a care plan, implementation, and evaluation. While successful as an educational tool, integrating it into clinical practice proved challenging. Nurses could complete assessments but found care planning more difficult; care plans were inconsistent, problems were poorly formulated, and time-consuming (de la Cuesta, 1983).

While the core idea endures, organisations increasingly use pre-printed, standardised care plans with options for individual tailoring. There is no inherent reason why pre-printed care plans cannot align with the nursing process, if one adopts a mass customisation model. However, apart from the Adult Generic Patient Assessment Booklet, which focused exclusively on safety risks, there was no formal requirement to document the nursing assessment and planning process in the official record. To the observer, care plan selection appeared largely routinised. For instance, there is no reference to the underlying rationale for a patient's plan of care, in the following fieldnote.

Staff nurse then takes the student through the care plans.

Staff Nurse (to student nurse): Hygiene, wound, constipation, successful discharge are the things people are on in the ward.

This example is particularly revealing, because it occurs in a teaching context.

Enacting patients through the formal admission process was an elaborate paper construction, which had performative value in constituting standards for the purposes of organisational and professional accountability. But nurses came to know patients as professional objects of practice through direct, embodied interactions during care delivery, and engagement with family members. These practical understandings centred on dynamic, situated concerns aligned with individuals' on-going needs and were shared and revised through the dialogic enactment of patients as intra-professional objects during nursing handover.

The following fieldnotes from handover illustrate these processes. In the first extract, a nurse describes the care of a patient recently transferred from another ward, noting a decline in mobility, increased drowsiness, challenges of managing her subcutaneous infusion, concerns about cognitive capacity, and wider behavioural issues affecting care.

Nurse: Bed twenty-three – [name] – eighty-six – came from Bedford Ward with fractured ribs seven to eleven. They apparently said she was mobilising independently, but when she mobilised to the toilet here, she was very unsteady and yesterday she was very drowsy. She's on subcutaneous fluids and it is very positional, but she won't let me touch it. We are just waiting for a (cognitive) capacity assessment. It was supposed to be yesterday but because she was drowsy, they decided to wait and do it today.

There is then a discussion about the patient's behavioural issues and the fact that the patient is refusing washes.

In this second extract, the nurse reports not waking a sleep-deprived patient for medication or food and also expresses concern for the patient's husband.

Senior Nurse: She's had about two hours sleep, and I decided not to wake her for drugs or food. So, she might be hungry later. She's still waiting for CRT (Community Resource Team) I said I would chase Tuesday. Her husband took a day off today. I told him not to come in and have a rest.

In this third extract, although the patient is in surgery, the nurse's handover highlights a family note, detailed plans for managing urinary retention and diabetes, and the patient's complaints of itching. There is no reference to routine postoperative care needs, though this will undoubtedly be a focal concern when she returns to the ward.

Staff Nurse: Left fractured neck of femur, a lot of medical history, gone to theatre. Her family came to see her and have written her a note if you can give that to her when she comes back. She goes into urinary retention and is only for in and out catheterisation. Orthogeriatrician does not want her catheterised. She drained one thousand one hundred when she was done earlier. Dip stick showed blood and so we've sent a specimen. She's on two litres of oxygen and sliding scale insulin. When she comes back the doctors want her on eight hourly fluids. This is the first time I have seen this lady, and she is complaining of itching. Doctor says she was like that yesterday too.

In these accounts, routine nursing care – as outlined in formal plans – was largely assumed. Instead, handovers focused on patients' unique, additional needs, based on embedded understanding of the patient's condition and context.

There are clear parallels here with studies of tinkering in healthcare practices (Mol, 2008; Pols, 2008). The concept of tinkering, drawn from Mol's work on ontological politics, foregrounds a practical ethics in which 'good care' is not predefined but worked out in the moment. Rather than following fixed protocols, practitioners respond to contingencies, making small, often improvised adjustments. The nurses' accounts powerfully illustrate this mode of practice. Leaving a patient to sleep, adjusting arrangements when a subcutaneous infusion is being resisted, or advising a worried husband to rest – these are small but significant acts of care. In contrast to the abstract, standardised patient of the formal care plan, these practices enacted patients as emergent objects of nursing practice, shaped through interaction, negotiation, and professional judgement. It was shared knowledge of these situated specificities that enabled good collective nursing practice.

Enacting Trajectory Objects of Practice

Object formation for clinical care and trajectory management were closely coupled in ward nurses' work. This interleaving is evident in the last three extracts in the previous section, where individual nursing needs are entangled with accounts of evolving care trajectories: a capacity assessment is being planned; a patient awaits CRT acceptance; and a postoperative patient is to receive eight-hourly fluids as prescribed. Trajectory management was not a separate activity or something layered onto care; it was embedded in nurses' gaze, disposition, and everyday practices. These examples again highlight the centrality of care trajectory narratives as ordering artefacts in nursing work. These two-part narrative constructions – combining clinical detail and trajectory plans – were routinely used to coordinate activity, orient colleagues, and respond to shifting needs. In this way, nurses enacted patients as both clinical and trajectory objects, oriented to the requirements of contemporaneous care, while also being positioned within a wider arc of anticipated interventions, assessments, and transitions.

While enacting patients as trajectory objects was ingrained in nursing practice, ward nurses were also tasked with completion of the Jenolan Admission Proforma. Designed to translate the patient into a trajectory object of practice for discharge planning, the first half focused on social circumstances: accommodation; relationships and caring responsibilities, any pre-existing support from social care services and community alarm arrangements. Nurses typically drew on existing records – ED CAS Card, EMS PCR, and the hip fracture Clerking Template – to populate these sections.

> Senior Nurse starts the new admission and begins by leafing through the notes that have arrived with him [...] She reviews the drug chart and starts transferring information on past medical history from the Hip Fracture Proforma to the Admission Proforma.

Senior Nurse: 'A lot of the information you can get from here, so you don't have to re-ask. They have already given the information for this and this form'.

The second half – the 'Unified Baseline Assessment' – was designed to inform the organisation of social care in the community (described in detail in Chapter 12, p. 240). The required information spanned clinical details and disease prevention, as well as personal care needs, activities of daily living, domestic support, relationships, mental health, mobility, and safety. While completion was required within 24 hours of admission, the form was poorly coordinative of nursing practice and compliance was poor.

Frailty Nurse: 'So, I need to know about the patients, what's their background, so I look at the admission sheet. Don't quote me on this but they're not always filled in'.

Part of the problem was the document required detailed discharge-related information within a day of admission. And yet, as I have described, nurses' understanding of patients and their social relationships and circumstances evolved over time. Recovery trajectories were variable and uncertain, moreover, and it was challenging to predict future social care needs at such an early stage in the hip fracture trajectory. Beyond this misalignment, the form also presented significant translational challenges. Unlike the Adult Generic Patient Assessment Booklet and the Hip Fracture Proforma, there were no explanatory guidelines or protocols to facilitate completion. Frailty nurses, familiar with the document's intent, described their various efforts to explain the documentation to the ward nurses.

> I've had some time with all of them … and I've broken it down into things that I wanted them to know. So, I started off with the admission documentation … I talked them through admitting the patient and there's all this information … but it's busy … but discharge planning starts on admission and if you don't know your patients, you can't discharge them. So literally went through every sort of domain that was there and explained why it was relevant … the sort of things they should be asking. […] And explained that … how can you send this lady home with a Zimmer frame (four-legged mobility aid) when she's got stairs to deal with and the toilet's upstairs? How's she getting that Zimmer up the stairs? So, you'll need to think about the facts, you'll need two Zimmers … one at the bottom of the stairs, one at the top of the stairs … you might need to start talking to the family about maybe we could put a second rail in, and the OT (occupational therapist) will address that.
>
> *(Frailty Nurse – Interview)*

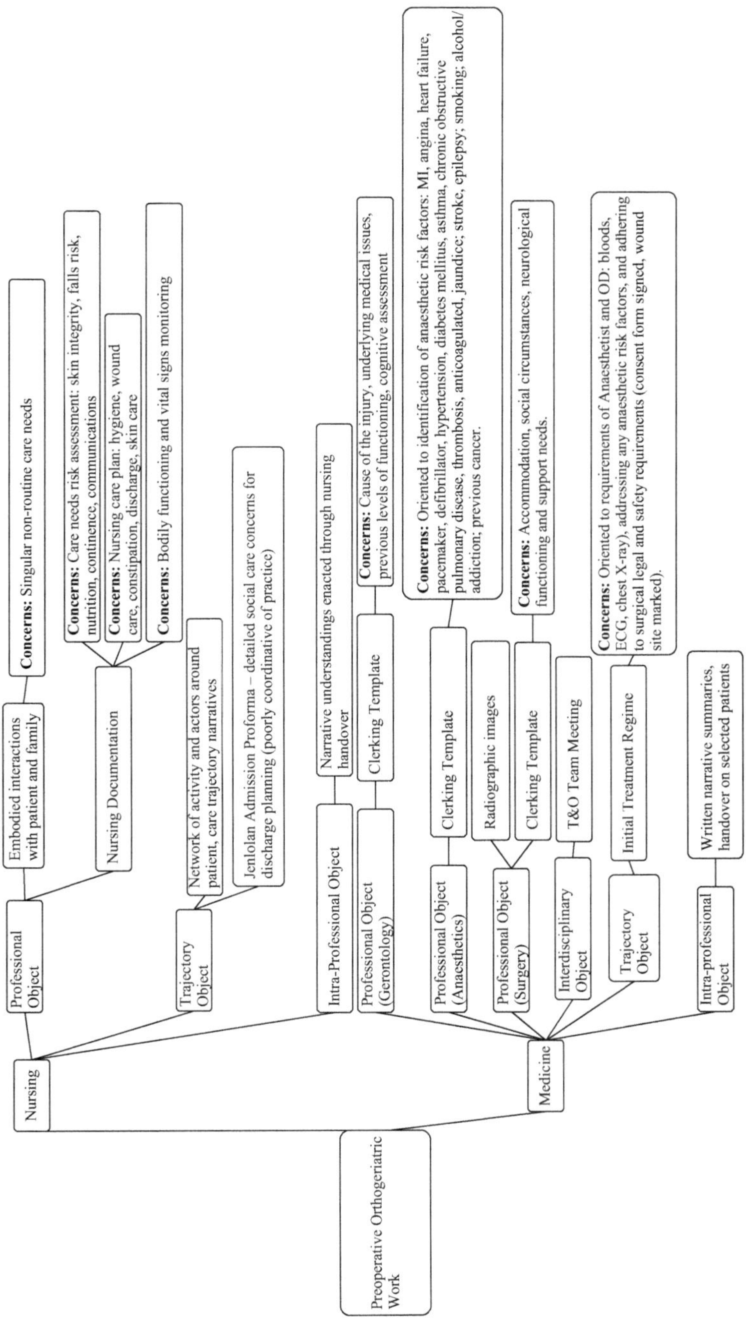

FIGURE 8.1 Object formation in preoperative orthogeriatric work.

As the frailty nurse acknowledges, staff capacity was a further factor contributing to non-compliance. Throughout the organisation and on social media, the volume of paperwork required of nursing staff was an ongoing source of complaint. Nurses prioritised patient care, often staying late to complete nursing documentation. Given these pressures – and the form's focus on the distant discharge concerns rather than immediate ward priorities, its limited power as a coordinating device in the preoperative period is unsurprising.

The version of the patient that emerged from the formal nursing admission process, was an object of practice for whom risks were assessed, preventative actions taken, care plans assembled to align with organisational standards, and discharge requirements foreshadowed (at least in part). Yet nurses really came to know patients as objects of practice through practice in their everyday embodied interactions, as they tinkered with the material reality of care. These understandings of the patient as a situated object of practice were enacted orally in handovers but remained relatively invisible in the formal record.

Summary

This chapter has examined how patients were enacted by resident doctors and nursing staff in preoperative orthogeriatric work. Driven by clinical and mobilisation logics, practice was mediated by formal artefacts designed to coordinate object formation around a wide range of concerns: details of the fracture and individual's medical history, risks and nursing care requirements, early indicators of recovery trajectory and discharge planning. These processes are summarised in Figure 8.1.

The Clerking Template effectively disciplined resident doctors' work, enabling them to enact patients into multiple objects of medical practice for surgical planning, while the Initial Treatment Regime served as prompts for care and intervention. Formal artefacts also coordinated nurses' work – particularly in risk identification at the point of admission – but were primarily aligned with organisational priorities and did not encompass the wider concerns through which nurses enacted patients in practice. The Jenolan Admission Proforma, intended to ensure that discharge planning started on admission, was poorly aligned with nursing workflow and in the face of the wider demands of the clinical environment, nurses prioritised preoperative care and surgical preparation.

Nurses' understanding of the patient evolved over time, through everyday interactions with them and their families. These situated, singular understandings were foregrounded in nursing work and surfaced most clearly in the nursing handover, whereas routine aspects of patient care tended to be taken for granted. Direct care was tightly interwoven with trajectory mobilisation, and care trajectory narratives were used to enact patients as dual clinical and trajectory objects. Communicated in handovers and negotiated through myriad daily interactions with the network of people involved in an individual's care, these narratives were central actors in the organisation of everyday work yet remained largely invisible in the formal documentation.

References

Allen, D. (2015). *The Invisible Work of Nurses: Hospitals, Organisation and Healthcare*. London and New York, Routledge.

De la Cuesta, C. (1983). 'The nursing process: from development to implementation'. *Journal of Advanced Nursing* **8**: 365–371.

Fox, N. (1994). 'Anaesthetists, the discourse of patient fitness, and the organisation of surgery'. *Sociology of Health & Illness* **16**: 1–18. https://doi.org/10.1111/j.1467-9566.1994.tb00138.x

Knorr Cetina, K. (1997) 'Sociality with objects: social relations in post social knowledge societies'. *Theory, Culture & Society* **14**(4): 1–30.

Middleton, M. (2018). 'Orthogeriatrics and hip fracture care in the UK: factors driving change to more integrated models'. *Geriatrics* **3**(3): 55 https://doi.org/10.3390/geriatrics3030055

Mol, A. (2008). *The Logic of Care: Health and the Problem of Patient Choice*. London, Routledge.

NICE (2011). *Hip Fracture: Management, Clinical Guideline CG124*. National Institute for Health and Care Excellence. https://www.nice.org.uk/guidance/cg124

Pols, J. (2008). 'Good care: enacting a complex ideal in long-term psychiatry.' *Medische Antropologie* **20**(1): 73–89.

Rheinberger, H.-J. (1997) *Towards a History of Epistemic Things: Synthesizing Proteins in the Test Tube*. Standford, CA Standford University Press.

Strauss A. (1988). 'The articulation of project work: an organizational process'. *The Sociological Quarterly* **29**: 163–178.

Strauss, A.L., S. Fagerhaugh, B. Suczet, and C. Wiener (1985). *Social Organization of Medical Work*. Chicago, IL, University of Chicago Press.

Walton, I. (1986). 'The nursing process in perspective: a literature review.' *Nursing Process Evaluation Working Group*. York, Department of Social Policy and Social Work, University of York.

9

BODIES AND MATERIALS

Operating Department Work

This chapter examines the organisation of patients, care, and treatment in the Operating Department (OD). For individuals with hip fractures, surgery is a pivotal event – one filled with hope: hope for a successful operation and the start of recovery, and hope that the risks outlined during consent do not materialise. Clearly bounded in time and space, 'going to theatre' marks a distinct phase in the acute care trajectory, where object formation is shaped by the corporeal-material demands of surgical work. The first part of the chapter explores the social world of the OD; the second analyses how patients are enacted for preoperative, intraoperative, and post-anaesthetic care.

The Social World of the Operating Department

This section explores the structures, organising logics, material resources, and interpretative repertoires that shape object formation and trajectory mobilisation in the OD. The patient trajectory unfolds across three phases – preoperative, intraoperative, and post-anaesthetic care – each with its own structure and logic. OD work follows a rational-linear approach, where formal tools, material routines, and shared interpretative frameworks are central actors. Activity centres on the patient's body and surgical intervention, and over a relatively brief five-hour trajectory, patients are enacted as multiple, phase-specific objects as care moves through the department.

Structures

The Department

The OD was a sequestered space within the hospital. Restricted access and the distinctive appearance of clinical staff set it apart from the rest of

DOI: 10.4324/9781003475019-16

organisational life. With a few notable exceptions (porters, receptionists and healthcare support workers who collected patients from the wards), everyone wore theatre scrubs, hair coverings, and specialist footwear. Unlike other areas of the hospital, there were no sartorial distinctions to signify status or profession; everyone dressed in the same attire, including visitors.

> I was shown by the receptionist to the ladies changing room and the racks where the scrubs were kept. The first challenge was deciding on which size to select, but the receptionist very kindly pointed me in the direction of 'small' which looked about right. The scrubs were kept in a public corridor outside the changing rooms, and I did not relish the prospect of getting undressed only to find that my selection was too small. In the event, and to my relief, the size was right. The next task was to help myself to a paper hat and cover my hair. The theatre hat was elasticated one side and not the other and I had a moment's panic when I could not think which way round this should be worn. Nobody was wearing a hat in the changing rooms to take a lead from. I did not want to amplify my outsider status by emerging from the changing room wearing the uniform incorrectly. I got there in the end, however, and found my way back to Reception, narrowly avoiding going into the men's changing room as I was completely disoriented, and the door did not have a sign on it. The receptionist directed me to the Trauma & Orthopaedic Theatre but, finding it hard to make any sense of my surroundings and fearful of entering an area which was out of bounds, I was thankful to spot the T&O doctor waiting for me in the back corridor behind the changing rooms.

The OD comprised two functional areas: Operating Theatres and the Post-Anaesthetic Care Unit (PACU), colloquially known as 'recovery'. Fifteen operating theatres were configured side-by-side along a single corridor; each linked to an Anaesthetic Room where patients were prepared for surgery. While not all OD departments have separate anaesthetic rooms, this is common in the UK. After surgery, patients were cared for in PACU until stable enough to return to the ward.

The Operating Department Team

The OD employed around sixty staff, including nurses, Operating Department Practitioners (ODPs), healthcare support workers, and receptionists. ODPs specialise in perioperative care, a role that has evolved from theatre porter to encompass anaesthetics (assisting the anaesthetist), scrub (assisting the surgeon), and recovery (supporting patients post-anaesthesia). Training has progressed from a Level 3 NVQ to diploma and, more recently, undergraduate degree. At the study site, nurses worked in the same roles as ODPs but were typically trained in only one area. Both groups were deployed in anaesthetic and scrub roles, but only nurses worked in post-anaesthetic care. Although this division of labour has previously been linked to blurred professional identities and boundary disputes (Timmons and Tanner, 2004), I observed little inter-professional tension and both nurses and ODPs held senior clinical leadership roles. Healthcare support workers contributed across all OD activities, and a receptionist managed patient flow. Despite their centrality to surgical work, anaesthetists and surgeons were not part of the OD's formal organisational structure, instead belonging to separate departments.

Work in the OD centred on the body. Its material and social organisation assumed patients to be insentient objects of practice. Facilities for addressing care needs beyond anaesthesia and surgery were minimal, and privacy was limited. Patients who did not conform to these normative expectations disrupted the department's smooth operation.

> The T&O surgeon said they have a lot of patients operated under spinal anaesthetic and having the patient awake changes the environment. He said it was necessary to modify the language used in communicating about the operation so as not to cause anxiety. He also said that in theatres the language used could sometimes be 'choice' and recounted an occasion on which the consultant surgeon under pressure unleashed a torrent of expletives forgetting that the patient was awake.
>
> Nurse said that she did not like patients remaining in PACU longer than was necessary as they were too awake [...] I observed such an occurrence today. Two women were in the PACU all morning, wide awake and watching carefully what was going on around them. Who could blame them – what else were they supposed to do? Nurse said that when they had 'awake' patients in the department, they had to keep putting the curtains around the beds which made work difficult as it circumscribed the space.

Organising Logics

Patient safety was a primary organising logic in the OD. It shaped the specialist division of labour and the progressive narrowing of focus through which patients were enacted for anaesthetic and surgical work. It was also evident in formal standards and policies which coordinated activity; in the monitoring and assessment of vital signs during surgery and recovery; in the careful handling and positioning of the anaesthetised body; in attention to bodily-material relations; and in strict infection control practices. It also governed the mobilisation of care across trajectory phases, with progression contingent on meeting specific clinical and procedural criteria.

Alongside safety, a mobilisation logic also drove activity. Operating theatres are costly resources, and the overarching aim was to manage patient trajectories efficiently. The department was subject to internal performance targets for operational processes, which had to be accounted for if unmet.

> Then as soon as they arrive, they ring that particular theatre and say your patient is in the bay and then there really should only be ten minutes between the last one leaving and the next one…that's what the computer's set for now. So […] when I press the button asking for the patient, to the time the porter presses the button to say he's going for the patient, that is only going to be ten minutes. If it's more than ten minutes, it comes up with a delay and you have to give a reason […] And then… they look at the porter leaving and arriving back and then from the porter arriving with the patient to the Anaesthetic Room and then they also look at the time this patient left and the last one's got into the Anaesthetic Room and if it's more than ten minutes you have to put in a delay reason.
>
> *(OD Clinical Leader – Interview)*

As the extract above illustrates, operating theatres were the primary drivers of departmental activity. Everyday practice was highly time-conscious and focused on managing patient flow. While some OD staff concentrated on ongoing surgery, others prepared for the next case.

> You can't be in the theatre all of the time because you have an Anaesthetic Room to look after also, you might be stocking it up, you might have to go to other areas of theatre or you're collecting equipment for the next case. So, we're never just concentrating on just the patient that's in the theatre because you'll also be thinking of what's coming next and because its only you, you have to be fetching, carrying and making sure its set up and that can be quite time consuming.
>
> *(OD Clinical Leader – Interview)*

> I want them (ODPs) sorting out the theatre, sorting out the Anaesthetic Room and being ready for the next patient so I encourage that because otherwise we'll have delays because you're not ready.
>
> *(OD Clinical Leader – Interview)*

Together, these clinical and mobilisation logics coalesced into a rational-linear mode of organisation. At each phase, the patient was enacted into precisely specified objects of practice oriented to safety standards, which structured trajectory mobilisation at critical junctures.

Interpretative Repertoires

Multiple formal artefacts structured OD work. The World Health Organisation Surgical Safety Checklist (WHO, 2009) was a central actor in the preoperative and intraoperative phases. Used globally, the tool aims to reduce errors and adverse events while improving teamwork and communication. It comprises three sections completed at key status passages: before anaesthesia ('sign in'), before incision ('time out'), and before leaving the operating room ('sign out'). Although research has documented resistance to its use (Russ et al., 2015; Wæhle et al., 2020; Treadwell et al., 2014), senior staff at the study site reported that, despite some surgeons' lack of enthusiasm and occasional ceremonial compliance (Meyer & Rowan, 1977; Vaughan, 1996, 1999), the checklist was largely seen as an important safety mechanism.

> We don't know the patient prior to theatre, so they're in our hands basically and everything we're doing for them we're doing blindly. We're relying on the information from everybody else, to allow us to do what we're doing correctly, and it's not till you're at the other end and you've done the hysterectomy (surgical removal of the uterus), and they were only having a hysteroscopy (visualisation of the uterus for diagnostic purposes) and you know, they're the vitals between good communication like the patient that lost the wrong kidney (reference to a major wrong site surgery event at Prince Phillip Hospital in Wales, 2000).
>
> *(OD Clinical Leader – Interview)*

> I can't say everybody thinks its meaningful, and maybe it can become a little bit ritualistic, but everybody participates in it regardless of what they think of it, so you do get an answer from everybody [...] and so at the beginning and the end of the procedure everybody generally knows what's going on or what's gone on so yeah I think it works well.
>
> *(OD Clinical Leader – Interview)*

In the post-anaesthetic phase, PACU nurses used a range of formal tools to assess, classify, and document recovery. For hip fracture patients, these included a pain scale; three consciousness assessment tools; and a structured framework for monitoring concerns specific to spinal anaesthesia recovery. A standardised PACU nursing care plan was also in place.

Materials

The Patient Record

Patient care in the OD was documented in an integrated 'Patient Care Record' (PCR). This was a 20-page A4 booklet organised into discrete sections aligned with the three phases of the surgical trajectory. In use for 15 years and revised to reflect evolving practice, it incorporated the formal interpretive repertoires described earlier and functioned as a coordinating, accumulating, and accounting device (Berg, 1997).

> The documentation is one that we protect ourselves and the more we write down the more we feel we protect ourselves because things happen so we tend to document as much as we can.
>
> *(OD Clinical Leader – Interview)*

The PCR had a highly structured tick box format, designed to enable meticulous documentation of the corporeal–material relations through which patients were configured as surgical objects. However, designed for all surgical cases, it encompassed a wide range of concerns. This universality posed challenges. While predefined fields and options can serve as a powerful prompt to action (Allen et al., 2009; Berg, 1997), the OD documentation was often time-consuming to complete, as many sections were irrelevant to specific patients. Its preformatted structure also constrained what could be recorded, limiting space for tailoring to individual cases. The following extracts from interviews with practitioners highlight these challenges:

> 'It doesn't leave us room to put everything that we have done, it asks very specific questions, and I think, yeah, well what about something else that is more important?'
>
> 'I think the boxes that we have to write stuff in are not always appropriate for what we've done, they're not relevant, or I think it just needs to be a blank box and for us to write in what we actually have done'.
>
> 'There isn't a huge amount of space for comments, and it is a generic one, isn't it? So, they are big, there's a lot of things you need to go through in that care plan and obviously that takes us time then.'
>
> 'They sort of put everything on there that you possibly will need for every sort of case […] and that's why it gets so big and time-consuming because it's for every patient'.

As an account of practice, the OD PCR primarily documented the activities of OD staff. Surgeons maintained a separate digital record, while anaesthetists – part of the Anaesthetics Department – used a distinct A4 anaesthetic record, identifiable by blue-striped margins. This form included sections for assessment, planning, and procedural documentation, and like the OD PCR, relied on tick boxes to produce a granular but highly technical account of care.

Equipment

Surgical work is sustained by an array of specialist equipment, and materials and ODs are technologically-rich environments. Anaesthetists used various devices to deliver anaesthesia, monitor vital signs, and ensure patient safety. A dedicated trauma and orthopaedics theatre – staffed by a long-standing team – was equipped with an airflow system, orthopaedic tables, traction devices, surgical lighting, and advanced imaging technology. Radiographers provided intraoperative imaging to confirm fracture alignment and prosthesis placement. In PACU, equipment supported continuous monitoring, including pupilometers, infusion pumps, piped oxygen, suction machines, and portable technologies for patient transfers.

Material Routines

Material routines – standardised configurations of artefacts, tools, and spatial arrangements – were key to coordinating OD work. The theatre stock room held T&O instruments (e.g. drills, saws, fixation devices) pre-assembled into standard sets for different kinds of surgery. This enabled efficient preparation between cases. The spatial organisation of the operating theatre, the sterile field, and surgical tools and equipment was also routinised to support turnover.

Coordinating Technologies

Across the OD, specialist proprietary software was used to coordinate and monitor activity. Used widely throughout the UK NHS, it supported theatre scheduling, resource management, patient tracking, and generated performance and utilisation data.

Operating Department Work

OD work followed a rational-linear organisation shaped by formal tools, material routines, and interpretative repertoires. Each phase of the patient trajectory was characterised by distinct organisational structures, logics, and spatial arrangements that shaped the division of labour, processes of object formation, and patient mobilisation through the department. Preoperative care encompassed the administration of anaesthesia, preparation of the patient's body, and the material arrangements for surgery. Anaesthesia was delivered in the Anaesthetic Room by the anaesthetist, supported by an anaesthetic practitioner. Following induction, the surgical body was configured in the operating theatre, led by the scrub practitioner and supported by the wider OD team.

Intraoperative care centred on the surgical intervention itself, including the maintenance of the sterile field, the procedure, and the reversal of anaesthesia. This phase involved anaesthetists and anaesthetic practitioners, surgeons and scrub practitioners, as well as circulating OD staff. In the post-anaesthetic phase, patients were cared for in PACU, where nurses led the monitoring and management of physiological recovery until patients were deemed stable for transfer back to the ward.

Making Patients and Mobilising Care

This section examines how patients were enacted as objects of practice in the organisation of care and treatment in the OD. It focuses on the concerns foregrounded as the patient trajectory moved through preoperative, intraoperative, and post-anaesthetic care. Object formation centred on the detailed corporeal–material relations of anaesthesia and surgery. Forensic attention was directed towards a tightly bounded set of considerations: the patient's body and the array of devices, technologies, and practices applied to it. Each stage of the OD trajectory involved specific processes of object formation, aligned with safety standards and mediated through formal interpretative repertoires. Trajectory mobilisation was punctuated by internal status passages that enabled movement between phases of care.

Object Formation in Preoperative Care

Object formation in preoperative care was distributed across the anaesthetist, anaesthetic practitioner, and theatre staff. It involved enacting the patient as two distinct situated clinical objects: one oriented to anaesthesia, the other to surgery. Beginning with the anaesthetic assessment on the ward, the process continued through anaesthesia administration in the OD and culminated in the theatre, where the wider team configured the patient for surgery.

In the Anaesthetic Room, the anaesthetist and anaesthetic practitioner worked together closely to enact the patient as an object of anaesthetic practice. The anaesthetist focused on the body; the practitioner managed the material arrangements. The anaesthetic plan, established in advance by the anaesthetist, guided the practitioner's preparation of equipment and drugs:

> Yeah, we need to know what their (the anaesthetist) plan is […] we need to provide the equipment, we need the keys to the drug cupboard, we need to prepare things, we need to get the right airway equipment ready.
>
> *(OD Practitioner 1 – Interview)*

> They may need spinal analgesia so you need the set-up for that, they might have difficult airway, so we need the set-up for that, so this is all equipment you have to prepare and it's not just a two-minute job. So, they might be having central access so they might need a line, arterial lines you know, so that's the communication and we do generally have good communication.
>
> *(OD Practitioner 2 – Interview)*

The first section of the WHO Surgical Safety Checklist – 'sign in' – was completed before anaesthesia. This preparatory threshold ensured that the patient was correctly identified, consented, and that key safety checks (e.g. airway risks, blood loss, imaging availability) had been completed. It also confirmed that the necessary equipment and drugs were in place.

> With the anaesthetic chart in his hand the anaesthetist asks the patient about allergies, antibiotics, asthma, whether he is fit and well. There is a brief conversation about how the injury occurred, which seems more conversational than clinically relevant [...] As the patient is telling his story, the anaesthetist is leafing through his medical notes [...] The OD documentation is opened at the Anaesthetic Room care plan.

While formally a discrete procedural moment, the 'sign in' was difficult to see in practice. It's activities were dispersed across time, space, and roles. Equipment checks and drug preparation often occurred between cases, and risk assessments were completed earlier as part of the initial anaesthetic assessment. Administering anaesthetic is an intricate cooperative activity (Hindmarsh and Pilnick, 2007). The 'sign in' acted not only as a safety mechanism but also a coordination device. It momentarily consolidated this distributed field of action into an enactment of the patient as a situated interdisciplinary object of practice, aligning the anaesthetist and ODP around the actions necessary for anaesthesia to proceed.

> The anaesthetist administers a block which will numb the patient's right arm. He does this using the ultrasound scanner to guide him. The anaesthetist and the ODP work together with the anaesthetist adjusting the needle and watching the ultrasound monitor and instructing the ODP on when to push on the syringe or draw back 'aspirate'.

Following anaesthesia, the patient was transferred to the operating theatre. The initial focus was on re-establishing anaesthetic arrangements – reconnecting breathing and monitoring equipment and managing the intravenous lines.

> The anaesthetist takes some time organising the IV (intravenous) lines. One is evidently not working correctly. She fiddles with the lines for a while and then discovers that the patient has her wrist flexed. I then observed the scrub nurse check whether she is happy for him to begin cleaning the surgical site.

Once configured as an anaesthetic object of practice, attention shifted to enacting the patient as a surgical object. Here again object formation is situated. OD staff positioned the body, attached supports and technologies, draped it in sterile sheeting, and prepared the surgical site with disinfectant. For patients under regional anaesthesia, a screen was erected to block their view of the operation. While these preparations were underway, surgeons scrubbed up and donned gowns and masks, and the scrub practitioner – already in sterile attire – organised instruments and materials.

> Several parallel processes are underway. The surgeon is scrubbing up. A theatre practitioner is attaching an extension to the operating table on which the patient's arm will rest. The anaesthetic practitioner is sorting out the anaesthetic tubing and attaching monitor leads to the patient's chest. The associate specialist applies a blood pressure cuff to the patient's arm, explaining that it will stop the blood flow, so the operation is easier. [...] I am introduced to the surgeon, who is now scrubbed, and he takes me to a screen on the back wall and shows me a 3-D image of the injury. Meanwhile the scrub practitioner has swabbed the entire arm with iodine, assisted by an un-scrubbed colleague holding the fingers with a swab. The patient is then fully draped – only the arm is visible – everything else is hidden under the blue sterile field. The surgeon is seated at the operating table with the patient's arm extended in front of him. The associate specialist surgeon takes a position on the other side of the table, and an OD practitioner moves a stool into place for him to sit on. Present too is a junior doctor. The scrub practitioner stands besides two trolleys laid out with surgical equipment.

> A young man is having screws removed following previous surgery. A different table – a traction table – is used to make sure that the patient's leg is in the same position as in the original surgery. The surgeon spends some time strapping the patient's foot to an L-shaped footrest, explaining as he does so that the technique of strapping the foot with wide tape was not technically very complex but nevertheless effective. The patient's left leg is abducted into what looks like a one-sided lithotomy position [...] At the other end, the anaesthetic practitioner is attaching monitors to the patient's chest and arranging the anaesthetic tubing, while the ODP adjusts the lights to shine on the operation site. The table surface under the patient's legs has been taken away and now his leg is suspended in mid-air. The scrub nurse is applying iodine to the surgical

> site. After this has been done, plastic sheeting is applied – this is stuck to the leg and then extended over a metal bar above the operating area creating a tent effect. Behind it sits an X-ray machine. The arrangement of materials creates a sterile field on the right side of the patient and a 'dirty' field on the left.

Through these well-rehearsed routines, the patient was transformed into a surgical object – configured into distinct sites of practice and visual fields around which roles, technologies, materials, and tasks were precisely aligned. Object formation involved not only the careful handling and positioning of the body and its material configuration, but also the detailed documentation of these actions in the OD PCR, formalising the team's responsibility for bodily care as an accountable component of surgical preparation.

Object Formation in Intraoperative Care

It is common to characterise healthcare as teamwork. Yet, although patients receive care from multiple professions, practitioners often work independently, with limited direct interaction (Allen, 2015). The organisation of intraoperative activity is distinctive, however. During surgery, multiple actors work simultaneously on the patient's body as a situated object of practice in closely coupled cooperative work. Workplace studies show that surgical work is characterised by embodied interaction, coordinated through talk, gesture and the spatial arrangement of bodies and tools (Heath and Luff, 2021; Hindmarsh and Pilnick, 2007; Mondada, 2014). In another example of situated tinkering (Mol, 2008; Pols, 2008), during surgery the patient is enacted through continuous adjustments across the team: the anaesthetist adjusts ventilation and drugs, the scrub team adjust instruments, surgeons adjust timing and technique.

While the temporal and spatial proximity of intraoperative work creates the appearance of unified teamwork, in practice however, even tightly coupled action rests on clearly demarcated professional accountabilities. The anaesthetised body is the anaesthetist's responsibility, and the surgical body is managed by the surgeon.

> As he works, the consultant explains that he is very close to an important nerve which effects fine movements in the hand, so he wants to be sure he does not 'clobber that'.
>
> *Consultant:* I can only relax when he can wiggle his fingers later.
> *Associate specialist surgeon:* He's had a block (nerve block).
> *Consultant:* He's had a block! (rolls eyes)
>
> The anaesthetist cheerfully confirms this is the case.

The consultant's concern – 'I can only relax when he can wiggle his fingers later' – indicates that postoperative motor function is a key signifier that no critical nerve has been damaged during surgery. While the nerve block – which temporarily inhibits motor function – ensures patient comfort and minimises the need for systemic anaesthesia, it delays the feedback mechanism the surgeon relies on to assess the impact of the operation. The surgeon's eye roll and the anaesthetist's cheerful confirmation underscores how a successful intervention from one professional standpoint may complicate another's accountabilities. This moment reveals the different professional jurisdictions of the anaesthetist and surgeon (Abbott, 1988) and how their respective clinical logics can interfere with one another. Beyond the division between anaesthetics and surgery, the OD team also had discrete responsibilities in supporting the anaesthetist, the surgical procedure, and caring for the patient during the operation. Thus, whilst intraoperative work is closely coupled, it is more accurately described as an interleaving of specialised roles, each with distinct accountabilities.

Intraoperative care began by enacting the patient as an interdisciplinary object of practice, through the second component of the WHO Surgical Safety Checklist. This stage – known as 'time out' – occurred after the patient was configured for surgery and immediately before skin incision, marking a shift in the patient's status from an object of preoperative care to an object of surgical intervention. It involved confirming team members knew one another by name and role, and agreement between the anaesthetist and surgeon on the patient's identity, surgical site, and planned procedure. The checklist also required displaying relevant radiographic images, and identifying anticipated critical events: for the surgeon, this might include blood loss, equipment needs or investigations; for the anaesthetist, patient's condition, potential complications, or monitoring needs; for the OD practitioner, issues with instrument sterility or equipment. The team also confirmed implementation of the surgical site bundle – evidence-based practices designed to prevent infections – including checks on antibiotic prophylaxis, hair removal, patient warming, blood glucose control, and anticoagulant medication. In some of the operations I observed, the time out was initiated by the surgeon, and in others OD staff.

> The consultant initiates the WHO checklist which begins with everyone introducing themselves. To which the consultant responds: 'Excellent!' Then in a formal way he introduces himself, names the patient and outlines the procedure. Someone asks a question about predicting any events, whether the patient is in receipt of antibiotics, whether thromboprophylaxis (interventions to prevent blood clotting) has been attended to.

In addition to the safety checks, the process temporarily paused practitioners' discrete activities and reoriented the team around a shared focus on the planned procedure, aligning their distinct roles and responsibilities in a collective articulation of surgical readiness.

Nowhere else in the hip fracture assemblage is the patient enacted with such intensity and focus than in the operating theatre. The sterile field is the most visible manifestation of this concentration. Except for the operation site, blue drapes cover the patient's body, and access to the immediate surgical area is restricted to the scrub practitioner, operating surgeons, and others by special permission. Here all attention centres on the surgery, conducted under the brilliance of the operating theatre lights with progress periodically checked with imaging.

> Other than the arm, the patient is completely hidden under the surgical drapes.
>
> I am encouraged to put on a mask so that I can enter the sterile field of the operation – where the airflow is moderated – and see more of what is going on. Both associate specialist surgeon and the consultant advise me to sit down and 'avoid anything blue' should I feel queasy.

> As the associate specialist surgeon works, he asks for X-ray films: Can I have a lateral please?

Beyond the sterile field, the anaesthetist monitored the patient's vital signs, and level of sedation. In cases where patients were awake under spinal anaesthetic – as with Megan, who had a respiratory condition – this also involved verbal reassurance and periodic checks on wellbeing.

> Megan coped remarkably well with the procedure and at intervals I observed the anaesthetist checking that she was OK and offering reassurance and praise for how well she was doing.

It is very hard to observe anaesthetic work; monitoring is continuous and technologically mediated, with adjustments to the administration of anaesthesia made as necessary. While essential to patient safety – in many cases the anaesthetist is literally keeping the patient alive – anaesthetic work only moved centre stage if a problem disrupted the surgery.

Throughout the operation, members of the wider OD team circulated at the periphery of the sterile field to support overall activity. They retrieved equipment and supplies, managed specimens, assisted the scrub practitioner with swab counts, recorded torniquet times and blood loss, and made entries to the OD PCR.

> It is then suggested that I stand back a bit as he is about to drill so that he has a straight edge on the bone, and this can sometimes spray everywhere. He starts this process and drills for a bit before requesting a new battery for the drill. The theatre ODP locates one for him.

On completion of the surgery the intraoperative patient was disassembled, with closure of the wound typically the trigger for action.

> Associate specialist surgeon and the junior doctor close the wound. The scrub practitioner opens an adhesive dressing but this proves to be too big and so she has to open another [...] Once the plaster is affixed the doctors remove the sterile drapes, the OD practitioner uncouples the patient from the blood pressure cuff, and the scrub nurse clears away the instruments.

At this point, the anaesthetist moved centre stage to reverse the anaesthetic. The patient had to be breathing independently before leaving the operating theatre; a decision based on the anaesthetist's professional judgment.

> [O]nce the surgeon has closed the skin [...] the anaesthetist takes over again. So, the anaesthetist then will give them a drug to wake the patient up.
>
> *(Clinical Leader – Interview)*

> Procedures are not over until your patient is reversed then out of theatre.
>
> *(Clinical Leader – Interview)*

Before the patient left the operating room, the final component of the WHO Surgical Safety Checklist – 'sign out' – was completed, marking the end of the patient's status as an object of intraoperative practice. This required the surgical team to confirm the correct procedure had been recorded; verify instrument, swab, and sharps count (ensuring nothing remained in the patient's body), removal of throat pack, correct specimen labelling, and identification of any equipment problems. The surgeon and anaesthetist must indicate any concerns regarding the patient's recovery and ongoing care. Like earlier stages, this was a brief but structured moment in which the patient was enacted as an interdisciplinary object of practice – not of imminent intervention, but of shared responsibility, temporarily stabilised at the point of closure.

While the WHO Surgical Safety Checklist instantiated the patient as a shared object of interdisciplinary practice at critical intervals in the pre- and intraoperative phases, this collective orientation was not sustained throughout the trajectory. Beyond these temporary stabilisations, clinical work proceeded primarily within professional domains, shaped by distinct responsibilities, priorities, and objects of practice. This was mirrored in the formal records, which documented distinct professional accounts rather than an integrated narrative.

Surgeons recorded procedural details on the 'operation sheet' within the OD PCR – a relatively unstructured section that allowed flexibility in how the operation was described and often accompanied by diagrams. These details were also entered into the T&O digital management system. Anaesthetic care was documented separately in the Anaesthetic Chart, focused primarily on pharmacological interventions, fluid balance, and technical aspects of anaesthetic induction. It included a graph to track vital signs and a tick-box section for significant intraoperative events. Although patients were continuously monitored, the anaesthetic record did not reflect this level of attentiveness.

> They're monitoring them continuously anyway but sometimes…but then writing that down and catching up. But I think generally, anaesthetists are notorious with not actually writing you know, an awful lot of stuff.
>
> *(OD Clinical Leader – Interview)*

The scrub practitioner recorded all other intraoperative care in a separate, four-page section of the OD PCR. This included devices used, skin integrity impacts from diathermy or defibrillation, confirmation of WHO checklist completion, wound closure, estimated blood loss, swab counts, and details of patient transfer from the operating table. A small free-text section provided for handover comments to the PACU nurse. Although designed to capture comprehensive details of the surgery under time constraints, the movement of patients often outpaced the scrub practitioner's capacity to complete it fully, especially in complex cases.

> You can have a patient who is very work intensive. I don't get time to do a thorough breakdown of everything that's gone on in there, and I'm often rushing into recovery afterwards to try and fill it all in…
>
> *(OD Clinical Leader – Interview)*

Object Formation in Post-anaesthetic Care

After surgery, patients were transferred to PACU, typically staying for around an hour. Staffed by nurses and healthcare support workers, PACU was a large open space, with a central nurses' station, and 14 post-anaesthetic care bays (12 adult and 2 child), each equipped with monitors and specialist equipment. Nurse provided one-to-one care, although this ratio was sometimes stretched under pressure. They remained at the bedside to enable continuous monitoring, while healthcare support workers assisted with comfort care and sourcing items for individual needs.

Patients arrived from theatre, accompanied by the anaesthetist and scrub practitioner, were allocated a space, and attached to monitoring technology.

> Almost immediately a new case arrives in PACU. The anaesthetist and scrub practitioner are greeted by the PACU nurse. Together they connect the

patient to equipment – oxygen tubing, chest drain suction, monitor leads, pulse oximeter, and blood pressure cuff. The scrub practitioner completes the 'final count' in the theatre care plan. The PACU nurse checks the monitor, adjusts the face mask. The patient is asleep.

PACU nurses received two separate handovers: anaesthetic details and relevant patient history from the anaesthetist, and details of the surgery from the scrub practitioner. Both were brief and focused on the immediate concerns of PACU care. This example relates to Megan.

Anaesthetist: This lady is [name] she's had a left DHS (dynamic hip screw hip surgery) [...] She's got COPD (chronic obstructive pulmonary disease) so her chest is quite bad. She has a bronchial inhaler. So, anything more than ninety-four (oxygen saturation levels) I am happy [...] She has a Fentanyl patch which she's used to, and she also takes Tramadol'.

Scrub Nurse: This is [name] she's had a left DHS. She has Mepore dressing wise, stitches on skin, blood loss two hundred mils. That's it from my side.

PACU care began with 'settling the patient': recording initial vital signs, checking attachments (IVs, drains), and responding as the patient woke – providing reassurance, removing airway devices, and addressing comfort (temperature, nausea, pain).

After the scrub practitioner and anaesthetist leave us, the nurse takes the patient's temperature and discovers this to be low. He requests a couple of extra blankets from the healthcare support worker. He then spends the next ten minutes or so writing an entry in the care plan. He transcribes vital signs readings from the monitor, makes periodic inquiries about the patient's pain and whether he feels sick, and on one occasion uncovers the patient's arms to check for IVs: 'Just one, nothing there?'. He looks under the theatre gown to inspect the elbow flexure. The patient stirs.

Patient: So, this is somewhere else entirely.
PACU Nurse: It's where everyone wakes up after surgery.
Patient: I had the dullest dream. All about DIY!

There was a discrete PACU section in the OD PCR. It included two complex observation charts which reflected the concerns through which patients were understood in the post-anaesthetic period. The first documented pulse, blood pressure, temperature, and respirations. The second captured a range of indicators – oxygen saturation, blood glucose levels, central venous pressure – and incorporated standardised assessment tools and scoring systems. Pain was graded on a 5-point scale; nausea and wound puncture sites were recorded, with bleeding flagged as a key concern. A large section of the chart focused on the level of consciousness, broken down into standardised categories: eye opening, verbal response, and motor responsiveness, each numerically coded. A separate section tracked signs of recovery from spinal anaesthesia, such as sensation and movement in the lower body. Through this documentation, patients were rendered as objects of PACU practice – made visible and knowable through structured observation, scoring systems, and categorical checklists. The chart translated bodily states into actionable data, aligning patient care with protocols of risk detection and recovery monitoring.

In addition to monitoring vital signs and attending to patient well-being, PACU nurses engaged in sensemaking to develop a fuller understanding of the patient beyond the brief handovers from the anaesthetist and scrub nurse.

Recovery Nurse:	I think most recovery nurses then, when they've got time, once the patient has settled, their airways settle and they are actually stable, for them it's like right let's find out a bit more about this patient. Because that's all you've had is a one- or two-minute handover from the anaesthetist ....so that's all you know about that patient, it's very little.

Understanding the broader patient's trajectory, was partly to support ward transfer (see Chapter 9), but also to manage the patient's recovery. In the following example, the nurse is trying to ascertain whether blood gases were taken in theatre so she can remove the arterial line, but this information is missing.

Recovery Nurse [to me]:	Did she take blood gases in theatre?
DA:	I saw a printout – like a large receipt – would that be it?
Recovery Nurse:	Could be. I want to take out her arterial line, but I haven't seen a blood gas. This is one of the many challenges we face. They should stick them in the anaesthetic notes. I might be able to get the reading from the machine. I was going to do a blood gas, but I've got nothing to compare it with. The trouble is if someone says it is OK, and I take it out and it's not .... I've done that!

In this case, the nurse asked me for clarification, as I had accompanied the patient throughout the operation. More commonly, sensemaking entailed contacting theatre staff for further information. Respondents conceded that the pressures on patient throughput could compromise record-keeping.

DA:	'Do PACU staff ever have to contact the theatre after the handover has taken place for additional information or clarification of stuff?'
OD Clinical Leader:	'Oh yes, frequently'.
DA:	'Is there any particular pattern to that?'
OD Clinical Leader:	'No, not particularly. Not a particular pattern as such, no it's just sometimes things do get missed and it might be that things if confused were confused before they remain so […] If they seem to be oozing a lot of blood, did they lose a lot in theatre because you didn't document that they have. Was that… is there anything we need to know? Sometimes they put wash out in and if they don't hand over that they've had washout in, you get what looks like a serious amount of fluid coming through and then you start to think oh gosh what's happening here? […] Or a surgeon, if we have a new surgeon and something is different, they might go and say why's he done this, and I'll see well he's a new one. Oh right, okay. And it's just the way he's going to do it from now on […] And we all miss things. And I'm no different to anyone else. Sometimes you do things, and you think I didn't write that down, but when you're under pressure to get another case on the table, you are going to miss things, but this way someone can come to you and say was such and such? Oh yes, didn't I document it, sorry'.

(Clinical Leader – Interview)

While monitoring activity was documented in structured, codified formats, other aspects of PACU care were recorded as free-text narrative entries. These were aligned with the PACU care plan, which comprised 12 categories:

1. Potential airway obstruction
2. Level of consciousness
3. Potentially unstable vital signs
4. Wound site
5. Wound drainage/urinary catheter
6. Intravenous infusion
7. Pain and restlessness

8 Nausea and vomiting
9 Nasogastric tube
10 External fixation
11 Limb observations following Lloyd Davis/ lithotomy position
12 Return to the ward.

As in the orthogeriatric ward (Chapter 8), the care plan functioned more as a performative display of nursing standards than a coordination tool. The 12 elements were internalised by PACU nurses, who rarely referred to the plan in practice. Moreover, reflecting the tension between standardised frameworks and relational care, nurses often grouped elements in their narrative entries.

> The entry into the notes is quite extensive and I asked PACU nurse about its content. He showed me the post anaesthetic care plan and how different aspects are numbered. These codes are used in the narrative entry to denote the element that the entry refers to. PACU nurse said that he often combined codes together – today this included 1+2; 7+8 and 3+11.

> She said that she frequently combined several of the coded areas together (1, 2, 11) as logically they hung together.

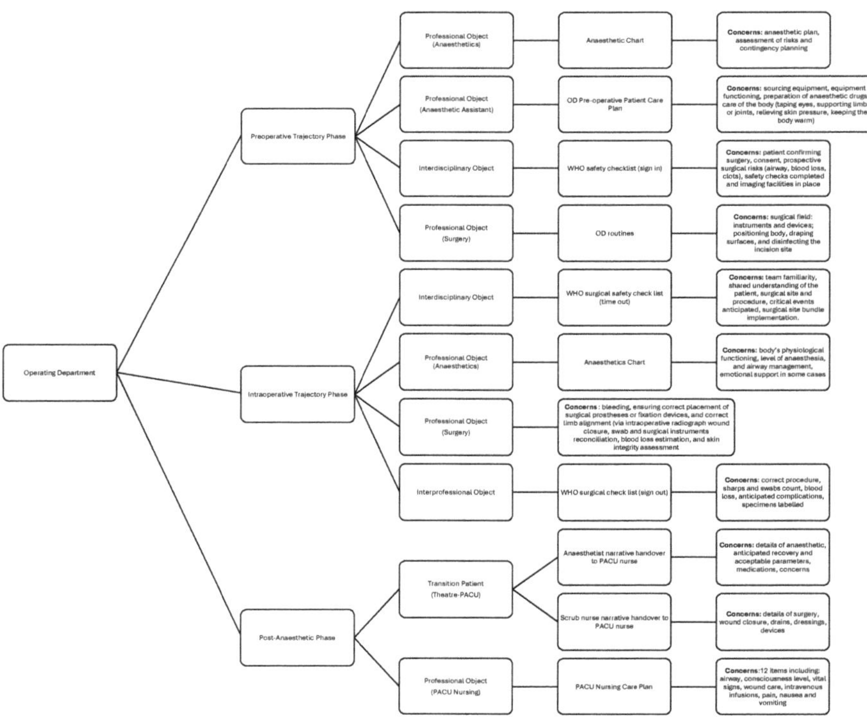

FIGURE 9.1 Object formation in OD work.

Patients remained in PACU until they were physiologically stable to return to the ward, the parameters of which were inscribed in formal standardised discharge criteria.

Summary

This chapter has described the social world of the OD and how patients were enacted for hip fracture surgery. OD work was characterised by a rational-linear organisation, with formal tools, material routines, and interpretative repertoires as central actors. Over a five-hour trajectory shaped by safety and efficiency logics, patients were translated into distinct objects of practice for preoperative, intraoperative, and post-anaesthetic care. Figure 9.1 summarises these processes.

OD work focused on both the body and the surgical intervention, with object formation centred on corporeal-material relations. Except for the PACU nursing record, documentation was highly reductionist, with forensic attention to a narrow set of concerns involving the body and its associated technologies. Trajectory mobilisation was punctuated by internal status passages, mediated by the WHO Surgical Safety Checklist, which coordinated activity and instantiated the patient as an interdisciplinary object aligned with safety standards.

Whereas other parts of the hip fracture pathway required receiving departments to enact the patient into their collective object of practice, the acute care assemblage required this work to be done upstream, on the orthogeriatric ward. The next chapter explores how this was accomplished.

References

Abbott, A. (1988). *The System of Professions: An Essay on the Division of Expert Labor*. Chicago and London, University of Chicago Press.

Allen, D. (2015). *The Invisible Work of Nurses: Hospitals, Organisation and Healthcare*. London and New York, Routledge.

Allen, D., E. Gillen and L.J. Rixson (2009). 'Systematic review of the effectiveness of integrated care pathways: what works, for whom, in what circumstances?' *International Journal of Evidence-Based Healthcare* 7(2): 61–74. https://doi.org/10.1111/j.1744-1609.2009.00127.x

Berg, M. (1997). 'Of forms, containers, and the electronic medical record: some tools for a sociology of the formal'. *Science, Technology, & Human Values* **22**(4): 403–433.

Heath, C. and P. Luff (2021). 'Embodied action, project, and institutional action: the exchange of tools and implements during surgical procedures'. *Discourse Processes* **58**(3): 233–250.

Hindmarsh, J. and A. Pilnick (2007). 'Knowing bodies at work: embodiment and ephemeral teamwork in anaesthesia'. *Organization Studies* **28**(9): 1395–1417 https://doi.org/10.1177/0170840607068258

Meyer, J. and B. Rowan (1977). 'Institutionalized organizations: formal structure as myth and ceremony.' *American Journal of Sociology*, **83**(2): 340–363.

Mol, A. M. (2008). *The Logic of Care: Health and the Problem of Patient Choice*. London, Routledge.

Mondada, L. (2014). 'The local constitution of multimodal resources for social interaction'. *Journal of Pragmatics* **65**: 137–156. https://doi.org/10.1016/j.pragma.2014.04.004
Pols, J. (2008). 'Good care: enacting a complex ideal in long-term psychiatry'. *Medische Anthropologie* **20**(1): 73–89.
Russ, S.J., N. Sevdalis, K. Moorthy, E.K. Mayer, S. Rout, J. Caris, J. Mansell, R. Davies, C. Vincent, and A. Darzi (2015). 'A qualitative evaluation of the barriers and facilitators toward implementation of the WHO surgical safety checklist across hospitals in England: lessons from the "Surgical Checklist Implementation Project"'. *Annals of Surgery* **261**(1): 81–91. https://doi.org/10.1097/SLA.0000000000000793
Timmons, S. and J. Tanner (2004). 'A disputed occupational boundary: operating theatre nurses and Operating Department Practitioners'. *Sociology of Health & Illness* **26**(5): 645–666. https://doi.org/10.1111/j.0141-9889.2004.00409.x
Treadwell J.R., S. Lucas, and A.Y. Tsou (2014). 'Surgical checklists: a systematic review of impacts and implementation'. *BMJ Quality & Safety* **23**:299–318.
Vaughan, D. (1996). *The Challenger Launch Decision: Risky Technology, Culture and Deviance at Nasa*. Chicago and London, The University of Chicago Press.
Vaughan, D. (1999). 'The dark side of organizations: mistake, misconduct, and disaster'. *Annual Review of Sociology* **25**: 271–305.
Wæhle, H.V., A.S. Haugen, S. Wiig, E. Søfteland, N. Sevdalis, and S. Harthug (2020). 'How does the WHO Surgical Safety Checklist fit with existing perioperative risk management strategies? An ethnographic study across surgical specialties' *BMC Health Services Research* **20**: 111. https://doi.org/10.1186/s12913-020-4965-5
WHO (2009). *WHO Surgical Checklist*. Geneva, Switzerland, World Health Organization.

10

CONSCRIPTED OBJECTS

Acute Care Transitions

This chapter examines how transitions are organised within the acute care assemblage, building on Chapters 8 and 9 to explore object formation and trajectory mobilisation at the interface between the orthogeriatric ward and Operating Department (OD). Acute care services were oriented to distinct collective objects of practice, and transition involved translational mechanisms of conscription, bracketing, and reconstruction, with formal processes and artefacts as key actors. The first half of this chapter describes and explains these arrangements. The second half illustrates transition processes in practice, focusing on the example of Megan, a hip fracture patient whose surgical trajectory I followed.

Transition Arrangements

This section explores how patients entered and exited the OD within the acute care assemblage. First, it outlines the transition interfaces between the orthogeriatric ward and OD, highlighting their distinct organisational logics and collective objects of practice. Second, it examines the socio-material infrastructure and mechanisms that managed transition, focusing on the interaction of formal tools and institutional roles. Third, it analyses how patients were enacted for transition and the qualities of transition objects at this stage of the trajectory.

Transition Interfaces

The two services in the acute care assemblage had widely divergent institutional functions. The orthogeriatric ward provided continuous care for hip fracture patients (and other older people with trauma and bone injuries) from admission

DOI: 10.4324/9781003475019-17

through to discharge, interleaving surgical preparation with wider patient needs. As collective objects of practice patients had a narrative quality – understandings that were sustained through the creation of working knowledge (Ellingsen and Monteiro, 2003). Doctors maintained narrative records of patients' care and treatment, while ward nurses used evolving care trajectory narratives to coordinate the shifting priorities and exigences of everyday activity.

In contrast, OD work focused on the requirements of anaesthesia, surgery, and post-anaesthetic recovery. It followed a rational-linear organisation, strongly oriented to patient safety and efficiency. The hip fracture trajectory in OD was condensed into five hours, with each stage – preoperative, intraoperative, and post-anaesthetic care – characterised by distinct object formation practices, and a clear division of labour, mediated by the WHO Safety Checklist. As collective objects of practice, OD patients had a technical quality: meticulous and detailed attention was directed at a narrow range of concerns aligned with the surgical intervention, the patient's body, and associated devices, technologies and practices.

Despite their differences, both services were enrolled in shared mobilisation and clinical logics: the orthogeriatric team was oriented to guidelines and national standards for timely surgery, and OD work was aligned with safe and efficient resource use.

Transition Infrastructures

Formal tools were central actors in the transition infrastructure. An Initial Treatment Regime (Chapter 8, p. 126) coordinated the work of orthogeriatric ward resident doctors, which was designed to enact the patient as a trajectory object oriented to the requirements of surgery. Although the anaesthetic department did not specify its own preoperative criteria, the threat of a cancelled operation gave it considerable power at a distance. The Initial Treatment Regime had been developed to obviate the risk of last-minute refusals by the anaesthetist.

> Trauma and Orthopaedic Surgeon: The NICE guidelines say they should be operated on in 36 hours and what can happen is you get there, and the anaesthetist can say, 'Hang on this hasn't been done'. So, the juniors, who are busy, can forget, or they do it, but they don't write it down. So, the checklist ensures you have thought about things, and they are done. We have seen a reduction in the cancellation of operations because of failures in the preoperative work up.

Beyond the Initial Treatment Regime, the OD Patient Care Record (PCR) incorporated two checklists – preoperative and discharge – designed to manage entry into, and exit from, the department. Checklists acted as obligatory passage points in mediating transition; they were a critical juncture that all actors had to pass through in order to achieve their goals (Law and Callon, 1992). Signed by actors from both services, the checklists fulfilled a gate-keeping function in the management of transition; patients could not be transferred unless certain criteria were met.

The agency of tools in the acute care assemblage was mediated by the wider network of socio-material relationships (Akrich, 1992; Latour, 2005). Frailty nurses used the Initial Treatment Regime to reflexively monitor the work of doctors to ensure all surgical preparations had been undertaken. Ward nurses and OD practitioners were formally tasked with managing the patient's entry into OD, while PCAU and ward nurses managed their exit. Tool use also relied on informal practices, by OD healthcare support workers and PACU nurses, to facilitate transitional processes at the ward–OD and OD–ward interfaces respectively.

While formal artefacts played a central role in coordinating transitions, discretion in their use was unevenly distributed. The capacity to adapt, bypass, or selectively engage with these tools was shaped by pre-existing professional hierarchies and institutional roles. Some actors were tightly enrolled in transition infrastructures through formal responsibilities and documentation practices (nurses, OD practitioners and healthcare support workers), while others operated with greater autonomy, either by virtue of institutionalised authority or professional standing (surgeons, anaesthetists).

Transition Objects

Transition objects in the acute care assemblage had a technical quality, centred on formal organisational criteria inscribed in the OD preoperative and discharge checklists. These documents condensed a range of extended activities into a reductionist format, enacting patients as specific, fixed, and ready-to-go objects. Once completed, the checklist rendered the patient as an immutable mobile (Latour, 1987) – a stable and transportable representation, which retained its form, enabling the patient to move across transition boundaries as a stable and authorised object of surgical practice. While technical transition objects mediated the mobilisation of trajectories into OD, they were complemented by a care trajectory narrative for the return journey. Generated informally by PACU nurses, these narratives were designed to translate the patient from the profoundly reductionist and fragmented objects of practice of OD work into an integrated account aligned with the collective objects of practice of orthogeriatric work.

Transition Processes

Transitions within the acute care assemblage were accomplished through conscription, bracketing, and reconstruction, and entailed complex processes of translation and object formation. Aligned around shared clinical and mobilisation logics, and bound together by institutionally mandated documents, services exercised reciprocal power to enact patients for transition (conscription). On entry to OD, the concerns of orthogeriatric practice were temporarily suspended (bracketing), as object formation centred on the corporeal-material relations of surgical work. OD practice was profoundly reductionist, with anaesthetists, surgeons, and OD staff working with discrete professional objects. Discharge entailed mechanisms of reconstruction to enable continuity of care on the ward. In illustrating these processes, the analysis traces how agency was distributed across human and non-human actors, examining both the capacities and constraints of tools in the management of transition, and the formal and informal practices that sustained their effects.

The Ward–OD Interface

Preparation for surgery began on admission with the medical clerking. As outlined in Chapter 8, resident doctors initiated standard investigations and assembled a medical history to identify conditions requiring management. Once the surgical plan was agreed, they were then responsible for preparing the patient for theatre.

> Well, all the investigations for the patient's general overall condition, it's down to the medics, you know. They'll do the investigations, they'll take the bloods, they'll take the X-rays. Chest X-rays, Echoes, whatever is required. I mean for the elderly patients, you know [...] quite often they're on Warfarin, you have to check their INRs (blood test which indicates how long blood takes to clot*)*. A lot of them can't have general anaesthetics because they've got chest problems, COPD (chronic obstructive pulmonary disease), emphysema or whatever [...] so you do a lot of spinal anaesthetics but then of course if your INRs not low enough you can't do a spinal anaesthetic so that is...is a problem occasionally, is trying to get the INR levels correct, low enough for them to be able to do a spinal anaesthetic [...] I think it's their job really to make sure that these hips are ready and...ready to come to theatre, you know, optimised to come to theatre.
>
> *(OD Clinical Leader – Interview)*

Activity was mediated by the Initial Treatment Regime, which translated the patient into a trajectory object oriented to the concerns of anaesthetists and the OD. This included standard preoperative investigations (full blood count, urea and electrolytes, blood group and save, chest X-ray, Electrocardiogram), and tailored tests (for example, blood coagulation, arterial blood gases), supported by two pages of clinical protocols and algorithms, to guide decision-making and junior doctor development.

> The house officers do it and part of the process of having stuff in the back (clinical protocols) … is they need to learn that […] This approach tells people how to get on so that the junior orthopaedic surgeons can both start treatment and learn about treatment and gain confidence in knowing that if they come across somebody later in their career […] they know how to do all the basic initiation.
>
> *(Orthogeriatrician – Interview)*

Resident doctors valued the proforma as a guide to practice but also highlighted its potential to constrain clinical reasoning.

> Senior House Officer said that she thought the downside was 'that they (proforma) stopped you from using your brain', but that the hip fracture one was helpful because 'you are dealing with a number of complex issues'.

> *F1 Doctor:* 'Because there are new doctors every four months, the proforma reminds you of what you should do. So, there's a column for Clexane (an anticoagulant) and DVT (deep vein thrombosis) prophylaxis. I was clerking patients on my first day and you might not know these things. So, it was a massive help – particularly the risk assessment section – and it does maintain the same level of care'.
>
> *F1 Doctor:* 'On the one hand they make you more thorough, on the other, they make it more mundane. If it's just a checklist you can end up just ticking the box rather than thinking. […] But it does remind you what needs to be done'.

While the Initial Treatment Regime was designed to coordinate medical practice, on it's own it was not sufficient. As described in Chapter 8, resident doctors' work was regularly disrupted. Frailty nurses, as permanent staff members, acted as a safety net – monitoring preparations and checking test results. In this context, the Initial Treatment Regime functioned as an accumulating device, which enabled frailty nurses to maintain awareness of trajectory progress.

> Frailty Nurse, who is reviewing the documentation, remarks: 'She's got no anti-embolic stockings prescribed! We have a protocol for TEDs (anti-embolic stockings) and Clexane (anticoagulant) which consultant orthogeriatrician developed for the doctors to ensure they stick to the procedures, but it does not always happen and occasionally people slip through. They have the whole procedure laid out here. See here he has ticked thrombo-prophylactic assessment but has not prescribed Clexane or TEDs!

Nurses have uncertain authority in care trajectory management (Allen, 2015), but frailty nurses worked closely with the orthogeriatric consultants, and resident doctors largely tolerated these interventions, at least in public.

Preparing patients for theatre was highly routinised in ward nursing work. This involved ensuring the patient was fasted, removing attachments, providing a theatre gown, and completing preoperative documentation. Designed to enact the patient as a transition object, the documentation had two parts: the OD Admission Proforma and Preoperative Checklist.

The OD Admission Proforma collated baseline clinical data: vital signs (pulse, blood pressure, temperature, respiration, blood oxygen saturation, the NEWS score, and Glasgow Coma Scale neurological observations) – which were necessary for assessing the patient's post-anaesthetic recovery; weight, height, and body mass index – used by anaesthetists to calculate drug dosages; details of skin integrity – which guided bodily care and enabled identification of intraoperative skin damage; sensory information (eyesight, hearing, use of aids) which was crucial for patient communication. A free-text section captured any relevant medical history.

The Preoperative Checklist included 22 requirements to preconfigure the patient for OD. The patient had to be starved to prevent asphyxiation, and their bladder emptied to ensure trajectory mobilisation was not disrupted by requests to use the toilet. The risks of developing a blood clot had to be assessed and preventative measures instigated, any allergies documented, all consent forms signed, and the surgical site marked by the doctor to prevent wrong-site surgery. All personal clothing, jewellery, make-up, hair gel and nail varnish, prostheses (wigs, hair pieces, dentures, spectacles, contact lenses, artificial eyes, and hearing aids) had to be removed and replaced with new attachments that facilitated OD work – a theatre gown and anti-embolic stockings (if prescribed). The patient also had to be accompanied by certain documentary attachments: images or X-rays, inpatient medication chart, anaesthetic chart, the inpatient medical record, and addressograph labels which were used to label charts and specimens in OD.

Checklist completion involved a systematic process of verifying each item, with responses marked as Yes, No, or Not Applicable (N/A). Although the Initial Treatment Regime and frailty nurse oversight aimed to ensure the readiness of patients, last-minute issues still arose. As the following extract demonstrates, the checklist fulfilled an important additional coordinating function.

> 10 am and senior ward nurse starts preparing a lady for theatre. The nurse referred to this as 'doing her checklist'. She finds a copy of the documentation and starts to complete some details. She is then called away to do something for another patient and answers a query from a doctor about someone else's discharge arrangements. The nurse returns to the checklist.

She scrutinises the anti-embolic stocking care plan. She turns from this to the admission booklet and reviews the thromboprophylaxis assessment. She shows the assessment to the ward pharmacist and observes, 'They've not filled this in properly. There's not a lot on this really'.

Ward Pharmacist suggests she checks the drug chart.

Senior Nurse: I am sure they said she had poor skin. I am not sure she should be on these (anti-embolic stockings). They've (doctors) written her up for them, but they haven't done the risk assessment. I wish I knew this when they were here (this is a reference to the doctors who have now left the ward) because they (OD) will not let her through the door.

[...]

Senior nurse applies the patient's wrist band and then asks me whether I can see any dentures. The patient is asleep with her mouth open, and no dentures are visible.

Senior Nurse: No earrings? (she checks the lady's ears) No rings? (she uncovers her hands and checks). Has she had any previous surgery?

She looks in the admission proforma and observes: No. That's impressive.

Senior Nurse: I wonder whether there is an arrow on her leg? Is the Thomas Splint (a form of traction) clue enough! Has she got a catheter? (looks at the end of the bed – she has). So, when did she last eat? (she writes midnight into the form). Midnight is the last time she could have eaten. Allergies? I'm not sure. I'll ask consultant orthogeriatrician if he will do the prophylaxis.

'Doing the checklist' involved sensemaking. In this example, the senior nurse drew on diverse resources to assess the distributed activities of nurses and doctors in enacting the patient as a trajectory object. Checklist completion condensed and stabilised this work, translating the patient into a transportable technical transition object aligned with the 22 prescribed concerns mediating entry into OD.

Patients were transported to OD by a healthcare support worker and porter. Action was triggered by the OD receptionist, notified via the digital management system (see Chapter 9) when the theatre was ready. The ward received no advance notice; nurses had to anticipate readiness based on the operating list, which was subject to change. Although in interviews senior OD staff described a formal handover between ward nurse and support worker, observations revealed otherwise. The ward–OD interface was mediated almost entirely through the Preoperative Checklist, which support workers used to assess patient readiness. Face-to-face interaction with ward nurses appeared largely incidental.

> We arrive on the ward, and the healthcare support worker retrieves the patient's medical notes from behind the Nurses' Station. She does not speak to anyone; she simply picks them up. We head into the four-bedded area, where she locates a surface on which to rest the folder while she 'check(s) that they have all the notes for us'. She checks the thromboprophylaxis risk assessment form, showing me as she does so that most patients have a white form – which our patient has – but that hip fracture patients also have the form included in the Hip Fracture Proforma, which she shows me on the back sheet. She looks at this to see that these things are completed. She also checks the drug chart to see that the anti-embolic stockings have been prescribed and Clexane, an anticoagulant. She checks the consent form has been signed and removes this from the medical notes folder.
>
> [...]
>
> The healthcare support worker approaches Megan, our patient. The relatives, who have been seated, stand up and move away from the bed area. She retrieves the OD PCR from the medical notes folder. She asks the patient for her name and date of birth and checks this information against the wrist and ankle labels. She also checks that the operation site is marked. [...] The healthcare support worker is looking through the patient notes and discovers there are no adhesive addressograph labels. She instructs the porter to locate some. She then picks up the yellow surgical consent form and asks the patient whether this is her signature. The patient says, 'My glasses are packed so I cannot see'. Healthcare support worker: 'I'll have to get them for you so you can check. You can leave your glasses here but if there is an issue downstairs I can confirm for you'.

OD performance targets required patients to be fully prepared when the team arrived to collect them; but this did not always happen. Checklist completion was interleaved with other nursing tasks, and elements could be overlooked – especially if an operation had been postponed, theatre lists had changed, or patients transferred between wards. Patients were not supposed to leave the ward if any preoperative requirements were incomplete.

> What happens is the healthcare support workers will phone up and say, 'They haven't got this done'. Because they're not meant to bring them, if an operation site hasn't been marked, if a consent form hasn't been filled in, and if the thrombolytic risk assessment form hasn't been done, they don't leave the ward.
>
> *(Senior Clinical Leader OD – Interview)*

A healthcare support worker I shadowed described her strategy when collecting patients: she first checked the items most often missed and likely to delay surgery.

> *OD Healthcare Support Worker:* 'You tend to go straight for the things we have lots of problems with – like the stockings, the anti-coagulants – because you know that's going to be the first hold-up. Then you've got to get the surgeon to come and sort them out'.

Although the checklist was intended as an obligatory passage point, respondents indicated that arrangements sometimes broke down, with healthcare support workers typically caught in the crossfire. Despite unresolved issues, surgeons, eager to undertake the operation, issued instructions to bring the patient to OD, overriding the formal process.

> So, the healthcare support worker will phone theatres and say this hasn't been done. Sometimes our surgeon will then take over and say, "Right. Bring them up to theatre", because all they want is to get them into theatre as soon as possible. "Bring them up, we'll sort it out when they're in theatre". So, and this has been a cause of confusion you know, because then the healthcare support workers will bring them up and they'll get into trouble from the senior nursing staff: "This patient should…but the surgeon told me to…I don't care, I shouldn't even leave the ward". But if the surgeon says and…it's very difficult so there's all this, you know, there's a bit of confrontation going on there.
>
> *(OD Clinical Leader – Interview)*

Here, the checklist's authority was unevenly recognised across professional boundaries. Surgeons, outside the OD line management structure, were prepared to bypass formal protocols in favour of expediency. This left healthcare support workers navigating conflicting accountabilities: expected to uphold checklist governance yet deferring to the authority of the surgeon. These dynamics were compounded by their ambiguous status. While playing a pivotal role in managing transitions this was an informal process. There was no documentation space for healthcare support workers to confirm checks had been completed, further complicating accountability.

Respondents indicated that using healthcare support workers to transfer patients to the OD was relatively unusual. Typically, patients are accompanied by a ward nurse, ideally the individual responsible for their care. Ward nurses were acknowledged to be busy and often unavailable to leave the ward, and this arrangement afforded OD greater control over patient flow. Consequently, interface management was wholly dependent on the circumscribed version of the patient available in the written documentation, with little opportunity for ward nurses who knew the patient to draw attention to any wider matters of concern.

> A lot of the patients who are brought to theatre, you have a porter and the healthcare support worker, and the healthcare support workers are actually very good, but they're only given very limited information, so then when ODP goes to check this patient in and you know in our waiting area they could be confused, Alzheimer's you know, or dementia – that makes it increasingly difficult for us to go through our checklist because the healthcare support workers from theatres have been given limited information.
>
> *(OD Practitioner – Interview)*

The journey to the OD was a significant event, yet these arrangements denied patients the psychological support of being accompanied by an individual with whom they had established a relationship, someone who could keep in play facets of identity beyond the corporeal concerns of operating work.

> It never will sit right with me that a ward nurse…because a ward nurse is the person who has started a relationship with that patient and then all of a sudden, a strange… two strange people turn up and whisk you down to theatre and then you're met with…by other strange people all dressed up. I've never agreed with that, and I really don't like it, and I really think that they should change but then I haven't got that power.
>
> *(OD Clinical Leader – Interview)*

On arrival at OD, the patient was taken to the Waiting Bay – a liminal space behind the operating theatres. Here, the patient's status was betwixt and between. No longer under ward care but yet to be formally accepted into the next phase of their surgical trajectory. Further checks were required before this could happen.

The patient was formally received by an anaesthetic practitioner, who explained next steps and repeated the preoperative checklist. At this juncture, checklist completion was a formally accountable process.

> We are greeted by the anaesthetic practitioner who introduces himself and explains that Megan will now be taken into the Anaesthetic Room. He asks her name, questions whether she is allergic to anything – to which she responds Penicillin. He asks about the nature of the allergic response, but she does not know, she just knows there were issues when she was a child. He asks about lose teeth, crowns, temporary fillings, confirms that the operation is to be on her left hip and asks whether she has a little arrow on there, but does not check this. He then explains that they are going into the anaesthetist where he will attach leads to her chest to monitor her heart and a cuff to her arm. He explains that the anaesthetist will put a 'block' in her leg, which will enable her to sit forward comfortably while the anaesthetic goes into her back. He explains that she will feel a cold spray. Accompanied by the healthcare support worker we push her bed down the long corridor to the Anaesthetic Room.

Anaesthetic practitioners performed the checklist process multiple times daily, and its questions had become deeply embedded in practice. While patient interactions followed a constrained, institutionally oriented question and answer format, the checklist itself was not always explicitly referenced. In the following example, the practitioner receives a hip fracture patient and covers many checklist items informally. He also asks about hip range of movement – information not required by the form but essential for safely positioning the patient on the operating table.

> Anaesthetic practitioner then engages with the patient and asks several questions. These include when he has last had something to eat or drink, whether he is wearing jewellery, whether he has been on dialysis at all, whether he has a good range of movement in all his joints other than the affected hip, whether he has a catheter. These questions appear to have come off the top of his head and they include questions I have not heard others ask. Anaesthetic practitioner pauses as if he is trying to remember something and then continues.

Anaesthetic Practitioner:	So, we are repairing your hip. Which side? Left? Is this your signature on the consent form?
Patient:	Yes.
Anaesthetic Practitioner:	Have they marked your leg? Can I have a look? OK and you have TEDS on the right leg (this is a reference to anti-embolic stockings). Has the procedure been explained to you?
Patient:	Yes.
Anaesthetic Practitioner:	OK – we'll go down to see the anaesthetist now.

> As he is talking, he is signing the preoperative check list section at the bottom of the page.

All the OD checklist processes I observed were completed without incident. Staff interviews indicated that this was not always the case, however, and that ward nurses did not always understand the rationale behind certain checklist items. Question nine – 'Does the patient have a prosthesis?' – was frequently cited as problematic. Its purpose was to alert surgical and anaesthetic teams to any pre-existing prosthetics or detachable items that could pose an intraoperative risk. OD staff highlighted this item was often inadequately completed.

> The one thing I find that people miss out on is terminology, the word prosthesis is very confusing for a lot of ward staff, they don't [...] really know what we need and the information doesn't translate through from the ward to us because the checklist isn't understood by everybody [...] I mean it's not a difficult document to complete because it's basically you know you can tick and sign [...] but it's the interpretation and obviously metal work for us in a patient is very important [...] because we use electro surgery and we don't want to electrocute them! And that's written as does the patient have any prosthesis and then it says hearing aid/contact lenses so the ward staff assume that they're just talking about that and then we find out they've two knees and two hips but that hasn't been indicated on the checklist, so there's a lack of transparency in – we're not telling them what we want to know.
>
> *(OD Practitioner – Interview)*

This example highlights the limitations of standardised forms in coordinating interdepartmental practice without shared understanding. While the checklist functioned as both a safety device and a tool of formal accountability, its effectiveness relied on an interpretive grasp of its clinical purpose. Completing the form 'correctly' required more than procedural compliance – it necessitated translation: the ability to connect the abstract categories on the page to their practical implications for OD care. In this context, the second preoperative check by OD practitioners acted as a practical safeguard, ensuring that the checklist's categories were not just completed, but correctly understood and clinically meaningful.

The OD–Ward Interface

As with entry to the department, discharge from OD was mediated by standardised, institutionally mandated criteria which prescribed the conditions under which a patient could transfer to the ward. These centred on physiological stability, patient comfort, and the division of labour between OD and ward teams. Physiological stability was precisely specified: the patient should be able to maintain their airway, be passing 1 ml/kg of urine hourly if catheterised, have blood oxygen saturations levels above 95% on air (or match preadmission saturations), have a respiratory rate between 10 and 24, stable cardiovascular observations within preoperative ranges, a core temperature above 36°C; and be neurologically oriented (or preoperative neurological compromise documented). All surgical drains and wounds had to be free of bleeding. Comfort criteria required that pain should be absent or within 'acceptable parameters' and the patient should be free of nausea or vomiting. Criteria related to the PACU–ward division of labour included ensuring an accurate fluid balance chart (including preoperative fluids and estimated blood loss), and prescriptions for postoperative analgesia, antibiotics, and thromboprophylaxis.

Alignment with these criteria was mediated by a 15-item discharge checklist, signed by the PACU nurse and countersigned by the ward nurse. The checklist enacted the patient's readiness for transfer by fixing clinical judgements into a standardised form that could travel across department boundaries. In one fieldwork episode, a PACU nurse went to great lengths to obtain an acceptable temperature reading to enact the patient in alignment with discharge criteria related to temperature.

> Nurse says he will check the patient's temperature before he returns to the ward. On entry to PACU it was 35.5°C and he put some extra blankets on the bed. He takes his temperature again and it is 35.3°C! He leaves the patient to find another thermometer, wondering whether his is faulty, but this comes up with the same reading. He then locates an alternative thermometer which takes a reading based on skin temperature – he referred to this as a temporal thermometer [...] Eventually he manages to get a reading of 36.0°C using the temporal thermometer. He says that he will bring this to the ward 'to show I am not lying'.

Not all discharge criteria applied to every patient, and some flexibility was permitted. For example, a patient with a pre-existing elevated temperature owing to infection might still have this postoperatively. Any departure from the criteria had to be accounted for (a section on the care plan entitled 'variance' (sic) was designated for this purpose) and typically required anaesthetist approval.

> *PACU Nurse:* 'It talks about patients' temperature, that their dressings are dry and intact or as they should be. It talks about their vital signs being within acceptable parameters because obviously they're different for everybody [...] So if their blood pressure is not within a normal limit, it could be that it's a normal limit for them and you document that this is their normal looking at the pre-op blood pressures and stuff, we accept that this is OK'.

> Nurse said that if the anaesthetist agrees it is OK for the patient to return to the ward where they do not meet all the criteria then the wards will have them back. I asked, 'But they won't accept it on a nurse's say so?' and Nurse said 'No'.

This illustrates how tools are embedded in broader relational networks that mediate their agency. In this case, the anaesthetist held institutional authority to override criteria. This contrasts with the earlier example, in which the surgeon by-passed policies without formal sanction.

Many discharge parameters referenced baseline measurements, recorded by ward nurses on the OD Admission Proforma. While these physiological details supported preoperative and intraoperative care, they omitted information critical to PACU – namely, the patient's demeanour and cognitive status. Cognitive impairment is common in hip fracture patients and was assessed during the initial medical clerking, and experienced first-hand by ward nurses. By bracketing off this information, the OD documentation made post-anaesthetic recovery assessment more challenging. Recovery nurses would typically contact the ward to obtain the information required to make sense of a case.

> *PACU Nurse:* With elderly people, if you need to find anything else out, we just phone the ward and ask the nurse'.

> PACU Nurse is concerned about her patient's drowsiness and calls the ward to establish what she was like before.

> *PACU Nurse:* Really chatty – oh dear! Well, she's just very sleepy.

The patient is evidently still quite different from how she was before she went to theatre and cannot go back. PACU Nurse said that the ward was reluctant to have her yet anyway because they had a lot of confused patients who kept climbing out of bed.

As in ED, discharge from OD was shaped not only by formal criteria but also by normative expectations about the division of labour between PACU and the wards. A key concern was reconciling OD and ward documentation to enable care continuity. This included extracting information from the intraoperative record and transferring it into formats used for ongoing care.

> *PACU Nurse:* 'I don't know if the ward nurses know how much we do down here to get the patient's ready. We keep them down here a long time and they go back with their fluid charts, drugs written up, blood transfusions completed. The wards just have to make them comfortable. We write reams. Often

> before you just noted that the patient was comfortable, and their pressure areas were intact. And whereas in the past as a ward nurse I'd be looking in the anaesthetic chart to see what drugs they've had, in theatre we do all that for them'.

PACU nurses also went to considerable lengths to translate the patient into an object of practice aligned with ward nurses' work. As described in Chapter 9, OD worked with a reductionist version of the patient, focused on the corporeal-material requirements of anaesthesia and surgery. Broader orthogeriatric concerns were bracketed off. Nursing documentation remained on the ward, and although medical notes accompanied the patient, they were not used intra-operatively. In theatre, the patient was divided into discrete clinical objects – anaesthetic, surgical, and OD – each documented separately. PACU nurses received separate handovers from the anaesthetist and scrub nurse. While the OD PCR and Anaesthetic Chart formed part of the cumulative medical record, most sections were structured through tick boxes, reflecting the need to document salient details of anaesthetic and surgical practice under time constraints. PACU nurses scrutinised this documentation to make sense of the case and reconstruct this fragmented technical information into an integrated narrative account of the patient's OD trajectory, which was documented in the PACU nursing record.

> *PACU Nurse:* 'Recovery really are the ones that actually write the document things, all the others just do tick boxes without actually writing'.

These narrative reconstructions were essential in translating the patient into an object of practice for transition.

Once the patient satisfied discharge criteria, preparations for transfer began. This entailed: disconnecting monitors, securing infusions and drains, gathering documentation and attaching portable technologies to support the patient in transit (oxygen e.g.). Unlike the patient's entry to OD, the PACU nurse who had cared for them accompanied them back to the ward and gave a formal handover to the responsible nurse. This included three components: a bedside discussion of the material care arrangements (wound, drains, lines, infusions), a narrative account of the OD trajectory, and sign-off of the discharge checklist.

> 17:15 – We leave for the ward.
>
> We are welcomed warmly by the staff nurse who asks 'Hello is this, Megan? She's going in the cube (cubicle)'. It is necessary to first move the bed out

and then we can move the patient in. We leave the bedside to do handover, as we do so I overhear the healthcare support worker making an introduction to the patient.

PACU Nurse: This is [name]. She had a fall and sustained a closed fracture of the left femur. She's gone down to theatre and had a DHS (dynamic hip screw). She has a spinal at T4-5. I've checked the block it's at T12. She can't move her legs. She's also had a left block […] She's had a litre of fluids and is now on IV antibiotics. Otherwise, no IVs in there. She's COPD and preop her sats were eighty-eight percent. Her chest is very severe, and the anaesthetist said it was very brittle. She was quite short of breath preoperatively but if you can keep her sats above ninety-four. In theatres it was about eighty-eight to ninety-seven. She's got an oxygen mask and says at home she gets headaches and short of breath. She takes oxygen intermittently for shortness of breath […] She has shortness of breath at rest, emphysema, prolapsed bowel, osteoporosis, uses a pillow at night. She lost two hundred mils (mls blood) […] So I took out the arterial line as any gases will be odd. Stopped IV fluids and started on oral fluids: she had a hundred and fifty mils downstairs. She has a Mepore dressing which is intact […] one cannula in hand. Cardio was OK, no pain and no nausea. Oh! She's allergic to Penicillin. She has her Ventolin inhaler with her.

It is instructive to compare the PACU nurse's handover to the ward nurse with my fieldnotes on the handover received by the PACU nurse from the anaesthetist and scrub nurse on this patient's entry to PACU (Chapter 9, p. 161). These are repeated here to illustrate the nurse's sensemaking work and narrative reconstruction in the management of transition at the OD-ward interface.

Anaesthetist: This lady is [name] she's had a left DHS (dynamic hip screw hip surgery) […] She's got COPD (Chronic Obstructive Pulmonary Disease) so her chest is quite bad. She has a bronchial inhaler. So, anything more than ninety-four I am happy […] She has a Fentanyl patch which she's used to, and she also takes Tramadol.

Scrub Nurse: This is [name] she's had a left DHS. She has Mepore dressing wise, stitches on skin, blood loss two hundred mils. That's it from my side.

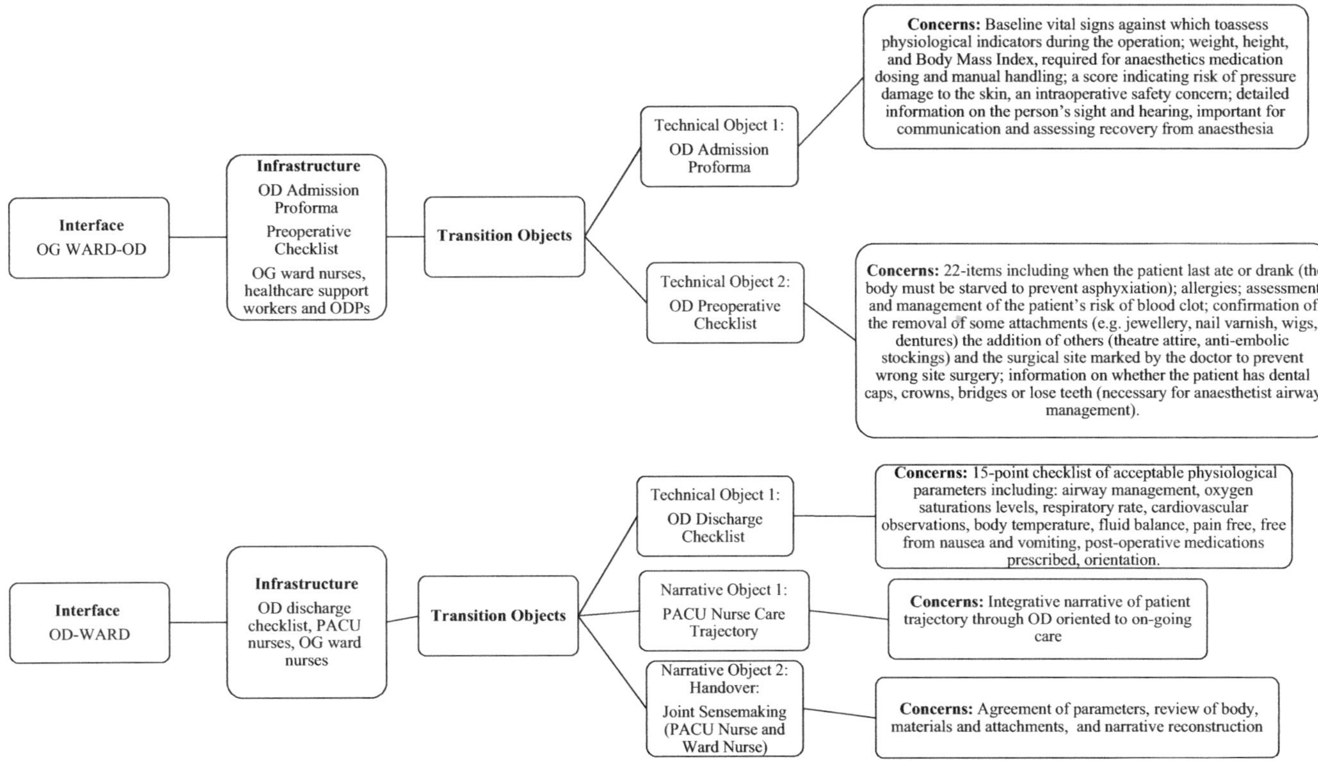

FIGURE 10.1 Transition arrangements in the acute care assemblage.

After handover, the ward nurse signed the discharge checklist to confirm transfer of responsibility. While transitions generally progressed smoothly, stories of interface management troubles and mismatched expectations circulated among PACU and ward staff.

> En route back from the ward, PACU nurse explained that the ward nurses could refuse to take a patient back if they were not happy with them and if this is the case then the PACU nurse must return to OD [...] PACU nurse said that in the past she has run into difficulties with ward staff if patients have not been prescribed the correct drugs. It was not uncommon for the trauma doctors to write in the patient's notes that they want three further doses of IV antibiotics but then do not write this on the drug chart. By the time they notice this in PACU the surgeons are back in theatre involved in another operation and cannot prescribe them. She said that if they brought patients to the ward without their drugs written up the ward nurses go mad [...] PACU nurse said that one nurse had kept her on the ward for twenty minutes and made her bleep the ward doctors to get them to come and prescribe the antibiotics. She had not managed to contact the doctors and said that she needed to go back to PACU.

These accounts serve as cautionary tales, revealing the contingencies that can destabilise even the most rational-linear of processes. The discharge checklist was intended to stabilise and transport the patient as an immutable mobile across organisational boundaries. Yet the frictions – missing prescriptions, unavailable doctors, contested responsibilities – offer a glimpse into the interpretive and collaborative practices that sustain these forms of organisation.

Summary

Transitions in the acute care assemblage involved complex processes of object formation and translation, reflecting the divergence between the collective objects of practice of the orthogeriatric ward and OD. In OD, detailed attention was directed at a narrow range of considerations focused on the patient body, and the materials, indicators, and practices associated with the surgical intervention. Matters of concern central to the objects of orthogeriatric ward practice – the circumstances of the accident, accommodation, dietary preferences, mobility, the situated tinkering arrangements to support care and comfort, social arrangements in the community, pets, carer responsibilities, falls risk – were not relevant for OD work. Trajectory mobilisation was a largely rational-linear process, accomplished through mechanisms of conscription, bracketing, and reconstruction. Formal processes enacted patients as technical transition objects, aligned with the concerns inscribed in the pre- and post-anaesthetic checklists. Centred on prescribed standards for entry into and exit from OD, they condensed the extended activities undertaken across the surgical trajectory, to constitute the patient into a transition object that was concrete, immutable and mobile. Signed by actors on either side of key interfaces, checklists were obligatory passage points, which carried the imprint of services' collective responsibility. Documents were strongly coordinative of practice but were enabled to act through the formal and informal efforts of human actors, and this agency was mediated by the wider network of professional relations and power. While effective in constituting the patient as a technical transition object of practice for OD work, it was human actors that performed the narrative reconstructions that facilitated transition back to the ward. These processes are illustrated in Figure 10.1.

References

Akrich, M. (1992). 'The de-scription of technical objects'. *Shaping Technology/Building Society: Studies in Sociotechnical Change*. W.E. Bijker and J. Law, Cambridge, MA, MIT Press: 205–224.

Allen, D. (2015). *The Invisible Work of Nurses: Hospitals, Organisation and Healthcare*. New York, Routledge.

Ellingsen, G. and E. Monteiro (2003). 'Mechanisms for producing a working knowledge: enacting, orchestrating and organizing'. *Information and Organization* **13**(3): 203–229. https://doi.org/10.1016/s1471-7727(03)00011-3

Latour, B. (1987). *Science in Action: How to Follow Scientists and Engineers through Society*. Cambridge, MA, Harvard University Press.

Latour, B. (2005). *Reassembling the Social: An Introduction to Actor-Network-Theory*. Oxford, Oxford University Press.

Law, J. and M. Callon (1992). 'The life or death or an aircraft: a network analysis of technical change'. *Shaping Technology/Building Society: Studies in Sociotechnical Change*. W.E. Bijker and J. Law. Cambridge, MA, MIT Press: 21–52.

SUMMARY OF PART 3

This part of the book examined the constitution and mobilisation of the definitive patient within the acute care assemblage, tracing the socio-material arrangements and practices that organised patients, care, and treatment within and across the orthogeriatric ward and the OD.

The two services had distinct institutional functions and collective objects of practice. Orthogeriatric work addressed a broad range of concerns spanning the pre- and postoperative trajectory, discharge planning, and the everyday specificities of care. While formal policies and artefacts were designed to initiate discharge planning at admission, in practice, the preoperative period centred on surgical preparation. Activity was distributed among ward nurses, frailty nurses, and resident doctors, incorporating both planned and responsive elements. Frailty nurses oversaw preoperative trajectory management, ensuring alignment with institutional standards, while ward nurses articulated everyday teamwork. Although some activities were formalised through documentation, many important aspects remained institutionally invisible but were nonetheless critical for trajectory progression.

OD work focused on the mobilisation of patients through preoperative, intraoperative, and post-anaesthetic care. Distributed between anaesthetists, surgeons, and the OD team, it centred on the corporeal-material relations of anaesthetic and surgical care. Embedded in formal routines, decision tools, and safety standards, care was coordinated through clearly demarcated trajectory phases. Formal artefacts mediated status passages, briefly constituted the patient as an interdisciplinary object, clarifying accountability and enabling professionals to coordinate action while remaining responsible for discrete domains of practice.

DOI: 10.4324/9781003475019-18

Transitions were organised through rational-linear mechanisms of conscription, bracketing, and reconstruction, conditioned by service alignment around shared organising logics. Formal artefacts were central actors: the Initial Treatment Regime disciplined junior doctors in enacting the patient into a trajectory object, oriented to the needs of anaesthetists and the OD team, while mandated checklists fulfilled a gatekeeping function in mediating entry into and exit from OD. Checklists functioned as obligatory passage points that bound services together and enabled reciprocal coordination of activity. They black-boxed the wide range of activities involved in preparing patients for surgery and supporting post-anaesthetic recovery, enacting patients as technical transition objects – concrete, fixed, and mobile. Signed across interfaces, checklists materialised the transition process, carrying the imprint of services' collective responsibility.

Documents were enabled to fulfil their functions by human actors. Frailty nurses monitored the work of resident doctors in preparing patients for OD, while informal work by OD healthcare support workers was essential for detecting failures of object formation at the ward level. Although checklists enabled mobilisation, their technical qualities were poorly aligned with the narrative-based collective objects of practice in orthogeriatric care. The care trajectory narratives generated by PACU nurses were essential for facilitating transition back to the ward, yet remained institutionally invisible and largely taken for granted.

Part 3 has illuminated the distinct yet interdependent social worlds of the orthogeriatric ward and the operating department, showing how patients were enacted and mobilised across services for the purposes of surgery. In Part 4, the focus shifts to the post operative period and the organisation of recovery and discharge.

PART 4

The Distributed Patient

The Recovery Care Assemblage

INTRODUCTION TO PART 4

Part 4 explores the *recovery assemblage*, tracing the socio-material relations that shape the hip fracture trajectory during the immediate postoperative period, the organisation of hospital discharge, and continuation of care in the community. The assemblage expands, and the patient is *distributed* – no longer confined to a single institutional locale but enacted across a dispersed ecology of professional and organisational boundaries, social relations, domestic spaces, and fragile care arrangements. At this point in the trajectory, the multiplicity of the patient is at its most pronounced (Mol, 2002).

Hospital discharge marks a critical status passage, yet recovery trajectories are uncertain, and post-discharge arrangements vary widely. Some patients returned home with short-term support from family or community rehabilitation services; others required long-term social care to live independently. For those whose needs exceeded what could be managed at home, discharge involved transfer to residential or nursing care facilities – either returning to a previous care setting or entering a new one. For some, discharge marked a new phase of recovery and the gradual resumption of everyday life; for others, it signalled increased dependency, biographical disruption (Bury, 1982) and rebuilding (Siegel and Krauss, 1991) and the reconfiguration of daily support.

Community health and social care in Wales is complex and fragmented, comprising multiple providers with distinct responsibilities. Services are commissioned by health boards and local authorities and span primary care, rehabilitation, interventions to prevent hospital admission, long-term care, day hospitals, and the residential and nursing home sector. Healthcare is publicly funded and free at the point of need; social care is means-tested. Most primary care practices in Wales operate as independent GP partnerships contracted by

DOI: 10.4324/9781003475019-20

health boards. Community nursing teams deliver geographically organised, home-based care, while local authorities are responsible for commissioning and delivering social care services. Local authorities also manage the interface with the care home sector, which includes residential, nursing, and specialist services provided by both public and private organisations.

Regional Partnership Boards offer a mechanism for pooling resources across health and social care by supporting jointly funded services. One such example – the intermediate Community Resource Team (CRT) – played a central role in supporting home discharge for hip fracture patients in the study site. However, like the rest of the UK, community services in Wales face mounting pressure from workforce shortages, funding constraints, and growing demand linked to an ageing population. Delays to hospital discharge are common, disproportionately affect vulnerable populations, exacerbating health inequalities.

While discharge arrangements in the hip fracture population were diverse, this analysis focuses on patients discharged home with short-term support from CRT. This choice was pragmatic: while I have aimed to reflect the diversity of discharge planning in the analysis, it was not feasible to follow every possible discharge trajectory in detail. Home discharge poses distinctive challenges from the standpoint of transition. In contrast to discharge into residential care – where patients move into pre-configured institutional settings – home discharge involves the organisation and assembly of caring infrastructures (Skovgaard et al. 2022). Studying these processes sheds light on the often-overlooked difficulties of transition at the hospital-community interface.

*

The analysis in this part of the book draws on ethnographic observation in acute and community settings, artefacts and documents, and staff interviews. On the orthogeriatric ward, I shadowed resident doctors, physiotherapists and their assistants, occupational therapists, the ward pharmacist, ward nurses, frailty nurses, and consultant orthogeriatricians. I observed ward rounds, nursing handovers, board rounds, discharge planning, and multidisciplinary team meetings. I also attended departmental meetings in physiotherapy and occupational therapy and shadowed the trauma and orthopaedic bed manager.

In the community, I observed the work of CRT over three full days, including home visits with therapists and pre-discharge screening by nurses. I attended two discharge visits – held on the afternoon the patient left the hospital – and interviewed health and social care leaders. I also observed referral meetings and multidisciplinary team discussions. This material was supplemented by 25 hours of fieldwork with a community nursing team; a day with digital hub call handlers who managed, among other tasks, referrals to district nursing; seven hours of shadowing St John Ambulance crews transporting patients home;

and observation of the hospital discharge lounge. I attempted, unsuccessfully, to gain access to a primary care centre, although I was able to interview a practising academic GP. Despite persistent efforts, I was also unable to negotiate access to shadow social carers. The bureaucracy involved was reminiscent of Dicken's Circumlocution Office in *Little Dorrit*, and I ran out of time.

This section begins with Chapter 10, which explores the complexity of recovery trajectories and how patients were enacted in the postoperative period on the orthogeriatric ward. Chapter 11 focuses on the work of the CRT, which provided intermediate, home-based support following discharge. Chapter 12 analyses the relationship between acute and community services and the organisation of transition.

References

Bury, M. (1982). 'Chronic illness as biographical disruption'. *Sociology of Health & Illness* **4**(2): 167–182.

Mol, A.M. (2002). *The Body Multiple: Ontology in Medical Practice*. Durham, NC., Duke University Press.

Siegel, K. and B.J. Krauss (1991). 'Living with HIV infection: adaptive tasks of seropositive gay men'. *Journal of Health and Social Behavior* **32**: 17–32.

Skovgaard, A.L., M.J. Jørgensen, T. Tjørnhøj-Thomsen, and M.T. Høybye (2022). 'Discharge readiness as an infrastructure: negotiating the transfer of care for elderly patients in medical wards'. *Social Science & Medicine* **312**: 115388.

11

RECOVERY AND DISCHARGE PLANNING

Postoperative Orthogeriatric Work

This chapter examines the organisation of patients, care, and treatment in the postoperative phase of orthogeriatric care. Unlike the narrow framing of the patient for surgery, the recovery assemblage was oriented to a much wider range of concerns. The team expanded beyond medicine and nursing to include physiotherapy, occupational therapy, and pharmacy, with patients and families becoming more prominent actors (see also Bishop and Waring, 2019). Professions worked largely asynchronously, each engaging with distinct objects of practice. Consequently, understandings of the patient were distributed across time, space, and disciplines.

This chapter first outlines the ecology of practice that conditioned postoperative orthogeriatric care. It then examines the multiple versions of the patient enacted in the mobilisation of care following surgery and the socio-material arrangements that enabled concerted action for discharge planning.

The Social World of Postoperative Orthogeriatric Care

This section explores the structures, organising logics, interpretative repertoires, and materials that conditioned care following hip fracture surgery. Unlike the time-critical coordination of the acute care assemblage, postoperative care unfolded more slowly across a wider array of actors, roles, and concerns. Work was shaped not only by clinical imperatives but institutional demands for discharge, and the realities of ageing, frailty, and uncertain futures.

DOI: 10.4324/9781003475019-21

Structures

The Orthogeriatric Ward

Postoperative orthogeriatric work is centred on recovery, rehabilitation, fracture risk management, and discharge planning. Recovery following hip fracture is variable and uncertain. NHS guidance suggests hospital stays from between one to four weeks, with full recovery extending over 12 months. Memory problems and frailty – common in this patient population and often contributory factors in the original injury – also affect rehabilitation. Many patients never regain their preadmission independence, which has significant implications for discharge planning.

Frailty Nurse: 'Few realise what a devastating injury hip fracture is. Ten percent die in a month, thirty percent in a year, sixty percent within five years, and seventy-five percent do not return to their pre accident state'.

Senior Nurse: 'Relatives think that because a patient was managing at home before they came into hospital, they will be able to manage when they get home [...] It's hard to get them to understand that they might not be as good as they were before'.

The Jenolan orthogeriatric team was highly skilled in managing these complexities. The Trauma and Orthopaedics (T&O) Bed Manager went to some lengths to secure a bed for hip fracture patients on the ward.

> We always say, it's important to have the right patient in the right bed at the right time [...] From the beginning [...] because we know how to deal with them, and we know how to deal with the elderly. And especially those that have got some degree of cognitive impairment [...] persuading them to get up and mobilise [...] And I think, if they're on the outlying, non-trauma wards, they've got their own patients, their own group of patients to look after, um, I think, perhaps they don't look after the trauma patients quite as well.
>
> *(Senior Nurse – Interview)*

The Postoperative Orthogeriatric Team

A wide range of actors were enrolled in the postoperative trajectory. Alongside medical and nursing teams (see Chapter 8), patients typically received care from a pharmacist, physiotherapist, and occupational therapist. A consultant orthogeriatrician led medical management, supported by resident doctors.

Orthopaedic surgeons were minimally involved beyond a weekly ward round, which focused on the surgery. Ward nurses provided ongoing care and coordinated daily activity; frailty nurses led discharge planning.

Jenolan had a designated pharmacist, a non-medical prescriber (a term used to refer to a healthcare professional, who is not a doctor or a dentist, who has undergone training to enable them to prescribe medication) with an extended role in osteoporosis management. A ward-based occupational therapist supported all hip fracture patients discharged home, focusing on supporting safe discharge and linking with agencies to organise appliances and adaptations. Physiotherapy was provided through a peripatetic hospital physiotherapy team. Physiotherapists typically worked with an assistant to support patients in mobilising following surgery.

Families and relatives were also central actors. Often already enlisted in ongoing care, they offered insights into the person's life before the injury and were able to appraise the viability of discharge plans, which could be contingent on their support.

Organising Logics

Ward activity was driven by mobilisation and clinical logics, which were sometimes in tension. Timely discharge was an organisational priority because of acute bed pressures. This was reflected in the mantra that discharge began on admission and in the organisation's investments in key roles, such as the frailty nurses and the T&O Bed Manager, who monitored bed capacity to ensure availability for ED admissions. Patients regarded as medically fit but unable to leave the hospital owing to downstream challenges were categorised as DToC (delayed transfer of care) cases. Frailty nurses and the bed manager worked closely to identify and resolve 'blockages'. DToC patients were 'matter out of place' (Douglas, 1966) and such was the emphasis on their management that I initially misheard the term as DETOX! The pressure to manage patient flows permeated ward activity, but was not always welcome by staff.

Senior Nurse: Before you go. Can I say, we went to Big Room which is where all the senior managers go and the reason we went was because of the progress we have made in managing our complex discharges, so a big thank you to everyone. We have a lot of patient throughput and this will continue; we are concerned with patient care, but that coincides with people getting the right treatment in the right place.

Nobody really responded to this. Staff nurse listened and then drifted off to get on with handover. I know from my conversations with people that there are mixed feelings about this.

Despite bed pressures and the institutional emphasis on patient flow, the team prioritised patient outcomes. Clinical activity was oriented to national evidence-based rehabilitation standards (NICE, 2011), which included a physiotherapist assessment and mobilisation on the day after surgery, early supported discharge, and consideration of bone health and falls prevention. Frailty nurses audited performance and submitted data to the National Hip Fracture Database. Beyond these external standards, there was a strong commitment to individualised patient care and promoting safe levels of independence through the 'least restrictive discharge option'.

> Social worker said that although they (the orthogeriatric team) were concerned with flows, they did not simply push people home who were not ready for it. 'Consultant Orthogeriatrician, when I started, said that he did not want a conveyor belt. We don't want to just churn people out'.
>
> 'Is this the right environment (in-patient hospital ward) to be telling people they can't go home and live on their own, in their own home?'
>
> *(Orthogeriatrician – Interview)*

This ethos was reflected in the use of the language of 'programme' rather than 'pathway' to describe the specialist frailty nursing role, a decision intended to underline the complexity of trajectory management over the linearity implied by the term pathway.

> I asked why they had not used the language of pathway. Orthogeriatrician said that a 'pathway' was a proforma 'one of these' (points to proforma in the notes) and it implies a single process whereas a programme is more tailored to the individual patients.
>
> Senior Nurse contrasted her previous work on elective pathways with the current role: 'Here we have none of the advantages of elective surgery, we have the apple cart that's been thrown up in the air and we have to try and put things back together again. It's frustrating but that's why it is so wonderful. Here this is about helping the patients, not length of stay, and doing all we can to ensure a safe discharge.

This clinical logic operated as a powerful countervailing mechanism in the context of wider organisational pressures to discharge or transfer patients.

Interpretative Repertoires

In the post operative period, the use of formal artefacts was limited to a Functional Assessment Tool deployed by occupational therapists for discharge planning and an Osteoporosis Screening Tool used by the pharmacist.

The Functional Assessment Tool – a double-sided A4 document – mediated the fine-grained assessment and documentation of the relationship between the person, their functional capacity, and home context. The Osteoporosis Screening Tool was designed to assess osteoporosis risk factors and identify candidates for bone-strengthening medication. It had a checklist-based format and drew on established tools like FRAX (https://frax.shef.ac.uk/FRAX/reference.aspx), but also incorporated site-specific concerns, reflecting its dual role in risk assessment and treatment planning.

Materials

The Patient Record

The 'medical' notes and nursing record were the only ward-based documents of patient care (see Chapter 8, p. 127). The pharmacist, occupational therapist, and physiotherapists contributed to the medical record but maintained separate formal records for clinical practice and professional accountability purposes, which were retained by their respective departments. Community health and social care services maintained distinct digital systems, which were inaccessible to acute sector staff, despite their relevance for discharge planning.

Coordinating Technologies

The team utilised a range of digital technologies to monitor recovery, including access to medical images and laboratory results. The clinical workstation also played a central role in this phase. In addition to the high-level information on patient trajectories used by nurses to organise their work (see Chapter 8), it included assessments of 'medical fitness' and a predicted discharge date. This data was monitored remotely by bed managers who intervened to expedite discharges, escalate DToC cases, and release bed capacity. To allow people the necessary time to recover and avoid management scrutiny, the team carefully curated this information. The first of the following extracts refers to how the definition of 'medical fitness', an organisational designation that indicated that an individual was ready for discharge, was stretched to legitimise continued hospital admission. The second extract illustrates how the team modified the predicted discharge date to give the patient more time to optimise their potential.

> Senior nurse explained that on the ward they operated with a broad definition of 'medical fitness' which extended beyond their physical well-being and included whether wider assessments had been completed.

Senior Nurse:	Rosemary Jones is not going to be today. Set it (predicted discharge date) for another week [...] Sarah Driver needs physio, but we need to go gently as this was the lady who arrested in theatre... keep the fifth. It might even be longer than that; she needs time to mobilise.

A patient status at a glance whiteboard (PSAGWB) was used to maintain oversight of patient trajectories, especially for discharge planning. PSAGWB are underpinned by the principles of visual management (Grief, 1991) and the idea that making issues visible provides a shared picture of operations and supports team decision-making. Each patient had a designated cell divided into two sections. The right-hand side contained clinical information: predicted discharge date, length of stay, medically fit for discharge status, observation frequency, NEWS Score if applicable, and specific care needs. The left-hand side focused on matters of concern for care coordination and discharge planning: 'Actions Outstanding' (e.g. dates of referrals to services), Social Worker (allocation, assessment, placement), tablets to take home (TTH), physiotherapy and occupational therapy referrals and equipment needs, Community Rehabilitation Team (CRT) referrals and screenings, and repatriation details (hospital, accepting consultant, and date).

All team members were required to update the PSAGWB in line with their respective activity, but practice was uneven, and this responsibility fell disproportionately to the frailty nurses.

Frailty Nurse:	You need to write the referral down in the box.
Physiotherapist:	Can I write in the other boxes? I only write in my box!
Frailty Nurse:	If you don't write when you have made a referral how do I know and not go and repeat it?

PSAGWB information was not digital and could not be accessed remotely by community or social services providers.

Postoperative Orthogeriatric Work

Nursing and medical care were continuous, whereas other team members worked weekdays, 8 am–4 pm. The physiotherapist and/or their assistant saw patients daily for mobilisation, the occupational therapist engaged intermittently with patients returning home, and the pharmacist visited three times weekly. Unlike the synchronous, spatially bounded work of the operating theatre, postoperative care was distributed across time and professions. Individual professions worked largely independently and operated with a different version of the patient, reflecting their specific work purposes.

Assessing recovery trajectories and discharge planning required the patient to be enacted as an interdisciplinary object of practice. Formal and informal coordination mechanisms were in place to support concerted action. Ward nurses articulated the daily network work of actors and activities around their patients, interleaving trajectory management with ongoing care (see Chapter 6, p. 95). Frailty nurses reflexively monitored recovery trajectories for discharge planning and liaised with the team. There was a weekly orthogeriatric ward round and multidisciplinary team meeting, and a three-times-a-week board round led by the frailty nurse, which focused on discharge planning. Dedicated discharge planning meetings were convened for complex cases.

Making Patients and Mobilising Care

Previous chapters have traced how, following a fall, an individual's undifferentiated troubles were translated into the objects of practice of Emergency Medical Services, and – through a progressive narrowing of focus – culminated in a definitive hip fracture diagnosis and the enactment of the patient in alignment with operating department safety standards to enable surgery. By contrast, the postoperative phase focused on a much broader range of concerns, oriented to the singular and non-standard needs of patients and their families. Issues prefigured at admission but bracketed off during the preoperative period, now moved centre stage. The understanding of the patient that emerged extended beyond the requirements of surgery and nursing care to include consideration of individual identity and the life world (Schutz, 1972). As Latimer (1997) observes, future persons are enacted according to a past, and a central concern in planning rehabilitation and discharge from the hospital was establishing the person's previous level of functioning. Details of the patient's mobility, independence, and cognitive capacity – documented in the medical clerking (Chapter 8, p. 130) – were important points of reference for assessing the recovery trajectory and determining a discharge destination.

This section describes how patients were enacted, and care was organised, through the differentiated work practices of the orthogeriatric multidisciplinary team. It examines the distinct constellations of concern shaping professional work and the coordinating mechanisms that enabled agreement on a discharge plan.

Object Formation in Medical Practice

Postoperatively, resident doctors worked at the interface between Orthogeriatric and T&O services. They addressed emerging issues, initiated tests, attended ward rounds, and engaged in ongoing sensemaking to enact the patient as an object of practice for continuous medical care.

Object formation was largely desk-based – reviewing test results, clinical documentation, and other data to construct an understanding of the evolving patient trajectory. This typically preceded and informed an in-person review of the patient. Undertaken alongside other work, sensemaking was often protracted and disjointed. The following field, illustrates these processes, extending over four hours as the doctor managed multiple demands.

> Her first job is to 'read about this new lady and update my list' […]. She begins with the Clerking Template and reads from the section on the presenting complaint. She then moves onto the social history section where an entry reads: 'Daughter lives locally, some issues with alcohol dependency'. It is unclear whether 'alcohol dependency' refers to the patient or the daughter. Doctor points out that the 'mini mental' (cognitive assessment test) has not been completed, but over the page the patient has drawn a clock correctly […] She continues to read through the medical notes, following the continuation sheets chronologically. 'This lady has had a tough post-operative recovery' (this refers to couple of entries in the notes from the critical care outreach team). Her HB (haemoglobin) was sixty-four. She must have lost a lot of blood. I am going to read the operation notes'. Doctor locates the pink printed operation document in the patient record but there is nothing about blood loss. […] She continues to skim through the notes and observes: 'They gave her more blood and her obs (vital signs observations) seemed to settle after that. Looks like she got pneumonia – they started her on IV antibiotics'. She reads on, 'Seems like her heart struggles, might be overloaded, plus, plus what does that say? Seems like she's been alright over the weekend, no crises. I am going to make a few notes and then look up her details on the computer'.
>
> The doctor locates a fresh continuation sheet and uses this to make a summary of the case. It is presented in a standard medical clerking format commencing with age, admission date and presenting condition. […] She makes an initial entry and then looks back to the operation notes asking: 'What did they do to the humerus?' She then flicks forward and locates a summary entry from an orthogeriatric doctor in the continuation sheets and appears to be extracting the past medical history from here.
>
> She goes over to the computer and assesses the patient's details on the clinical portal. She skims through letters from secondary to primary care – there are 16 in total. One is a letter from a cardiologist to the primary care doctor. Doctor: 'Ok, she's an ex-smoker' (this information was not in the current medical notes, or at least she did not locate it there when she was reading through). 'She's got quite bad angina too. They're giving her a spray and oral trinitrate as well. I am not surprised she has a degree of heart failure.'

She finds another letter, which refers to a discussion having taken place with the patient about her daughter's alcohol dependency and mental health issues. This helps to clarify the ambiguous entry in the hip fracture clerking proforma. There is also a letter from the Trauma and Orthopaedics Service concerning an earlier fracture. Doctor expresses surprise that she is not in receipt of preventative treatment for osteoporosis.

[...]

Doctor then has a look at the patient information on the clinical workstation, observing that sometimes things are included here which are not put in the medical notes.

At this point we are interrupted by the need to attend a Trauma and Orthopaedics team ward round.

[...]

Following the ward round she returns to the review of the patient she says: 'They (trauma and orthopaedics team) are expecting to send her home. Do they know all this I wonder? They can't send her home; it is completely inappropriate. Let's look at her home situation'. She turns to the section on the hip fracture Clerking Template – 'So she lives in a house, well this will be a problem'. She writes this onto her sheet. Doctor: 'She does her own shopping and mobilises with a frame and a wheelchair. [...] So those blood gases are normal for her. People have been doing blood gases as they are worried about her lungs, but that gas is probably normal'.

We are interrupted again by the need to attend another ward round, re-write some medication charts, and go to the Trauma and Orthopaedic Clinic to take blood. Having started the patient review at 0730, it is after 11 am before the doctor has an opportunity to attend to the patient in person.

Doctor: I hear you had nasty fall at home.
Patient: Not at home. I had gone round to a neighbour.

The patient then talked in detail about the purpose of the visit to the neighbour, the mechanism of the entrance doors and how they came to knock into her. She was then evidently on the floor for some time, and because of the position she was in, the ambulance crew could not get her up. There then followed discussion of the difficult postoperative recovery but how markedly improved she now is.

Doctor asks about her home arrangements, and the patient informs her that she lives alone in a downstairs flat (this is contrary to the information on the hip fracture clerking proforma which states that she lives in a house).

Doctor:	And your daughter lives nearby?
Patient:	Yes, she does but she is totally dependent on me.
Doctor:	She's totally dependent on *you*!!!
Patient:	Yes, she has mental health problems. She's agoraphobic and has not left the house for eight years, a total recluse.
Doctor:	It sounds as if you have a lot to deal with.
Patient:	It's too much now. I knew that when I had a fall last year but that was nothing compared to this. It is awful because she has nobody, but I definitely can't do it. She must accept help and that's what my grandson is doing now.
Doctor:	Who does the shopping?
Patient:	Me. I go out every day.
Doctor:	How much help do you have?
Patient:	I have lots of friends, and I can get on the phone or text people.

Doctor asks whether there are any adaptations in the house. The patient says she has handrails, toilet rails and a perching stool which had been provided for her late husband and which she has retained since his death. She says the only issue is the bathroom which requires a step up which is 'a bit scary'.

The discussion moves on to her medical problems and it emerges that the patient has been smoking up until this admission – albeit secretly. The doctor refers to her underactive thyroid and the patient asks: 'Is it underactive? I thought it was over!'

Doctor:	It says underactive here.

The conversation shifts to the patient's previous fracture, and the circumstances surrounding this. As she is talking the doctor is making an entry in the notes and reviewing the observations charts.

Doctor then asks to 'take a little look' at the patient and having closed the bedside curtains, listens to her chest, heart, and examines her ankles. She notes that the patient has an indwelling urinary catheter and says she will get that removed as 'it is one less thing to worry about'.

Doctor also removes the dressing – with the patient protesting that she does not want to see the wound as she is frightened to look. After some soothing words of reassurance, she is persuaded to let the dressing be removed.

In this fieldwork episode, the doctor deployed diverse information to construct the patient's trajectory. Some sensemaking practices were systematic – starting with the hip fracture Clerking Template (see Chapter 8, p. 126), she carefully consulted various sources, knowing that pertinent information was distributed across different systems and documents. Some aspects of her searches were driven by her emerging understanding of the case; for example, she sought out the operation notes to ascertain whether the patient's low HB could be caused by surgical blood loss. Records were sometimes ambiguous (e.g. it was unclear whether the reference to alcohol dependency related to the patient or her daughter) or key information was missing (e.g. the results of the 'mini mental'), or the written record differed from the patient's account (e.g. details of the accommodation). Through a process of cross-referencing between different human and non-human data sources and iterative recontextualisation, the doctor made sense of individual evidentiary fragments and the overall patient trajectory.

This example illustrates how at this stage of the hip fracture trajectory object formation in orthogeriatric doctors' work extended beyond biomedical concerns to include social context and future prospects. Clinical matters intersect with trajectory management and discharge planning in the doctor's practices. The patient was understood not only in terms of physiological recovery, but also their capacity to resume everyday life. The doctor questions a discharge decision taken during the ward round, noting that it overlooked the patient's home situation. This moment reveals the tension between the clinical logics of the orthogeriatric and T&O specialities outlined in Chapter 8. While the latter focused on the surgical event and the healing of the fractured bone, the former embraced a more holistic understanding of the patient, integrating social, functional, and cognitive factors.

Doctors documented assessments in comprehensive free-text summaries in the medical record, capturing the history, current plans, and future goals. These narratives stabilised the evolving trajectory and served as intra-professional reference points. Unlike nurses, doctors did not have a formal medical handover for all patients. These summaries enabled clinicians to articulate their reasoning and provided others with an accessible and up-to-date account of the case, sparing them from having to undertake their own extended sensemaking processes.

Registrar: 'It is a way of summarising the current state of affairs, identifying any issues – one, two, three – and then the plan and aims. I have a poor memory so it's useful to have the plans in context, which is important in four years if there is litigation. Also, it's good to see, so when you go to the notes you know that this doctor knows what they are doing. It's also a good idea to know what the plan is so if I am on call then I make sure that I work with the plan rather than making a different decision'.

Object Formation in Pharmacological Practice

The ward pharmacist's role focused on medication management and correcting any prescribing or dose discrepancies. On Jenolan, this centred on two primary concerns: reviewing preadmission medications to mitigate falls risk and assessing the clinical history for undiagnosed osteoporosis. Polypharmacy – the simultaneous use of multiple medications – is associated with a higher falls risk in older adults and is becoming more common due to the increasing prevalence of comorbidities and long-term conditions. Osteoporosis is the leading cause of hip fractures. Since formal screening is costly, bone-strengthening medication was prescribed when the clinical picture was strongly suggestive of the condition.

As with resident doctors, object formation began as a desk-based activity and was followed by an in-person consultation. The pharmacist used a structured A5 proforma to support their work. The first side recorded basic personal details, reason for admission, medical history, and a comprehensive 'medication history' (allergies, adverse drug reactions, prescribed medications, and changes during admission). The second side contained the Osteoporosis Screening Tool – a checklist of risk factors including fragility fractures, family history, renal function, milk intake, smoking, alcohol, early menopause, hysterectomy, endocrine disorder, height, weight, Body Mass Index, oral steroids (more than three months), previous treatments, medication compliance problems, or possible contraindications. A small section captured the prescribed treatment and comments.

Object formation typically began with reviewing the hip fracture Clerking Template, followed by consultation of other information sources to build a comprehensive understanding of the patient.

> He begins by looking at the patient record and goes straight to the Clerking Template.
>
> [...]
>
> *Pharmacist (reading):* 'Fell somewhere between ten pm and eight am – well that's a bit vague. OK, advanced dementia, wandering for some time. That might explain why its vague'.
>
> He shifts his attention to the social history section and establishes that the patient was admitted from home which, according to the record, she shares with someone else.
>
> No information has been entered in the medication section on the hip fracture Clerking Template other than an indication that there are no allergies. Pharmacist said it was not clear whether this meant she was not on

> medications before her admission or whether the information has been omitted. [...] There is a reference in the clerking document that the patient was accompanied by her daughter to the ED and the pharmacist questions why the daughter was not asked about her medications. Pharmacist said he could call the GP or try and find out the medication history from the family. He then flicks to the EMS PCR (emergency medical services patient care record).
>
> *Pharmacist:* 'I often look at the ambulance chart. They were at the scene. Sometimes people have a list of their medications on the fridge and the paramedics are trained to look out for that sort of thing. Look they have written here that she has hypertension and is on Bendrofluazide (a diuretic which increases urine production) and also antibiotics'.
>
> *Pharmacist:* 'I use all the information available to me. I've had a look at the bloods, and she seems a bit dry. I wonder why she is on antibiotics'.

Sensemaking was iterative. When the patient's preadmission medication history was missing from the Clerking Template, the pharmacist consulted the ambulance EMS PCR – a favoured resource. In this instance, it yields useful information, but the pharmacist noted that the patient's primary care doctor and family could also be contacted if necessary. Mediated through the distinctive prism of medication management, the pharmacist pieced together evidential fragments to form a provisional understanding of the patient. For example, having noted the prescription for diuretics, the pharmacist seeks out blood test results, which indicate the patient is 'a bit dry'. Dehydration is a potential side-effect of diuretic use, and because it can cause light-headedness, dizziness, and fainting, it is a medication of interest in the context of a clinical history of hip fracture. In the next extract, the pharmacist has established a history of previous fractures and is concerned that certain medications, which he infers are prescribed for chronic pain, may be contraindicated from a falls prevention perspective.

> The lady in question has previously fractured her shoulder and her wrist. Pharmacist said that this should have triggered an osteoporosis screening referral, but it has not [...] He is also concerned to review her regular medications to see whether any are suboptimal from the perspective of falls prevention. He identifies two problematic medications: Amitriptyline which he explains can cause postural drop (blood pressure drops suddenly on standing), dry mouth, blurred vision, and constipation, and another drug – I didn't catch the name – which is a pain killer. Pharmacist says that these two drugs in combination point to chronic pain.

> [...]
>
> What was fascinating was how the pharmacist was able to make sense of and assemble a picture of the patient based on the medication profile. When I shared these observations with him, he was clear that these were simply inferences but that they would be used to shape the questions he asked the patient.

After assembling a provisional object of practice through desk-based sense-making, the pharmacist met the patient in person. This was an opportunity to elicit further information, explore working hypotheses about medication needs, and agree on a plan. In the following extract – continuing from the previous case – he begins by discussing the patient's pain and recommends stopping Amitriptyline as it increases fall risk. He also explains his plan to commence bone-strengthening medication.

> We go to the patient. She is deaf and the conversation is mediated through an interpreter [...] Pharmacist begins a line of questioning designed to establish whether the patient has a history of chronic pain. However, she speaks mostly about the events leading up to the fall. Pharmacist tries another strategy; having removed the box of Amitriptyline from the bedside locker and presented the patient with the box, he asks what she takes these for. The patient is uncertain and states that her doctor had prescribed them. Pharmacist explains that he would like to stop them because they are more likely to make her fall. The patient says that she sometimes feels as if the room is spinning. Pharmacist returns to the question of pain and this time the patient refers to pains in her back. Showing her the other box of medications – the pain killers – he says, 'We will keep these as they help with the nerve pain but stop these. I'd like to stop you from falling and breaking anything else'. The patient then says she thinks she might need a walking stick and pharmacist says that the physiotherapists will work with her on that.
>
> [...]
>
> The pharmacist asks whether the patient likes milk (she does) and how much she drinks typically. The patient says she has it in tea, but otherwise she drinks water as she often has a dry mouth. Pharmacist explains that milk contains calcium which is good for her bones. He also tells her that the Amitriptyline will make her mouth feel dry.
>
> Pharmacist shows the patient another container of medications and says: 'We would like to give you these – they are calcium and vitamin D for your

bones. Just one a day. We'll ask your GP to give them to you when you go home'. He then goes on to explain that, 'We also want to give you a bone strengthening treatment in a couple of weeks [...] It makes the bones stronger and halves the risk of a fracture if you fall. You've already had a broken wrist and a broken shoulder, so you probably have osteoporosis, and your bones aren't so strong'. The patient says, 'It is just old age. I'm not worried I have had a good life'.

A few further questions follow about steroids, alcohol, and bowel issues. According to the pharmacy proforma, the patient has a long history of diarrhoea but when he questions the patient on this point, she describes constipation followed by loose stools.

[...]

Back at the Nurses' Station the pharmacist asks the senior nurse about the patient's history of diarrhoea, retelling the patient's account.

Pharmacist: While she's here we can sort out a few things with her meds (medication) that might be causing constipation. She's got back pain – or at least that's my interpretation of it – and why she's taking [name of medication]. She didn't know why she was on it – that's me putting two and two together.

What emerged from this process was an understanding of the patient refracted through a pharmaceutical lens. In assessing her fall risk, it was the patient's medications that were foregrounded as matters of concern, not her mobility, the layout of her home, or any other factors that may have been implicated in the original injury. While focused on bone health and fall prevention, the admission allowed for a broader medication review. In this case, the pharmacist proposes to reassess prescribed painkillers, which may be causing constipation. As a non-medical prescriber, the pharmacist was able to independently adjust medications; however, he also attended the weekly medical ward round, where medication management was a focal concern.

Many healthcare professionals deployed secondary documents for object formation, but the pharmacist was relatively unusual in keeping meticulous details on data sources. The proforma included a tick box section listing the range of sources pharmacists used to enact patients for their work: patient, relative/carer, patient's old notes, GP letter/fax, GP repeat list, GP surgery, nursing/residential home administrative record, community pharmacy, and other.

Object Formation in Physiotherapy Practice

Physiotherapy object formation focused on a narrow set of concerns. To support postoperative mobilisation, physiotherapists needed two key pieces of information: surgical details (especially weight-bearing status) and the patient's preadmission functional and cognitive status. This information – readily available in the OD PCR and hip fracture Clerking Template – enabled immediate treatment without extensive sensemaking.

> I asked what information the physiotherapists needed to do their job. Physiotherapist: 'It's very simple, it's the post op guidelines, the pink form in the medical notes that tell you what they've had and what they need. Most important is their weight bearing status; then we're off. That's all we need. Then there's the hip fracture proforma and what you find out about what's happened and the history. You make a judgement. For example, [name] and [name], if I had reviewed them then before their operation and they were both doing their shopping so I would aim to stand them with a frame the day after theatre, but I would not do that with the Parkinson's guy. He said that the other important information was the clock face exercise (an assessment of cognitive functioning).

Physiotherapy care was recorded in the ward-based medical notes and a separate 'physiotherapy treatment card', used hospital-wide. The structured front page captured personal data, intervention type, equipment, outcomes, and discharge tasks (e.g. referral letters). The remaining pages were for free-text entries.

The Chartered Society of Physiotherapy, the professional body and trade union for physiotherapy in the UK, mandates a patient 'database' as standard professional documentation. Colloquially known as 'carding', this task could only be undertaken by physiotherapists or physiotherapy assistants with the relevant qualifications. The format was not formally prescribed, but the examples I observed mirrored the medical clerking, focusing on concerns such as complaint, history of complaint, past medical history, medications, social history, assessment, and intervention.

In hip fracture care, however, this database was largely performative – serving as a professional artefact that accounted for physiotherapy practice, rather than informing immediate care. The process primarily involved transcribing information from other records, often after the patient had already been seen. Although an institutional requirement, it was experienced by staff as time-consuming and of limited practical utility.

> Later in the morning I observed the technician meticulously copying the typed ward round entry. She was tracing her finger under each word and appeared to be copying it verbatim.

> The physio 'carding' is done after the patient has been seen, but the form the entry takes, mirroring the format of a medical clerking, gives the impression of a prior assessment and then subsequent treatment. This does not happen in practice. They tend to eyeball the notes, particularly the pink operation sheet, find out about the patient's cognitive ability, often from talking to the nurse, get the patient out of bed and help them to mobilise and then write the cards up afterwards. As far as I could see the technician did much of this paperwork, with the physio then being asked to sign off the entries.

The physiotherapist saw patients daily after surgery. Outside these sessions, nurses sustained rehabilitation, with activity woven into the routines of ongoing care. In the context of staff shortages, physiotherapists withdrew active input once a patient was deemed to have reached their rehabilitation potential – sometimes resulting in no further physiotherapy before discharge.

Object Formation in Occupational Therapy Practice

The occupational therapist was responsible for organising the material infrastructure needed for patients to manage safely at home after discharge. As such, their professional objects of practice were inherently future-oriented, centred on the intricate interplay between the patient, the affordances and constraints of the home environment, and interventions required for daily living. While nursing and medical staff documented social circumstances and living arrangements during admission, and physiotherapists addressed general mobility, occupational therapy involved a more granular and relational understanding of these concerns and their practical implications.

> *Occupational Therapist:* The nurses do a brief summary – in there it just says she lives at home and has a stick. What we do is more detailed.

> Occupational Therapist said that [...] the physio had a narrow technical approach to care compared to the holistic approach they worked with.

Rather than treating home circumstances as background, occupational therapy involved understanding how the patient's everyday life – domestic routines, environmental constraints, and available support – might interact with their current and projected capabilities. This involved translating general indicators into situated questions of feasibility: Can the person manage stairs? Prepare a meal? Access the bathroom? In this way, occupational therapy moved beyond preliminary estimation, producing a more detailed and practical basis for assessing discharge options.

Object formation in occupational therapy followed a three-part process: an admission interview, a home environment assessment, and a ward-based assessment before discharge. These concerns were documented in an Occupational Therapy Treatment Card, a structured A4 proforma used to inform and account for professional practice. The front page captured basic personal and medical information, which was extracted from existing documentation, in a 'carding' process, which, like physiotherapy, was regarded as laborious. The reverse side contained a standardised discharge plan covering key activities to support functional independence in the home: bed transfer, chair transfer, toilet transfer, domestic activities of daily living (i.e. meal preparation), and physical activities of daily living (i.e. washing, dressing, and personal care). The rest of the page was blank for free-text entries.

The initial admission interview was mediated by the Functional Assessment Tool, which supported a fine-grained understanding of the relationship between the person, their functional capacity, and home context. It included predefined fields focused on detailed features of the physical environment, performance skills, and activities of daily living, and was designed to facilitate the detailed documentation of needs (see Table 11.1).

TABLE 11.1 Functional Assessment Tool Categories of Concern

Environment	
Physical Environment	
Type of Dwelling	House, Bungalow, Flat
Ownership	Private, Council, Housing Authority, Sheltered Rented
Access	Steps, Rails, Stairs, Stairlift, Banisters (Left/Right)
Heating	Rugs/Mats, Fire (Gas/Electric/Coal), Temperature Control
Bedroom	Upstairs, Downstairs
Bed	Single, Double, High/Medium/Low, Soft/Firm
Chair	High/Medium/Low, Soft/Firm
Bathroom	Upstairs, Downstairs
Bath	Yes, No
Shower	Cubicle, Over Bath, Level Access
Toilet	Upstairs, Downstairs, Outside
Commode	Yes, No
Kitchen	Table, Chair/Stool, Cooker/Microwave, Freezer, Trolley
Social Networks	
Lives With	Alone, Spouse, Dependent, Relatives
Health of Cohabitee	Independent, Assisted, Dependent
Employment of Cohabitee	Full-time, Part-time, None
Support Services	District Nurse, Day Centre, Home Care
Additional Carers	Relatives, Friends, Neighbours, Home Care

(*Continued*)

TABLE 11.1 (Continued)

Performance Skills	
Sensory and Communication	
Hearing	Intact, Impaired, None
Vision	Intact, Impaired, None
Smell	Intact, Impaired, None
Touch	Intact, Impaired, None
Speech	Intact, Impaired, None
Aids and Equipment	Information on sensory and communication aids (hearing aids, glasses, etc.)
Motor Skills	
Handedness	Left-handed, Right-handed
Mobility	Supervised, Independent
Assistive Aids	Frame, Crutches, Sticks, Wheelchair
Walking Distance	<5 m, <10 m, <15 m, Unlimited
Managing Steps	Independent, Supervised, Assistance with 1, Assistance with 2, Dependent
Stairs	Independent, Supervised, Assistance with 1, Assistance with 2, Dependent
Transfers	Independent, Supervised, Assistance with 1, Assistance with 2, Dependent (from Bed, Chair, Bath, Shower, Toilet, Wheelchair)
Cognitive Skills	
Concentration	Independent, Requires Prompting, Dependent
Memory	Independent, Requires Prompting, Dependent
Orientation	Independent, Requires Prompting, Dependent
Comprehension	Independent, Requires Prompting, Dependent
Initiative	Independent, Requires Prompting, Dependent
Continence	Independent, Dependent

Physical Activities of Living	
Personal Care	
Washing	Independent, Supervised, Assistance of 1, Assistance of 2
Dressing	Independent, Supervised, Assistance of 1, Assistance of 2
Undressing	Independent, Supervised, Assistance of 1, Assistance of 2
Grooming	Independent, Supervised, Assistance of 1, Assistance of 2
Feeding	Independent, Supervised, Assistance of 1, Assistance of 2
Drinking	Independent, Supervised, Assistance of 1, Assistance of 2
Toileting	Independent, Supervised, Assistance of 1, Assistance of 2
Adjusting Clothing	Independent, Supervised, Assistance of 1, Assistance of 2
Domestic Activities of Daily Living	
Preparing Drinks	Independent, Supervised, Assistance of 1
Preparing Snacks/Meals	Independent, Supervised, Assistance of 1
Carrying Items	Independent, Supervised, Assistance of 1
Cleaning	Independent, Supervised, Assistance of 1
Laundry/Ironing	Independent, Supervised, Assistance of 1
Shopping	Independent, Supervised, Assistance of 1

The patient assessment interview was described by the occupational therapist as 'a way of getting to know the patient, set the scene, and assess their cognition'. I observed several of these encounters. All examples of institutional talk, they followed a question-answer format that largely reflected the structure of the assessment form. As a generic tool, not all sections were relevant to every patient, and there is an interesting repair in the following example, in which the occupational therapist self-corrects after asking whether the patient was left- or right-handed, a category of concern relevant to arm injuries, but not hip fractures. Despite the prominence of the tool and the routinisation of the process, assessments also included individually tailored segments, oriented to specific details of the patient's story and the wider concerns of discharge planning. In the following extract, for example, having established the patient already has a range of assistive devices following a previous hospital admission, the occupational therapist also asks about a key safe – which would enable carers to access the home, how confident she feels, and whether she has an alarm pendant – none of which were included in the formal tool.

Occupational Therapist:	Do you live on your own?
Patient:	Yes.
Occupational Therapist:	House?
Patient:	It is a maisonette.
Occupational Therapist:	Ground floor or first?
Patient:	First.
Occupational Therapist:	Right so there are stairs to think about.
Patient:	I've got a double handrail.
Occupational Therapist:	The steps to go up the maisonette – are they inside or outside?
Patient:	The handrails go up the path and I manage to get up with handrails.
Occupational Therapist:	Do you only get up with help from family?
Patient:	I do manage to get up on my own.
Occupational Therapist:	Have you got central heating?
Patient:	Yes.
Occupational Therapist:	When you are inside is everything on the same level?
Patient:	I have handrails on the landing and bathroom, and I have a seat to lower me down into the bath.
Occupational Therapist:	So, someone has been out to assess?
Patient:	Yes, when I came out of hospital before I had carers but that has finished now.
Occupational Therapist:	Have you got a key safe?
Patient:	There's an entry code.
Occupational Therapist:	So, if someone visits, they can open the door?
Patient:	Most know the code.

[...]

There is some discussion about family support and the patient talks about where her son and daughter live. There is also a reference to her niece.

Occupational Therapist:	Do you have a commode?
Patient:	No.
Occupational Therapist:	Do you have the right height for the toilet?
Patient:	It's quite new; I can go quite easily.
Occupational Therapist:	Have you got any equipment to make it higher?
Patient:	I have a handrail to hold on to. That's quite good.
Occupational Therapist:	Before you came into hospital did you have any support apart from the carers?
Patient:	A nurse came to put a dressing on my bottom because when I came out of Swallow Hospital, I had a sore. It was very painful.
Occupational Therapist:	Do you wear a lifeline?
Patient:	A pendant? Yes.
Occupational Therapist:	Are you able to wash and dress yourself?
Patient:	Yes, I manage.
Occupational Therapist:	And you are able to make a cup of tea?
Patient:	Yes, and I have Valley Foods and can use the microwave to warm them up.
Occupational Therapist:	In the kitchen have you got a table and chairs?
Patient:	Yes.
Occupational Therapist:	So how do you carry things?
Patient:	I have a trolley.
Occupational Therapist:	How do you manage with your shopping?
Patient:	Mostly my son does it for me.'
Occupational Therapist:	'What about cleaning and laundry?
Patient:	I am not able to do a lot of cleaning, but I am arranging for a cleaner to come in quite soon and have help once a week.
Occupational Therapist:	Are you right or left-handed?
Patient:	Right.
Occupational Therapist:	That's a silly question and more relevant if you had broken your hand! When you were at home before did you use a stick or a frame?
Patient:	Stick and I would also go to Meadow House two days a week.
Occupational Therapist:	Like a Day Centre and have something to eat and meet with friends?
Patient:	That's right.

Occupational Therapist: Can you normally get in and out of bed?
Patient: Yes, until I fell!
Occupational Therapist: How did you fall?

Patient then describes how she had removed her lifeline and had fallen getting into bed. The lifeline was out of reach, and she was unable to get up, spending all night on the floor. She was discovered by her niece.

Occupational Therapist: How do you feel about going back home? Do you feel confident? We could always think about getting support of a longer-term package to get you stronger and back on your feet.

Following this initial assessment process, the patient was enacted as a provisional object of practice, centred on their home environment, social network, and functional support needs. In this example, the home was well-adapted, but others required further arrangements to support safe discharge. In many cases, this involved an in-person visit – either by the occupational therapist or a technician – to assess environment features such as access, stairs, door widths, room proportions and layout, and furniture height. Family members were also called upon to furnish this information.

As discharge approached, ward-based functional assessments were conducted to determine the need for assistive devices. Assessments were undertaken in the hospital context and involved improvisation and translation to anticipate how arrangements would materialise in the home context. In the first example, the therapist asks the patient to imagine she is in a normal bed, so that she can assess the need for a bed lever. In the second example, a patient who is reluctant to accept a toilet raise is reminded that hospital toilets are higher than those at home.

Occupational Therapist is instructing the patient so she can observe transfers: Pretend you are in a normal bed without the back rest bit. So, without pulling on anything bring yourself up to sit. [...] We need a bed lever.

Occupational Therapist: I wonder if you mind if I see you in action. You might need something for the toilet.
Patient: No, I don't think so; if I need one, I can get one later.
Occupational Therapist: You're quite an independent lady.
Patient: Yes.
Occupational Therapist: I can tell. The toilet is higher in hospital than it is at home. It is three inches higher. So, we can give you a seat.

Patient: I don't really want one!

Occupational Therapist: But if you need it, it's best for me to give it you now. Let's have a chat. Is there room in the bathroom for a chair for you to have a wash? I can bring a chair in for you to have a look.

The professional objects of occupational therapy practice in hip fracture care were inherently trajectory-oriented and deeply relational. The patient, as enacted through this three-part process, was understood through the interdependencies between their functional capacity, the unique affordances and constraints of their home environment, and the ensemble of equipment and assistive technologies needed to support independence after discharge.

Object Formation in Nursing Practice

Enacting the Patient in Ward Nurses' Work

As discussed in Chapter 8, orthogeriatric nursing involves generating multiple objects of practice. While standardised care plans and the Jenolan admission documentation provided an institutionally mandated enactment, nurses came to know patients through the embodied routines of care and the dense web of daily interactions – with doctors, allied health professionals, family members, technologies, and materials – that unfolded across their trajectory. Nursing work was thus mediated by three overlapping objects of practice: a formal, performative, and predominantly technical, object grounded in risk assessments and care plans; a situated object shaped by patients' immediate and evolving needs; and a narrative trajectory object oriented to the coordination and anticipation of ongoing care (Allen, 2015a).

Real-time nursing notes recorded nursing interventions and accounted for practice, but unlike resident doctors, nurses did not write narrative summaries of patient trajectories. Instead, patients were enacted as continuous intra-professional objects through twice-daily oral handovers. Each handover, led by the outgoing nurse, followed a similar rhythm: bed number, name, age, and reason for admission, followed by an overview of individual needs, any changes in their treatment plans, and information relevant to wider trajectory management. Handover had a recipient design (Heritage, 1984), with the reporting nurse establishing how well the team 'knows' the patient, to adjust the level of detail. The following extract contrasts two handovers: one for a new patient, which is more detailed, and one for a patient known to staff, which is more concise. As noted in Chapter 8, an intriguing feature of the handover is the omission of routine nursing care, in favour of the singularities of individualised needs and trajectory management.

Staff Nurse 1: This lady has got vascular dementia. She's from [...] nursing home. Past medical history – non-insulin dependent diabetic, asthma, hypertension, deaf, vascular dementia, macular degeneration, she's blind in the left eye, she has an old CVA (stroke), pneumonia, UTI (urinary tract infection) and back pain.

Staff Nurse 2: How old is she?

Staff Nurse 1: Eighty-five. She had a left DHS (dynamic hip screw surgery) yesterday. I've got one set of obs (physiological observations) off her that I am happy with but she's resistive. She's been eating her tubes. She was unwell post op... she's got a Fentanyl patch. She does spit out her tablets and the only thing I could give was Paracetamol. We've got some liquids, but she spat them out. When I checked, her pressure areas were fine. Dressing in-tact. I can't think of anything else.

Staff Nurse 2: Oxygen?

Staff Nurse 1: No, not on oxygen. Sats (blood oxygen saturations) are fine.

Staff Nurse 1: [Name] She's been refusing to be turned all day and when I turned her this evening she's got a broken area there on her bottom.

Senior Nurse: Is it new? Have you done an incident form?

Staff Nurse 2: She had an old one there, it looks like a bit of a scuff.

Staff Nurse 1: Nobody told me.

Staff Nurse 2: It might be an old one. I'll have a look.

As these extracts illustrate, despite being called a handover, information flow was rarely one-way. Rather, issues were typically discussed collectively, often leading to new understandings and/or the identification of areas of uncertainty requiring clarification. The result was a modified intra-professional understanding of each patient's care, non-routine care needs, and specific activities to be undertaken during the shift.

Enacting the Patient in Frailty Nurses' Work

Ward nurses articulated immediate bedside care but had limited capacity to proactively manage discharge planning. Frailty nurses had been appointed to fill this gap. They reflexively monitored recovery trajectories and coordinated discharge planning.

Allied Health Professional: 'You notice when frailty nurse is not here as she always keeps on top of things [...] She knows exactly what is going on better than the junior doctors and she coordinates the ward. She's more in tune with the patient's pathway and generally a dynamic person'.

Unlike ward nurses' embodied understandings of the patient, frailty nurses relied heavily on documentary resources and artefacts for object formation. These understandings were refined through their interactions with other team members and, less frequently, with patients, to generate a version of the patient centred on recovery and the evolving discharge plan.

To support the complex demands of discharge planning, frailty nurses had adapted an existing audit instrument into a more expansive, informal tool. Printed on a single sheet of A4, it served a dual function: collecting data for the National Hip Fracture Database and care trajectory management. The audit component comprised fields on standard categories – patient identifiers, admission and assessment details, treatment specifics, discharge timelines, and 30-day follow-up indicators. The frailty nurses had expanded the form with additional fields – critical to rehabilitation and discharge planning – that reflected the wider scope of their practice. These included the mechanism of injury, fall history, comorbidities, medication and osteoporosis screening, and detailed social histories. Functional assessments of activities of daily living – cooking, dressing, washing, shopping – were documented alongside notes on carers and the involvement of social workers. By embedding these elements within a single document, the nurses transformed a retrospective data collection tool into an accumulating and coordinating device for trajectory management. Carried on a clipboard, the form was portable and could be quickly updated by adding a written note. As with the Assessment Unit nurses' handover form (Chapter 6), this was very much a working record (Fitzpatrick, 2004), intended to support frailty nurses' practice, rather than a formal document of the patient's care, and was discarded once audit data had been entered at the end of the in-patient admission.

The frailty nursing role was widely valued by the multidisciplinary team; however, its working arrangements were not without tensions. Several participants expressed concern about the separation of discharge planning from clinical care.

Staff Nurse: The frailty nurses now do all the discharges, make the referrals, go to the panel meetings and things we don't know about. The OTs (occupational therapists) refer to CRT (community resource team) whereas we used to do that too.

Occupational Therapist: We have an MDT (multidisciplinary team meeting) on a Wednesday, and the ward nurses do not speak; the Frailty Nurse leads the meeting.

Senior Nurse observed: I don't see how they (frailty nurses) maintain their NMC (Nursing and Midwifery Council, the professional regulator) registration. All they do is discharge planning and make phone calls, they don't have any clinical contact with patients.

Staff Nurse: But not everyone wants to do it (frailty nurse) as its not being a nurse.

Frailty nurses did not attend nursing handover, so their understanding was primarily derived from documentary sources. This contrasted with ward nurses' embedded and relational knowledge – forms of knowing that were relatively invisible in the formal record. These different sensemaking practices produced divergent understandings of the patient that needed to be reconciled in practice.

> Frailty Nurse is liaising with the nursing staff and appears to spend more time telling them what she has found out rather than using them proactively as an information source. On a number of occasions, it is evident that the nurses are well-informed about patients even if the information is not in the notes. In fact, sometimes they are better informed and offer an important alternative understanding of the patient than the frailty nurse has managed to glean from the notes.
>
> A little later I observed Frailty Nurse informing the staff nurse about the patient's mental health issues. Staff Nurse is very causal – disinterested even – about receiving this information and makes it clear that she is well aware of his history. She is also able to offer some additional information that Frailty Nurse is unaware of, which is that his wife does not want him to return to the residential home he was in and believes he would be better suited to an EMI (dementia unit) facility.

These observations highlight the trade-offs involved in redistributing responsibilities within the nursing workforce. The frailty nurse role addressed ward nurses' limited capacity to engage in forward planning while delivering immediate care, but introduced new boundaries between forms of nursing knowledge. Both were essential to keep patients moving safely through the system, and making sense of the patient as an intra-professional object of practice required ongoing negotiation between these modes of knowing.

Object Formation for Collective Decision-Making

> Once they've been to theatre, it's working out where they're going. Are they going back to where they've come from? Are they safe to go home? [...] Do I need to put any sort of services in? [...] If they can't go home, where's the next place? Do they go into residential care? Do they have capacity to accept that?
>
> *(Frailty Nurse – Interview)*

Discharge marks a critical trajectory threshold that leads to markedly different futures. For some, it signalled the end of acute care and the gradual resumption of everyday life; for others, increased dependency following injury required new support arrangements. Discharge planning was accomplished through 'match-making' (Allen, 2015a, 2015b), a process of aligning the patient's evolving recovery trajectory with a prospective future, balancing independence with safety. This involved enacting the patient as a two-part collective object of practice: an interdisciplinary object, focused on recovery, and a trajectory object, oriented towards possible discharge destinations.

As Mol (2002) observes, healthcare practices often sustain different enactments of the patient in parallel, without conflict, provided they do not interfere with each other. In hip fracture, discharge planning disrupted this equilibrium. It brought previously parallel forms of knowing the patient – clinical, functional, relational, institutional, personal – into direct interaction, where they had to be negotiated and, at times, reconciled. Enacting the patient as a collective object of practice for discharge planning was a complex and emergent process, undertaken in conditions of existential disequilibrium and uncertainty, with different scenarios explored by the team, patient, and family to arrive at a workable plan.

Concerns about the person's functional abilities before the injury – foreshadowed at admission – moved centre stage. Understanding 'what the person was like before' was essential for setting realistic rehabilitation goals, appraising recovery, and envisioning supportive arrangements required after discharge. This was not straightforward: patients eager to return home could underplay previous difficulties, and key actors could hold different perspectives on the situation.

> Occupational Therapist said that this was an interesting case, because Stan had described his life before admission as one in which he was managing independently. Occupational Therapist: This was true, to an extent. But when we spoke to his daughter, she said that they had noticed a decline in his mobility and that he was shuffling more.

> Social worker said that it can sometimes be difficult to assess a case, as people often give you half a story: 'They tell you what they know they need to say to get what they want, but this can be misleading'.

Memory problems, common among hip fracture patients, further complicate discharge planning. If a patient was assessed as lacking the capacity to contribute to the planning process, then decisions were made on their behalf – typically involving discussions with the family, at a Best Interest Meeting, a formally constituted event in the UK NHS. However, cognitive status was often unclear, and capacity assessments became entangled with disagreements about the feasibility of discharge plans. The following ward round extract relates to a lady with uncertain cognitive capacity who has previously insisted she does not require support to be discharged home, a proposal considered to be unsafe by the team.

> Orthogeriatrician sits on the bed and starts talking to the patient. She is perfectly lucid and coherent and says she realises she needs help to manage at home and is willing for carers to come in. As the conversation unfolds the other team members on the round are incredulous.

Resident Doctor 1:	She's like a new woman. That's not what we had yesterday!
Orthogeriatrician:	Is that normal?
Staff Nurse:	No!
Orthogeriatrician:	Well, based on what I have seen today, we need to plan for discharge with a package.
Resident Doctor 1:	But she won't accept it.
Orthogeriatrician:	But it's the least restrictive thing to do. She's not been in a home previously and we shouldn't institutionalise her.
Resident Doctor 2:	Would you not start with community resource team, so they have chance to assess her?

> Orthogeriatrician says that this is certainly an option, but that there is a need to be clear that she will need ongoing support and not just a short-term rehabilitation. 'If she will accept a package of care, then we can safely discharge her. If she will not, then she will have to go into a home.'

Resident Doctor 2:	Are you sure she has capacity?
Orthogeriatrician:	If she agrees to a package of care then she does!

The most complex trajectories arose if the patient wished to return to their home, but staff and/or family had concerns about safety or sustainability. In such cases, two primary mechanisms were used to align perspectives: discharge planning meetings and ward-based trials.

Discharge planning meetings varied in composition – sometimes including both patient and family, and sometimes the family only – and enabled detailed discussions about the person's needs and support required for safe care. In the following example, a meeting was arranged with the patient and their family. Having previously managed in her own home, the patient has agreed she needs to move into residential care. By the time of the meeting, however, she is wavering.

> The frailty nurse had organised the meeting in the belief that after much deliberation the patient had reached the decision that she needed to move into a residential home. However, when we started the meeting, it was clear that she had once again changed her mind. Her emotional turmoil was palpable and on numerous occasions she repeated that she did not want to go into a home, while at the same time apologising for 'messing you all around'. There was a lengthy discussion in which different members of the team tried to underline the reality of a home discharge – i.e. that she would not be able to mobilise over long distances because of her cardiac problems and so would be limited to transferring from chair to commode and bed to chair, she would receive support from a four times a day care package provided by social carers, but in between visits she would need to open her nebuliser ampoules as apparently social carers are not permitted to do this and she also needed to be able to take the top off a flask so that she would have coffee available throughout the day. The district nursing service cannot provide this support. At various points there was some suggestion that she did not fully grasp how restricted her movements would be at home, indeed her daughter observed: I don't think she understands that she will not be able to move from room to room.

This extract underlines the biographical and emotional challenges of discharge planning decisions and how the practical reality of home-based care contrasts with ideals of independence associated with home.

In addition to formal discharge planning meetings, staff used ward-based trials to simulate the home care conditions and assess whether patients could manage with the available support. These trials evaluated patient capability but also operated as a form of negotiation – testing assumptions, surfacing ethical tensions, and, at times, prompting patients and families to reassess their expectations – with the aim of bringing about an alignment in collective understanding of the patient and their future trajectory. The following extracts illustrate how these practices unfolded in everyday ward work:

> Healthcare Support Worker emerges from the 9-bedder and informs Staff Nurse: [name] is asking for the toilet. She's only supposed to have four (number of episodes of assistance) isn't she and this is the third.

Staff Nurse: Yes, it is the third, but ethically we cannot refuse if she needs to go. The family are aware that if she needs assistance more than four times then going home is never going to be feasible.

Frailty Nurse: But after a long process we think he has capacity and that he has expressed a wish for a placement in a residential home. We did a trial care package on the ward which didn't go well and made him realise he needed help.

Senior Nurse: She was adamant she was going home. So, we tried it this weekend, and it has not worked […] That's what I had hoped; that we would show her over the weekend how hard it can be.

Multidisciplinary team meetings are recommended for collaborative planning in complex patient populations, but the Jenolan team found the weekly meeting insufficiently agile. Instead, a key mechanism for organising discharge was a board round, a concise, 30-minute multidisciplinary meeting held three times a week.

> On a ward round when you've got one minute per patient, you don't have a decision-making structure … you start making presumptions … "On my recollection, I think she was doing … and I think the prognosis was …" but actually that's not fed with information by having not been round since last Tuesday. So the decisions are made slightly on the hoof and to some extent, we get them right, but they are challenged on a daily basis now … so if it doesn't feel right, people will flag it up the next day or the same day or during a meeting … whereas two years ago, we had a meeting once a week and you'd make the same mistake or assumptions … we're trying to shoehorn people into the right box.
>
> *(Orthogeriatrician – Interview)*

Board rounds, led by the frailty nurses, were key to the translational work necessary to reach a consensus on recovery trajectories and prospective discharge destinations. Each patient's progress was narrated as a care trajectory, enabling team members to contribute to a shared enactment of the patient oriented towards recovery and future discharge. While drawing on diverse understandings of the patient across the wider team, these narratives involved more than aggregation. They entailed sensemaking and synthesis, generating a collective object of practice that was 'more than one but less than many' (Mol, 2002). This shared understanding was not formally documented in the patient record.

> We talked about the board round […] Consultant Orthogeriatrician 2 said that it was important as it ensured momentum and was a mechanism for

reaching an understanding of individual cases. He said that much of the information generated during these sessions would not be found in the medical record as it was 'opinion' and 'subtleties of understanding'. 'We all know about the patient, but we don't know what we know until this is brought together, and this is more than you get in the notes, with individual entries [...] Our job is sorting out people's lives and you can't write about a lot of that in the notes'.

'You need to be able to put together a story [...] a simple synthesis of what's going on ... what makes this situation tick and where the impediments are [...] That's where the frailty nurse is staggeringly effective [...] Nobody will tell you something's wrong if you haven't expressed what's going on. So, getting a very simple, working model of this individual expressed and spoken in front of people who know they can say 'No that's wrong' is, I think, the most efficient way of running that process'.

(Orthogeriatric Consultant 1 – Interview)

Combining an understanding of the person's recovery trajectory with the equivocality and complexity of the individual's lifeworld, patients, as objects of collective practice, took on the qualities of epistemic objects (Knorr Cetina, 1997): open-ended, emergent, and in flux. This indeterminacy is evident in the following board round extracts, where patient trajectories are shaped through interdisciplinary deliberation and partial alignments of professional judgement, patient preference, and institutional constraint. In the first example, the team works to reconcile the patient's stated desire to return home with professional concerns about her safety and functional ability – surfacing tensions between patient autonomy and clinical judgment, and revealing how decisions remain provisional, contingent on further negotiation and functional improvement.

Frailty Nurse:	[name] there are issues about her not being able to go back to where she came from.
Doctor 1:	Usually, she was living alone in a flat. She can't go back as she is.
Doctor 2:	She knows that, but she wants to return to her flat.
Frailty Nurse:	Would she be agreeable to a placement?
Doctor 2:	We haven't discussed that.
Physio:	She was slow to get going.
Doctor 1:	She wants to get back to her flat.
Physio:	We're dealing with an old CVA (stroke) too so there are good reasons for her being slow. She's still responding to physio, and she is still making improvements.

In the second example, the patient is not only an object of clinical and social assessment but also of ethical deliberation. Questions of who has the authority to decide – professional, patient, or family – are complicated by fluctuating patient preferences and contested interpretations of capacity. The discussion reveals how emotional strain, institutional boundaries, and legal responsibilities converge, confounding decision-making.

> The conversation then moves on to patient [name]. Frailty Nurse raises the issue that Resident Doctor has overheard a very frank conversation taking place between the patient and her daughters in which they were pressing the residential home issue. Frailty Nurse suggests that Resident Doctor should document it in the notes.

Resident Doctor:	Well no. To be honest it is exactly the same conversation I can imagine having with my parents.
Senior Nurse:	The family have a point. They are at the end of their tether but what can we do if she refuses? She's deemed to have capacity.
Frailty Nurse:	She wanders though.
Senior Nurse:	We can't know that.
Frailty Nurse:	At the meeting she agreed to residential and today she has changed her mind.
Orthogeriatrician:	The more we push the more she clams up. Its Friday today: let's leave it over the weekend, no one is going to be doing anything, let's leave her to calm down and review things after the weekend.

> Frailty Nurse says family have written an 'essay' on the carers' perspective of UAs (unified assessment form) and dispute the DOLS (deprivation of liberty assessment) view that she has capacity.

Orthogeriatrician:	Capacity assessment is my responsibility and not DOLS and based on what I saw on Tuesday she has capacity, but we know that if she wants to go home this is not without risks.

What is visible in these examples is a form of coordination that involves negotiating uncertainty, distributed responsibility, and shifting patient preferences. More than aligning tasks or mobilising action, this was a collective effort to bring together partial, situated knowledges in an evolving reference point, in order to construct a generative understanding of the patient and their

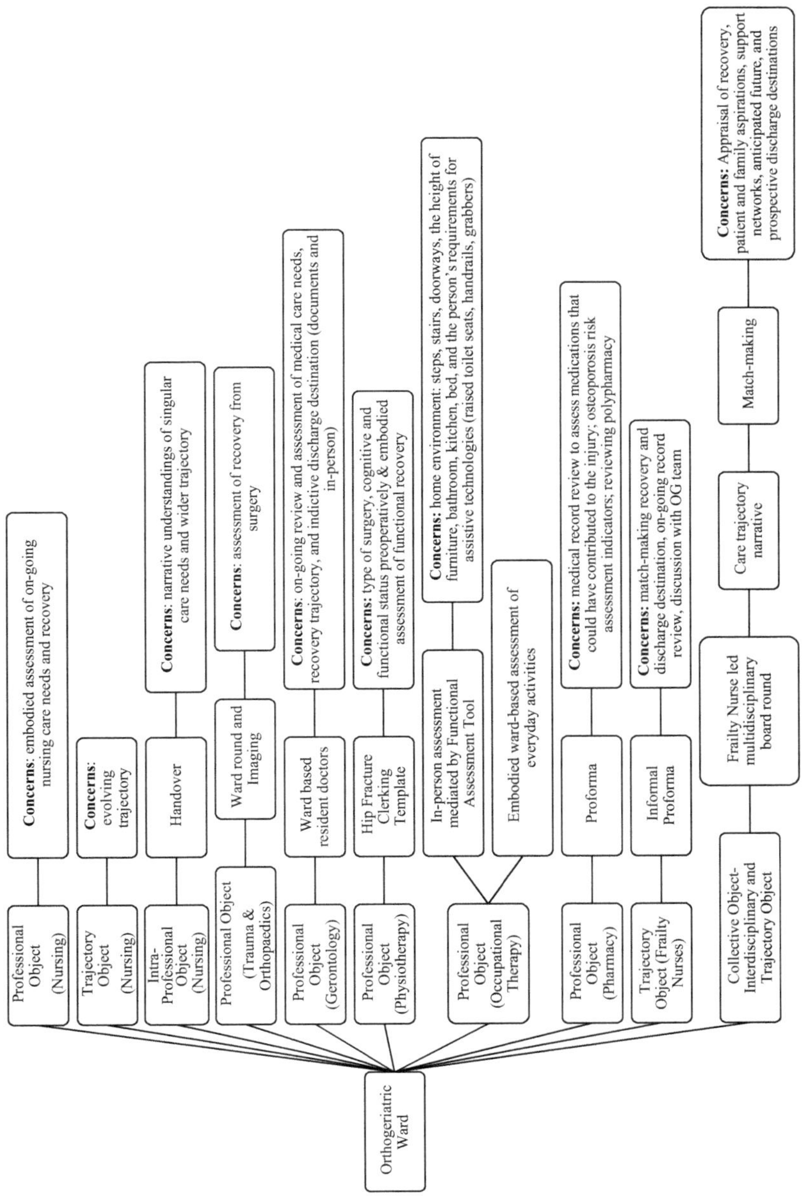

FIGURE 11.1 Object formation in postoperative orthogeriatric work.

situation. While the concept of epistemic objects is well established in science and technology studies (Knorr Cetina, 1999) and clinical ontology (Mol, 2002), I propose the notion of *epistemic organisation* to describe this distinctive organisational form. This framing enables us to distinguish between modes of organisation that aim to deliver interventions and those that aim to generate understanding.

As discharge plans crystallised, the patient evolved from an emergent epistemic object of practice – open-ended and indeterminate – to a more settled narrative object, encompassing their aspirations, functional capacity, the home environment, social support networks, and the intricate network of infrastructural arrangements needed for safe discharge and continued progression to independence. These narrative understandings functioned as boundary objects (Star and Griesemer, 1989), enabling team members to progress their respective responsibilities in discharge planning. As I will describe in Chapter 13, as plans progressed, issues could surface, and the patient as an object of practice once again became open and indeterminate. As the discharge plan began to crystallise, however, the patient was further transformed from an integrated narrative object of practice into a reductionist technical object (Rheinberger, 1997), defined by the time-critical tasks of discharge.

Summary

This chapter has examined the organisation of patient care and treatment in postoperative orthogeriatric work. Within a significantly expanded assemblage, the patient was enacted into multiple objects of professional practice, oriented towards a diverse range of concerns – from the relatively narrow priorities of the pharmacist and physiotherapists to the broader, holistic approaches of physicians, ward and frailty nurses, and the occupational therapist. Despite these varied understandings and the distributed nature of work, all actors were united by a shared goal: to support the patient's recovery and develop a discharge plan.

Recovery trajectories were often uncertain, unfolding in an environment marked by existential disequilibrium. Reaching consensus on a discharge was an extensive and complex task, which involved enacting the patient as a dual object of collective practice: an interdisciplinary object focused on recovery, and a trajectory object concerned with discharge destinations. This dynamic process enabled the team, patient, and family to explore and negotiate options through iterative match-making. Frailty nurses played a pivotal role, reflexively monitoring trajectory progress and leading the translation effort necessary to support collective decision-making. Figure 11.1 summarises these processes.

References

Allen, D. (2015a). *The Invisible Work of Nurses: Hospitals, Organisation and Healthcare*. London and New York, Routledge.

Allen, D. (2015b). 'Inside "bed management": ethnographic insights from the vantage point of UK hospital nurses'. *Sociology of Health & Illness* **37**(3): 370–384. https://doi.org/10.1111/1467-9566.12195

Bishop, S. and J. Waring (2019). 'From boundary object to boundary subject: the role of the patient in coordination across complex systems of care during hospital discharge'. *Social Science & Medicine* **235**: 112370. https://doi.org/10.1016/j.socscimed.2009.05.002

Douglas, M. (1966). *Purity and Danger: An Analysis of Concepts of Pollution and Taboo*. Abington, Oxon, Routledge & Kegan Paul.

Fitzpatrick, G. (2004). 'Integrated care and the working record'. *Health Informatics Journal* **10**: 291.

Grief, M. (1991). *The Visual Factory: Building Participation Through Shared Information*. New York, Productivity Press.

Heritage, J. (1984). *Garfinkel and Ethnomethodology*. Cambridge, Polity Press.

Knorr Cetina, K. (1997). 'Sociality with objects; social relations in postsocial knowledge societies'. *Theory, Culture & Society* **14**(4): 1–30.

Knorr Cetina, K. (1999) *Epistemic Cultures: How the Sciences make Knowledge*. Cambridge, MA, Harvard University Press.

Latimer, J. (1997). 'Giving patients a future: the constituting of classes in an acute medical unit'. *Sociology of Health & Illness* **19**(2): 160185 https://doi.org/10.1111/1467-9566.ep10934396

Mol, A.M. (2002). *The Body Multiple: Ontology in Medical Practice*. Durham, NC, Duke University Press.

NICE (2011). *Hip Fracture: Management, Clinical Guideline CG124*. National Institute for Health and Care Excellence. https://www.nice.org.uk/guidance/cg124

Rheinberger, H.-J. (1997). *Towards a History of Epistemic Things: Synthesizing Proteins in the Test Tube*. Stanford, CA, Standford University Press.

Schutz, A. (1972). *The Phenomenology of the Social World*, Evanston, IL, Northwestern University Press.

Star, S.L. and J.R. Griesemer (1989). 'Institutional ecology, 'translations' and boundary objects: amateurs and professionals in Berkeley's Museum of Vertebrate Zoology, 1907-39'. *Social Studies of Science* **19**(3): 387–420. https://doi.org/10.1177/030631289019003001

12

REABLEMENT AND INFRASTRUCTURES

Community Resource Team Work

This chapter examines the work of the Community Resource Team (CRT), which delivered short-term, home-based health therapies and social care. Supporting most patients discharged home after hip fracture surgery, the CRT provided daily living assistance and physiotherapy to aid rehabilitation. It coordinated the dynamic relationships between individuals, their functional capacity, and the infrastructural arrangements of home and community. This chapter outlines the social-material arrangements that characterised the social world of CRT and then explains how patients were enacted in CRT work and the mechanisms that enabled safe transitions from hospital to independent living.

The Social World of the Community Resource Team

The CRT operated within a distinct social world at the intersection of health and social care. Positioned between hospital and home, it played a key role in managing the arrangements needed for safe transitions. This section explores the structures, organising logics, interpretative repertoires, and material arrangements that conditioned the provision, organisation, and coordination of post-hip fracture home care.

Structures

Service

Jointly funded by the regional University Health Board and Local Authority, the CRT was an integrated health-social care service based in the grounds of a former psychiatric hospital. It served 2,000 people, offering short-term 'step-up'

DOI: 10.4324/9781003475019-22

and 'step-down' home care. 'Step-up' care aimed to prevent hospital admission or further decline, typically via primary care referrals. 'Step-down' care supported independence post-discharge, with referrals from secondary care. Based on a reablement model, service access depended on an individual's potential for independence. Social care was available for up to six weeks, health therapies for up to 12, with services gradually withdrawn in partnership with patients and families.

The CRT Team

The CRT team included nurses, healthcare therapists (occupational, physiotherapy, dietetics, speech and language), support technicians, home care managers, and social carers. Nurses, therapists, and technicians were employed by the Health Board, while home care managers and social carers worked for the Local Authority.

Team involvement varied by patient need – some required only social care, others therapy, and some both. Hip fracture patients typically need support with daily living and physiotherapy; occupational therapists assess the home environment and make recommendations about daily routines and social care planning.

Though nurses were part of the team, CRT did not provide community nursing. CRT nurses screened new service referrals and managed complex cases, such as when an individual's needs were changing or care needed stepping up, or where there was a need to support medication management. Specific nursing intervention required a separate referral to the community nursing service. Internal referrals could also be made to the dietician or speech and language therapist.

Delivering integrated home care was not without its challenges. Unlike the hospital, care was discontinuous, and social carers' scope of practice was limited and tightly regulated. CRT could advise on additional public and private services, but gaps were common – and often had to be filled by family or friends.

Organising Logics

CRT work was driven by demand management and safety logics. Like elsewhere in the UK, community health and social care services were over-extended, and the CRT caseload was tightly controlled. All new referrals were reviewed to assess alignment with service functions, and patients were only accepted when there was sufficient capacity. Patients in receipt of step-down care, such as hip fracture patients, represented a third of the service's caseload. Because hospitalised patients were considered to be in a place of safety, step-up care cases were prioritised, and there was typically a waiting list for step-down care referrals.

CRT screened new cases immediately before discharge to ensure the infrastructural arrangements were in place for safe transfer. The service also dedicated significant resources to a 'discharge visit' on the day patients returned home, in part for object formation purposes, but also to assess infrastructural arrangement safety and mitigate any risks. All cases were reviewed after four weeks; if independence hadn't been achieved, a long-term package of care – provided exclusively by the Local Authority and means-tested – was organised.

Materials

The Patient Record

CRT patient records were maintained in separate digital systems for health and social care. Initial discharge assessments were completed on paper forms, which informed the creation of digital case records in each system. Subsequent assessments by CRT professionals – social care managers, occupational therapists, physiotherapists – generated distinct objects of practice which were used to develop care plans for home carers and physiotherapy technicians.

Although the official record was digital, social carers and therapists lacked mobile ICT access. Instead, they used a shared paper record kept in the patient's home, detailing care provision, service plans, medication management, and continuation sheets for documenting their respective activities. This information was later digitised.

While separate record systems were seen by some as a sign of poor integration, coordination challenges were partly offset by team colocation, enabling ongoing dialogue about shared patients, and by the duplication of digital and paper records.

Infrastructural Arrangements

Unlike a hospital, where the caring infrastructure is established, home discharges require care arrangements to be assembled de novo. As discussed in the previous chapter, the occupational therapist had a key role in assessing needs and organising assistive technologies or adaptations to support independent living during recovery. Home care infrastructures are finely balanced ensembles. They rely on finely tuned interactions between people, technologies, routines, and services, and are inherently unstable; shaped by unpredictable bodies, fluctuating needs, the limits of technologies, service constraints, and the shifting dynamics of family and support networks. CRT invested significant effort in managing these interdependencies – coordinating equipment, care packages, family involvement, and changing patient capacities – often improvising to sustain safe, workable home environments.

Occupational Therapist: So much of what we do is organising and sorting things out: food, equipment, referrals to certain services, liaising with the family.

One of the team is trying to locate a deep bucket for a commode. A patient is drinking a lot because it is summertime and voiding large amounts of urine. The therapist wants to reduce a three-times-daily care package but can't because the commode can't handle the volume.

CRT Therapist: We do well – we are flexible, and we have to sort out a lot of things for people that are referred and that takes a long time.

At one level, 'sorting things out' entailed tinkering with arrangements in response to evolving need (Pols, 2008; Mol, 2008; see Chapter 8, p. 141). At another level, however, it also involved interventions to stabilise care infrastructures at the point of discharge. Acute sector staff went to great lengths to prepare for discharge, but most cases required situational adjustments to ensure safety once the patient returned home.

Interpretative Repertoires

CRT work involved multiple formal interpretative repertoires. Central among these was the admissions folder, used at the initial visit to enact the patient into a provisional object of collective health and social care practice. It contained risk assessment tools (home safety, nutrition, falls, lone worker) and a Unified Baseline Assessment of care needs template, designed to enact patients into the objects of practice of social care work. Because health and social care providers were separate services, the folder also included a consent form for sharing care information.

Social care was further mediated through additional formal protocols. The Service Delivery Plan specified the levels of support provided to the patient, including the tasks, length of call, and time of day. The Medication Administration Scheme Needs Assessment, a 40-item risk assessment tool, determined how medication support would be managed – by the patient, social carers, or family. The Service Users Guide, retained by the patient, explained the service's purpose, defined carers' activities, and described complaints procedures, quality assurance, and staff management.

CRT Work

Nurses and therapists worked core hours; social carers followed a rota with scheduled calls extending from 7 am to late evening. CRT nurses divided their time between screening referrals and case management, with someone always available for urgent step-up care. Except for occupational therapists who initially collaborated with social carers to advise on how best to support patients, team members largely worked independently.

There was an 'allocation meeting' to consider new referrals, attended by nurses, therapists, an administrator, and social care managers. Time was also assigned in the afternoon for discharge visits on new step-down cases.

Staff shortages was a persistent issue, frequently discussed during fieldwork. Team members expressed concerns about waiting lists and the difficulties of providing adequate support for active cases. As one physiotherapist put it:

> We are all supposed to be efficient these days but when does efficiency shade into poor care? When you have insufficient staff and time constraints, it effects communication. The NHS relies on good will: nurses going home late, therapists doing visits to see if people are safe at the end of the day.

Targets, such as discharging patients within three days of referral, often clashed with staffing realities – particularly in social care. In practice, discharge timelines stretched to seven days or more. During fieldwork, reference was made to one individual who had waited 19 days.

Making Patients and Mobilising Care

Object formation in CRT began the day the patient returned home, with the generation of a collective object of practice. Conducted during the discharge visit, this initial assessment created a provisional understanding of the patient which was used to stabilise care arrangements. It was later supplemented by more specific enactments, translating the patient into distinct, professionally accountable objects for social care, occupational therapy, and physiotherapy. While team members worked largely independently, formal and informal mechanisms supported collective monitoring of patient progress towards independence.

Object Formation and Collective Practice

The patient was enacted as a collective CRT object during the discharge visit, typically led by an occupational therapist and a social care manager. These visits were resource-intensive, often taking half a day, including travel and documentation. Object formation involved three components: a risk-assessment-mediated interview, negotiation of initial social care needs, and appraisal of functional independence in the home. These processes were interwoven with efforts to stabilise infrastructural arrangements. Two discharge visits were observed during fieldwork: Andrea, a woman discharged after hip fracture surgery, and Geoff, a man discharged after elective knee replacement.

Discharge visits typically began with office-based sensemaking to develop a preliminary understanding of the case. The following field note relates to Andrea – widowed, living alone, and having been diagnosed with a lung malignancy post-admission, which was being managed palliatively. Here, the occupational therapist is puzzling over a discrepancy between the information included in the referral, which makes no reference to the lung condition, and the screening documentation, in which there is a reference to palliative care.

Occupational Therapist 1: This referral is pants (not good quality) and the worst part of it is that an OT (occupational therapist) has done it! It has the past medical history as the NOF (neck of femur, i.e. hip fracture) only.
Occupational Therapist 2: Where is the palliative issue?
Occupational Therapist 1: I don't know, it doesn't say. They may have discovered it when she was in.

Occupational Therapist 1 links in with Nurse 1 who is in the admin office and asks whether she can access the portal (national digital health record) for her. Therapist says that there is nothing in the hospital referral about palliative care.

Nurse: That's strange. I wonder whether she's been told she's got cancer on the ward.

Nurse looks through a few case notes and eventually locates a chest X-ray. Standing behind her, I can see that there is a clear section on the report that states 'Conclusion: which points to a right upper lobe carcinoma'.

[...]

Occupational Therapist 2: Do we know whether it was a pathological fracture?
Nurse: (looking at hip fracture X-ray) It doesn't say.
Occupational Therapist 1: Probably assume it was a fall.

The nurse is now looking at the Emergency Department entry – 'She was admitted with a fall'. When you said hip fracture I wondered if we had got the right woman.

Patients referred for CRT step-down care had varied medical, surgical, and health histories. In this example available documentation was insufficient for the occupational therapist to make sense of the case. This uncertainty threatened the therapist's professional identity. As she explained, 'It is so difficult as we should know these things. It makes us look incompetent'. By accessing the clinical portal and reviewing Andrea's X-rays and Emergency Department record, the team deduced that the discrepancy in CRT documentation had arisen because of the changed clinical picture between the original referral and the pre-discharge screening process, and that the hip fracture was associated with a fall at home and unlikely to be pathological (i.e. caused by the cancer). The team established that Andrea's referral was for short-term support following hip fracture surgery. While the discharge visit would clarify these assumptions, this initial formulation shaped the occupational therapist's initial orientation.

The visit began with the assessment interview mediated by formal artefacts. Although the admissions folder included multiple risk assessment tools (home safety, nutrition, falls, lone worker, care needs), my observations showed that home safety and care needs assessments were prioritised. In both visits, I observed, questions about falls and nutrition were designed to identify any immediate risks, rather than constituting comprehensive assessments. This selective use of assessment protocols reflected a concern not to overwhelm patients immediately after their return home, as well as the practical limitations of time constraints during the visit.

> Occupational Therapist said that the discharge meeting involved loads of questions and when people had just returned home from hospital it could be a bit over-whelming.

More broadly, however, CRT work was embodied and context-sensitive and object formation tended to rely less on structured tools and more on observational assessment and situated sensemaking.

Three fieldnote extracts from Andrea's discharge visit illustrate the relative agency of the formal assessment tools in mediating the interaction. Participants included an occupational therapist, a social care manager, Andrea, and her two adult daughters. The occupational therapist led the process and completed the assessment proforma; the social care manager was also actively engaged and made her own separate records.

In the first field note, the Home Safety Checklist is a central actor. This single-sided A4 form assessed key safety considerations and was organised into discrete sections: equipment needs, medication management, community alarm information, access to the property, food provision, weight loss, and 'any other concerns'. The structure and organisation of the checklist shaped the flow of the assessment conversation, with topics emerging in the order they appeared on the form. The interview began with an explanation of the service, followed by a question from Andrea about the disposal of (incontinence) pads, then shifted to focus on checklist-related issues, introduced by the therapist's question: 'Has she got access to one toilet?'.

Occupational Therapist begins by asking whether they know anything about the CRT. They do not.

Occupational Therapist:	OK. Well, anyone you would have seen on the ward we have here: occupational therapist, physio, dietician and a doctor should you need it. We have social care manager here who will explain to you in a minute about social care. I am afraid I am going to ask lots of questions to find out what you need from us. Do you have any questions?
Andrea:	I am wearing pads – would you be able to dispose of them?

Occupational Therapist looks a bit confused.

Daughter 1:	Mum does not have a rubbish collection.
Occupational Therapist:	They would normally go in the black bags. Do you have a district nurse allocated?
Daughter 1:	Not to my knowledge.
Occupational Therapist:	Would you like me to speak to the district nurses to see if we can get some bags?
Andrea:	Hopefully it won't be long. It was caused by being in hospital.
Occupational Therapist:	Has she got access to one toilet?
Daughter:	She'll use the one on this floor. It's all designed for her to live here.
Occupational Therapist:	Have you anything to help you get in and out of bed?

There is no response.

Daughter:	No. Mum's a bit deaf.
Occupational Therapist:	Sorry I will speak up. Did the doctors give you a list of medications when you left hospital?

Daughter gets up and brings a bag of medications into the room.

Occupational Therapist:	Do you know if they are all there?
Daughter 1:	There's just what's in the bag. I have checked.

Occupational therapist spends some time checking the medicines – noting that 'it is a relatively simple prescription'.

Daughter 1:	Are there any instructions on how to take them?
Occupational Therapist:	It normally says on them. (Reading): Codeine and Aspirin every day. Can you apply the patches?
Andrea:	Yes.
Occupational Therapist:	So, nothing complicated in there. Are you happy to organise these yourself as we can get the pharmacy to put them all together. Do you know the Dossett Boxes?

Daughter 1 gets up and picks up a box from the side.

Occupational Therapist:	OK you have one. But we can get pharmacy to set this up if you don't want to do it yourself. Have you got an alarm?
Andrea:	No.
Occupational Therapist:	Have you considered one?
Andrea:	I looked at them in the Saga magazine and the price was outrageous!!
Occupational Therapist:	There are other suppliers. I will leave you the information for some.
Daughter 2:	How much?
Occupational Therapist:	Don't quote me but I think it's only a couple of pounds a week.
Daughter 2:	How does it work?
Occupational Therapist:	You can have different services. You can have an emergency response where when the alarm goes off a family member is contacted or a premium service where the call goes into a call centre, and they come out. Obviously, that's more expensive.
Daughter 2:	I think that's a good idea.
Andrea:	Do you wear it around your neck?
Occupational Therapist:	Yes, or on your wrist like a watch.

(There is a reference to Age Concern and how they could come out and offer support)

Occupational Therapist:	You have got a key safe? Are you happy to give us that number and notify us if it is changed?
Daughter 1:	OK.
Occupational Therapist:	How are you fixed for food?
Daughter 2:	OK. Well, we're just going out now as we emptied the cupboards when Mum was admitted. Mum normally goes online, and they deliver it

	and carry it all in for her. Mum has a lady to clean and if necessary, she can help out with the shopping and my sister lives in the city.
Occupational Therapist:	Any recent weight loss?
Andrea:	No.
Daughter (out of sight of the patient and sotto voce):	Yes!
Occupational Therapist:	If you feel it is a problem then you could see the dietician.
Andrea:	I've had an upset tummy since I've been in hospital.
Daughter 1:	So, we'll see how she gets on with home cooking.
Occupational Therapist:	OK but bear in mind you can access the dietician.

Mediated by the Home Safety Checklist, the first part of the interview was designed to enact the patient aligned with a delimited range of issues. While immediate concerns for CRT, the daughters' interjections and off-script disclosures highlight a disconnect between institutional priorities and what mattered to the patient and family.

The interview then shifted to the Brief Falls Assessment, structured into sections covering falls history, the person's functional status, and their need for support with activities of daily living. While the tool could trigger a more detailed assessment if a threshold risk score was reached, this was not necessary in Andrea's case. As with the Home Safety Checklist, the tool's structure shaped the therapist's questioning, with each domain introduced sequentially to guide the conversation.

Occupational Therapist:	Have you had any falls in the last six months?
Daughter 1 (with a hint of sarcasm):	Apart from the obvious one!
Andrea:	Yes. I broke my hip and my toe.
Occupational Therapist:	And before you went into hospital you were managing independently?
Andrea:	Yes. I had some help with the house and some help with the garden.
Occupational Therapist:	Personal care?
Andrea:	No problems.

The assessment tools deployed by CRT were generic, designed to enact a broad patient population in alignment with institutional standards and concerns. The occupational therapist's failure to adapt her line of questioning to Andrea's recent fall – known to all present – elicits a sarcastic response from the daughter, bringing into view the tension between the demands of standardised practice and the ethos of individualised care.

In the third part of the interview, the therapist's questions broadly followed the structure and content of the Unified Baseline Assessment tool, a double-sided A4 document used to evaluate care needs and inform the social care plan. Also incorporated into the Jenolan Admission Proforma (see Chapter 8), the tool was organised into 10 'domains', each associated with a category of concerns. These included:

- **Clinical background** (allergies, weight, medical history, falls, recent hospitalisation, breathing difficulties)
- **Disease prevention** (blood pressure monitoring, nutrition, alcohol, and tobacco use)
- **Mental well-being** (cognition, dementia, substance misuse, mental health)
- **Personal care and well-being** (pain, oral health, footcare, mobility, continence, sleep)
- **Activities of daily living** (washing, dressing, toileting, transfers, eating, decision-making, equipment needs)
- **Sensory needs** (sight, hearing, speech, communication)
- **Relationships** (carer support, caring responsibilities)
- **Safety** (abuse, personal safety, manual handling)
- **Managing in the home** (meal prep, hot drinks, housework, heating, shopping, home care)
- **Immediate environment and resources** (accommodation)

The following extract begins with questions on clinical background and disease prevention, moves on to considerations of personal care and well-being, through immediate environment and sensory needs.

> The questions go on and include issues such as allergies – 'shellfish and feathers', smoking and drinking – 'Twenty cigarettes a day and a glass of whisky at night'. Occupational Therapist requests that Andrea does not smoke when care staff are with her.
>
> *Occupational Therapist:* Have you got any pain?
> *Andrea:* Just in my hip.
> *Occupational Therapist:* Is it stopping you at all?
> *Andrea:* I haven't moved much today.
> *Occupational Therapist:* Is it stiff?
> *Andrea:* Yeah, quite stiff.
> *Occupational Therapist:* Be aware of the need to keep moving about.
>
> Further questions follow about teeth.

Occupational Therapist:	How do you manage your toenails?
Andrea:	They did them for me when I was in hospital.
Occupational Therapist:	Be aware that you can't do them now.
Andrea:	I assume someone can do that for me.
Occupational Therapist:	Well, the NHS list is quite long – six weeks.
Andrea:	I'll have in-growing toenails by then!
Occupational Therapist:	So, it might be better to go privately.
Daughter 1:	Would they come to the house?
Occupational Therapist:	Yes.
Andrea:	How soon until I can bend?
Occupational Therapist:	Six weeks minimum but we will see how you go. Any pressure areas, sore skin?
Andrea:	No.
Occupational Therapist:	No. You usually use the Zimmer frame?
Andrea:	No! It's an aberration! I had a stick before.
Occupational Therapist:	Would you like to get back to that?
Andrea:	Preferably.
Occupational Therapist:	Stair-wise are you OK?
Daughter 1:	She was OK this morning. She walked up those stairs with the ambulance crew coming behind.

[…]

Occupational Therapist:	What about the stairs here?
Andrea:	Yes, but I don't need to use them.
Occupational Therapist:	Do you go out?
Andrea:	Not really.
Occupational Therapist:	You said about the pads. Are there any bowel issues?
Andrea:	Only in hospital.
Daughter 2:	When mum was in hospital, they gave her Codeine which made her constipated and then they gave her loads of laxatives, and this had the reverse effect. So, she doesn't really want to take Codeine.
Andrea:	I used to take Nurofen which was OK as long as I didn't take it with Aspirin.
Occupational Therapist:	If that's what they have prescribed you should really take it.
Daughter 2:	Yes, but if the Codeine causes constipation, then it will need to be reviewed.
Occupational Therapist:	The nurses can come out and review the medications.
Andrea:	The nurse said you can get a pain patch.

Occupational Therapist: OK. Right.
Andrea: But I've not tried yet.

The daughters then say that for the next couple of weeks they will ensure that one of them is with their mother overnight, so she is not on her own.

Occupational therapist asks about glasses and hearing aid.

Andrea: I can't bear hearing aids. I hate anything in my ears.

The therapist's line of questioning largely follows the architecture of the Unified Baseline Assessment tool, advancing through predefined domains that enacted the patient in institutionally recognisable terms. While this structure ensured alignment with standards, it also constrained the conversational flow, flattening complexity and sometimes sidelining the patient's own sense of what matters. Andrea's remarks – by turns dry, resistant, and pragmatic – along with her daughter's interjections, subtly push back against this framing, reasserting the specificity of her situation and priorities.

This extended example offers a rich illustration of how institutional talk unfolds in practice. The occupational therapist set the tone early on, warning the family, 'I am afraid I am going to ask lots of questions to find out what you need from us.' This prefaced an assessment process that was structured, routine, and mediated by universal tools. Yet, as the interaction progressed, it became clear that the patient was not only enacted through the categories and concerns inscribed in the forms, but also through the active interventions of Andrea and her daughters. Their contributions reflected different agendas and priorities, contesting, reinterpreting, or redirecting the institutional script. These moments revealed both the limited scope of the assessment interview as a mechanism of object formation and the asymmetries of agency embedded within it. Whilst the therapist retained structural control – directing the flow and framing what counted as a legitimate concern – the family's responses introduced alternative perspectives and priorities.

Although the assessment tools structured much of the interaction, they were not followed slavishly. The occupational therapist exercised discretion, glossing over components that seemed less relevant or better addressed through other means. For instance, she spent little time on equipment needs listed in the Home Safety Checklist, did not work through the Brief Falls Risk Assessment in detail, and moved quickly through the 'activities of daily living' and 'managing in the home' sections of the Unified Baseline Assessment. These areas were earmarked for more formal evaluation during the functional assessment later in the meeting. In some cases, such as the mental well-being and safety domains, the therapist relied on observational assessments rather than formal questioning. Thus, while the assessment tools were powerful actors in structuring the interaction, therapists did not treat them as rigid scripts, but as prompts that mediated professional practice by prescribing what was institutionally accountable.

Despite the dominant question-and-answer format, the interview also included more discursive and collaborative moments. These typically revolved around the sharing of advice and information, helping the family think through and adjust care arrangements. The occupational therapist offered suggestions on managing medications, setting up community alarms, and accessing chiropody services, while the daughters shared details of existing support for shopping and cleaning. These exchanges not only informed but also enrolled the family into the care infrastructure, positioning them as active participants in bridging gaps in formal service provision.

Medication was a key safety consideration. The therapist took time to confirm that Andrea's prescriptions had been dispensed by the hospital and that her daughters were comfortable supporting administration. Although concerns later surfaced about the Codeine prescription, Andrea's regimen was considered 'relatively simple' for CRT purposes. If patients required social carers to assist with medication, the social care manager was responsible for conducting a detailed needs assessment and developing an administration plan – a complex process often too time-consuming for the initial discharge meeting. In such cases, family members were typically expected to provide interim support.

The second part of the visit focused on agreeing on the level of support required from social carers. Carers could visit up to four times daily (morning, lunchtime, evening, and bedtime) to assist with meal preparation and personal care. Unlike the standardised format of the assessment interview, this stage was underpinned by a person-centred approach to enable the tailoring of services to individual requirements. Yet, while the previous part of the visit highlighted the tensions between standardisation and individualisation, a striking feature of both Geoff and Andrea's visits was the challenges they faced in articulating their specific needs when given a choice. These difficulties were founded on several sources of uncertainty. Most immediately, having been discharged from the hospital in the morning, they simply did not yet know how they would manage. In the first of the following extracts, the discussion centres on Andrea's meal-time support, and in the second extract, it concerns Geoff's personal care.

Occupational Therapist:	What about lunch time?
Andrea:	I don't bother with lunch.
Occupational Therapist:	So, are you happy you could get yourself a drink if you wanted one?
Andrea:	I don't know. I haven't tried yet.

Occupational Therapist:	You could ask the carers to make you a flask when they are here in the morning.

The daughters exchange glances and clearly think this is a good idea.

Andrea:	But I really want to get back on my feet again.
Occupational Therapist:	What about your evening meal. Have you been cooking for yourself?
Andrea:	Well, yes, but I don't know what will happen now. I want things to be as normal as they can.
Occupational Therapist:	Would you like someone to come in and help?
Andrea:	I don't know.
Occupational Therapist:	They can be flexible and if you find you don't need them, then they can withdraw.
Social Care Manager:	Would you be looking for help with washing and dressing?
Geoff:	I don't think so, but I can't tell you now from sitting here on the first day home.
Occupational Therapist:	That's why the team are here, to support you and find out what you can do.

[…]

Geoff:	When I have a history then we can discuss, but right now I have no history.
Occupational Therapist:	What about the shower; is that walk in?
Geoff:	Yes.
Occupational Therapist:	Do you shower daily?
Geoff:	I used to, but I don't know about that now. I couldn't in hospital because I could not take these stockings off.
Social Care Manager:	The carers could help with that.

Andrea and Geoff, in their own ways, expressed uncertainty about the support they would need. Andrea reflected on what she had been able to do before her injury, expressing a desire to return to normal, but was unable to articulate her current needs. Geoff's reference point is the hospital; he highlights the effects of context in mediating his capacity and asserts he cannot know about his capacity to manage at home – his ability to shower, for instance, as this is entirely untested. Both examples highlight the challenges of planning care without an experiential reference point. Neither Geoff nor Andrea had inhabited their postoperative bodies in the home environment. Recognising this uncertainty, the professionals do not press for a definitive answer but offer flexible and responsive arrangements.

Another layer of uncertainty concerned how social care services would be delivered. The management of visits is a well-known concern in home-based care, and much of the discussion in Andrea's case centred on scheduling and organisation. In the following extract, after the occupational therapist reinforces the aim of support as fostering independence, Andrea and her daughters raise concerns about the consistency – particularly the timing of visits and continuity of carer.

Occupational Therapist:	Because this is about rehab then we expect you to do as much as you can. But we could get the carers to come in and help you dry your feet.
Daughter 1:	What is the length of visit?
Social Care:	They can do between seven and nine or after nine.
Occupational Therapist:	But they will stay with you as long as is needed.
Andrea:	Will they come the same time each day?
Social Care:	We can't say a time: it will be between seven and nine or after nine. Do you get up early? Because if we say seven to nine, they have to start somewhere, so it could be seven.
Andrea:	As long as I know when to expect them.
Daughter 2:	Will it be different carers?
Social Care:	They work a rota so there will be different carers because they can't come in the morning and then again in the evening.
Occupational Therapist:	So, they will come out anytime between seven and nine but they will tell you about the day before what time they will be coming the next day. What about lunch time?
Daughter 1:	When will we know their names?
Social Care Manager:	When they come, they will introduce themselves and they will write their names in the book.
Daughter 2:	A common complaint is that there are too many different carers.
Social Care Manager:	You shouldn't get too many different ones.

This exchange illustrates that Andrea and her daughters were not only navigating the logistical aspects of care but also anticipating the emotional and relational impacts of interacting with unfamiliar carers. The occupational therapist's assurances about the flexibility of schedules are juxtaposed with the family's desire for predictability and familiarity, suggesting a deeper unease about being subjected to an impersonal service. This highlights how the presence of carers in the home, while necessary, also serves as a reminder of the tensions between institutional service provision and the status of the home as a private, personal space.

Beyond these uncertainties, CRT's person-centred ethos represented a significant normative shift from the standardisation and routines of acute hospital care. After an extended hospital admission, Andrea and Geoff were unaccustomed to choice.

Geoff: They were so very busy in hospital. It's all automated. They have a, b and c to do. They don't have time to think about the things you are talking about.

The CRT team acknowledged that discharge meetings could be overwhelming for patients, and in practice, the typical response to this uncertainty was to plan high levels of support initially, with the occupational therapist working with home carers on the day after discharge to undertake a formal needs assessment and advise on strategies and aids to foster independence.

Occupational Therapist: Social care manager needs to know when he (Geoff) needs a wash, how to support it, where he does it, and how he needs support for breakfast. But he didn't know, and we will have to go back.

This approach acknowledged the provisional nature of care planning and the need for ongoing adjustment as patients began to inhabit their postoperative bodies at home.

The final part of the discharge visit involved evaluating the patient's functional independence within the home. It involved enacting the patient as a situated object, and focused on mobility, access to essential areas like the toilet and bed, and transfers between bed and chair – key elements for daily safety. Here, object formation was interwoven with practical interventions, including material adjustments and advice, to stabilise the home care infrastructure. In the first extract, we begin with Andrea's functional assessment.

Occupational Therapist tells Andrea she needs to see her walk around. Andrea says she feels very stiff, and this becomes quite evident as she tries to get up from the sofa.

Andrea: I can't get up. I can't manage it!

The effort of standing is clear, and Occupational Therapist has to steady the Zimmer frame and assist Andrea to stand by supporting the small of her back.

Occupational Therapist:	Move the frame forward.
Andrea:	I just need to catch my balance for a moment.

Andrea is clearly unsteady.

Occupational Therapist:	How are you feeling?
Andrea:	Not secure.
Occupational Therapist:	What's the matter?
Andrea:	My knees feel as if they are giving way.
Occupational Therapist:	Have you had this before?
Andrea:	No. Oh, my back's hurting. I've got to sit down I'm afraid.
Occupational Therapist:	Nice and slowly.

What follows is a very uncontrolled descent into the chair.

Occupational Therapist:	Your knees weren't a problem before?
Andrea:	No but I've been in hospital.

There is then a conversation about the need to raise the sofa and how this might be achieved until risers can be fitted tomorrow. The daughter is despatched to find towels and blankets which the Occupational Therapist says are better than cushions as they tend to be 'less squidgy'.

Andrea:	I should be alright. I've just got cold and stiff.
Occupational Therapist:	Shall we try again?

This time things go more smoothly, and Andrea walks from the sofa into the bathroom and then the bedroom. Social Care Manager follows, and Occupational Therapist walks closely with the patient.

Occupational Therapist:	Have you got a long way to walk?
Andrea:	You'll see.
Occupational Therapist:	I am just thinking it might be a good idea to have a stop chair in case you get tired.

Daughter says this is a good idea.

[…]

Daughter 2:	There are so many things to think about. On Monday they told her she was not coming out as she could not stand up well enough.

DA:	What changed things?
Daughter 1 (who has re-entered the room):	I cried, and she cried, so they said we could go.

I asked Daughter 1 how things had gone in the bedroom. She said that the bed was too low, and Andrea could not get up from it, but they have resolved the issue by putting the mattress from 'dad's bed under hers'.

[...]

Daughter 1:	There's no room for a commode in the bedroom and the Zimmer frame.
Social Care Manager:	It's very different in the hospital as the nurses are on hand and everything is the right height.

In this example, the mediating effects of context on Andrea's functional capacity are clear. Notwithstanding her overall stiffness (having sat in the chair since returning home in an ambulance), the low height of the sofa and bed negatively impacts her mobility. Geoff had a similar experience. His discharge was predicated on the assumption that he could use the stairs to access the bedroom and bathroom. Although assessed in hospital, he was unable to manage the stairs at home, which his son described as 'looking like Mount Everest'. In each scenario, the occupational therapist had to take remedial action. She improvised with blankets and a mattress to raise the height of Andrea's chair and bed, and advised Geoff's family to bring a bed downstairs and made alternative arrangements for personal hygiene.

Andrea and Geoff required significant adjustments to their infrastructural arrangements to ensure their safety. For Geoff, some challenges reflected the unanticipated impacts of the home environment on his mobility, but in both cases, there were clear shortcomings in discharge preparations. For example, equipment had been provided, but neither Geoff nor his family knew how to use it – revealing a fundamental information gap in the discharge process.

Occupational Therapist:	I see you're walking on crutches, but have they also given you a frame?
Geoff:	I dunno!
Son:	Yeah – here.

He gets up to look and actually returns with a frame to go over the toilet and not a walking frame which is what the therapist is referring to. The therapist later observed that the family had been given the toilet frame but had no idea what it was or what they were supposed to do with it.

Andrea's case, too, reflected limitations in discharge planning. The initial visit identified several issues which needed addressing – arrangements for disposing of incontinence pads, accessing private chiropody services, and reviewing her Codeine prescription. More notably, there were conspicuous gaps in the physical adaptations to the home.

> Occupational therapist is unimpressed by the lack of arrangements that have been made in Andrea's case. Nothing in the house has been measured and this should have been done prior to discharge either by the family or by a technician. I asked whether they have done the access visit. Occupational Therapist said that if they had done the access visit then there should have been a form. And if they have done it then there is a wider question of why the issues which have been identified today have not been flagged. Occupational Therapist said that ward-based staff often order too much equipment to cover their back and then they have to send items back. This is certainly true in this case. Andrea has been sent home with a commode, but this will not fit into the bedroom and allow space for a Zimmer frame and is probably unnecessary as the toilet is only a short distance anyway. The perching stool in the bathroom blocked the door as there was not enough space.

While all discharge arrangements involved inherent uncertainties, the shortcomings in Andrea's discharge arrangements puzzled me, given my familiarity with the orthogeriatric team and the occupational therapist's role in discharge planning. CRT acknowledged variability in discharge planning quality across the acute sector, but Jenolan was highly respected. There is, however, a reference in Andrea's fieldnote which points to a discharge decision taken at short notice – 'I cried, and she cried, so they said we could go'. Similar indications were present in Geoff's case, which may explain some of these omissions.

Beyond the structured technical components of the visit, object formation also depended on situated sensemaking. CRT staff were highly attuned to reading salient features of the home environment to inform their assessments. Although the admissions folder included multiple detailed proforma, not all were obvious actors in the discharge visit. Rather, their concerns had become integrated into providers' professional vision (Goodwin, 1994). With the exception of the request that Andrea should not smoke when carers were in the house, the Lone Worker Assessment tool (intended to ensure provider safety) was absent from the formal process. Similarly, matters relevant to the Falls and Manual Handling assessments were addressed through the functional capacity evaluation.

> On return to the office the Occupational Therapist said she would now write up the unified assessment, make a case note, fill out a Lone Worker Assessment which 'I have done mentally', complete the 'FROP-Com' (the formal falls assessment tool for older people in the community) – 'I know the falls risk and I have seen his mobility. I'll do a manual handling form too'.

Health and social care providers used these technical and situated enactments of the patient to generate their own formal case records in their respective digital systems. The process was estimated to last about an hour. In the days that followed, the patient was subsequently enacted into the individual professional objects of practice of CRT therapists and social carers.

Object Formation in Occupational Therapy Practice

Occupational therapists typically led the discharge visit, giving them a provisional understanding of the patient and their care needs. Patients were subsequently translated into formal objects of professional practice the day after discharge, through situated, embodied assessments of support needs in daily activities. These enactments were recorded in the healthcare digital system and used to advise social carers on how best to support the patient.

Object formation in CRT occupational therapy differed from that in the acute sector in several ways. As discussed in the previous chapter, orthogeriatric therapists focused on organising socio-material arrangements for discharge, but these relationships were largely untested. In contrast, CRT therapists worked with relational and situated objects of practice. The patient, as an object of practice, was closely tied to their social and physical environment, and the occupational therapist's professional focus was aligned with the real-world connections between the person's needs and the affordances of the home context. Furthermore, whereas the hospital-based OT was focused primarily on immediate discharge plans, the CRT therapist's focus included consideration of longer-term needs, extending beyond CRT provision.

Occupational Therapist 1: 'We are good at thinking beyond the next step [...] these people need someone to take the longer view. So, we look at 3rd sector and Otago involvement and look at what we can do to reduce their need for our help'.

Occupational Therapist 2: 'We have links with Age Connect – their role is to act as a voluntary service broker and look for voluntary and third sector options that could provide services that CRT normally provides. For many the problem is loneliness and isolation. There's also a directory of third sector services, so the idea is to link people into local lunch groups and activity groups such as the stroke association'.

Object Formation in Physiotherapy Therapy Practice

People recovering from hip fracture surgery also received support from CRT physiotherapists. Like their acute care counterparts, they created a database (see Chapter 11) on each new patient. Object formation began with provisional sensemaking, reviewing the initial case entries derived from the discharge meeting, but also the clinical portal. As in the acute sector, details of the surgery were significant matters of concern, and it was important to establish accurate information before planning care.

> Physio 1 said that she would often go back and look at the operation notes. Physio 2 has said this too. Physio 1 said that this would tell her useful things that could have a bearing on her practice. Physio 1 said that one of the most useful information sources was the clinical portal. She said, 'There are not many therapies reports on there, but you get lots of letters and sometimes patients can be poor historians and can't remember what the doctor told them about weight bearing for example'.

The physiotherapists typically carried out an initial in-situ assessment and developed a mobilisation plan. If cases were not complex, then subsequent visits would be delegated to a technician.

> As we walked back to the car, the physio observed that the patient had some degree of cognitive impairment which the Occupational Therapist had picked up on. 'He struggled to process certain things'. But she thinks that the exercises will help him. These will be undertaken by the technician. I asked whether it was normal for the physio to do the assessment and the technician the treatment. She said, 'This is the efficiency of the system. To be fair the techs are good they are band four and five and if it was complex or if there were other things going on, I would go in'.

Object Formation in Social Care Practice

Home care managers formally enacted the patient as an object of practice for social carers. Unlike health settings, where care was organised around nursing plans, social care was framed as a service contract. Managers translated provisional assessments into a Service Delivery Plan, codifying needs, objectives, and preferences into measurable units – visit length, time bands, and specific tasks. Patients signed this documentation, which detailed what carers could and could not do. Patients were thus enacted not only as care recipients but as parties to a formal agreement defining service scope. Similarly, if medication support was needed, managers conducted a detailed assessment using the

Medication Administration Scheme Needs Assessment proforma, leading to a medications administration plan which also required the patient's (or a proxy's) signed consent. Additional documentation was used to define and delegate responsibility for medication support – either to a care worker or, in some cases, to a named family member identified as 'the person liable for medication administration'.

These documentary processes enacted the patient as a *contractual object of practice*, oriented to concerns related to risk, responsibility, and liability. Within this framing, the patient and/or family were positioned – albeit ambiguously – as authorised participants in the organisation of care. While required to sign off on plans, this authority was shaped by the institutional need to distribute liability and standardise tasks. The home care manager occupied a unique role in this process: not simply coordinating services but actively constructing a risk-managed plan of action in which tasks could be safely delegated to non-professional workers within tightly bounded terms. In this way, as an object of social care practice, the patient became the central figure around which both care – and institutional risk – were organised and distributed.

Because I was unable to observe the work of social carers directly or access their completed documentation, I could not follow how these formal enactments were materialised. While the documentary architecture of home care planning reveals a distinctive mode of coordination – one that seeks to stabilise care arrangements through contractual clarity – it is likely, as with ward-based nursing, that care in practice was more responsive, negotiated, or adaptive than the documents suggest.

Object Formation for Collective Decision Making

There was no formal mechanism of team coordination, such as a daily handover, and CRT staff worked largely independently. Nevertheless, a form of loose, dynamic collaboration was sustained through ongoing, informal interactions, enabled by colocation. These interactions enacted the patient as an interdisciplinary object of practice. Social carers regularly reported progress by telephone to social care managers, and participants described a general pattern of shared awareness and continuous conversation.

> *Occupational Therapist:* They are discussing patients all the time; they are all in one building and all on the same floor.

> I went out with the physio on her second visit of the day. The patient in question had already been seen by the Occupational Therapist who'd done both the discharge visit and then a follow up visit. Physio: I've already had a chat with Occupational Therapist about him, and she's picked up a few issues.

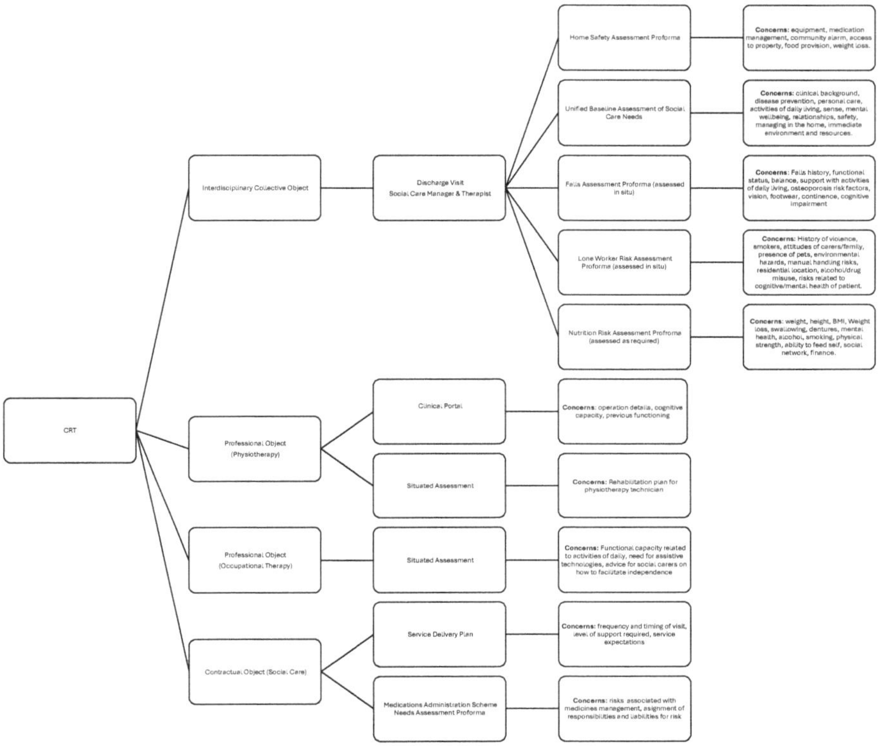

FIGURE 12.1 Object Formation in CRT Work.

Interdisciplinary object formation was fluid and centred on the individual's progression towards independence. Because of capacity limitations, the emphasis was on reducing and withdrawing support as soon as it was safe to do so. A weekly meeting reviewed all cases to determine whether support could be scaled back or whether a longer-term social care package was needed. In this context, object formation for collective decision-making was centred on evolving patient needs within the institutional constraints of the service.

Summary

This chapter has explored the work of CRT, which provided short-term intermediate support for individuals discharged home after hip fracture surgery. CRT's role involved managing the social and material arrangements necessary for a safe transition to independent living. Object formation was incremental. The process began by enacting the patient as a collective object of practice, centred on the relationship between the patient, their functional capacity, the home environment, and social support networks. It was mediated through formal assessment documentation and situated evaluations of the patient's abilities in the home context but also shaped by ongoing negotiations with patients and families as professionals sought to reconcile institutional standards with the specific concerns, preferences, and practical needs of patients and their families. This approach allowed for a preliminary assessment of the discharge plan's safety and the implementation of interventions to stabilise these arrangements as needed. While laying the ground for CRT collaborative work, further, more detailed enactments of the patient were required to support the specific practices and professional accountability requirements of home carers and healthcare therapists. In social care, these enactments were shaped by a distinctive contractual logic, framing care in terms of tasks, time bands, and delegated responsibilities. Figure 12.1 summarises these processes.

CRT work was characterised as 'sorting things out'; and the cases explored in this chapter have highlighted the difficulties of predicting patient need in the home care context, and the complexity and precarity of discharge planning processes.

References

Goodwin, C. (1994). 'Professional Vision'. *American Anthropologist* **96**(3): 606–633.

Mol, A. (2008). *The Logic of Care: Health and the Problem of Patient Choice*. London, Routledge.

Pols, J. (2008). 'Good care: enacting a complex ideal in long-term psychiatry.' *Medische Anthropologie* **20**(1): 73–89.

13

UNSTABLE OBJECTS

Recovery Care Transitions

This chapter considers the organisation of home discharge at the interface between hospital and community services. Home discharges are appreciably more complicated than transfers to institutional environments, because assembling the care infrastructure is integral to the management of transition. This complexity is compounded in hip fracture by the unpredictability of recovery trajectories, uncertain impacts of home environments on need, fragmentation of community provision, and capacity pressures across services. Home care infrastructures involve numerous finely balanced interdependencies. In the hospital, discharge plans often needed adjusting as they evolved, and in the community, further refinements were typically necessary to ensure safety and stability. Transition from hospital to home entailed significant organisational challenges, challenges the infrastructures in the study site were inadequately designed for. The first half of this chapter describes and explains these transition arrangements; the second half illustrates processes in practice.

Transition Arrangements

This section explores the arrangements that mediated trajectory mobilisation and care transfer for home discharge. It begins with the hospital–community interface and the relationships between the orthogeriatric ward team and community providers. It then outlines the complex infrastructure shaping transition, tracing the diverse formal artefacts and processes, and highlighting system gaps. Finally, it examines transition object formation, focusing on the translational work needed to reconfigure the patient from the emergent narrative object of orthogeriatric practice into the discrete technical objects required by community services.

DOI: 10.4324/9781003475019-23

Transition Interface

Transitioning from hospital to home involved managing multiple interfaces with community services. Primary care doctors, responsible for ongoing medical management, were involved in all cases. Many patients also received support from community nurses, particularly for wound care or injections. For most hip fracture patients, however, the primary point of transition from the orthogeriatric ward was the Community Resource Team (CRT)

While both hospital and CRT aimed to support recovery and promote independence at home, their institutional priorities diverged. The orthogeriatric team prioritised returning patients home rather than prematurely recommending residential care, while CRT focused on mitigating home care risks. In the context of delayed discharges, acute sector staff framed the hospital as potentially hazardous – patients decondition and are at risk of a hospital-acquired infection. But for social care providers, compared to intermittent community care, the hospital represented a place of safety. These differences in orientation were a source of tension even *within* the CRT.

Senior Healthcare Leader CRT: 'So, they (social care) do all these safety and risk assessments when healthcare is trying to support people in the community, and this is a source of conflict which comes across in all we do here. We focus on getting people out of hospital and we're under pressure to take people and for social care their priority is keeping people safe and admitting them to hospital is one way of doing that'.

Both sectors faced capacity constraints. In the hospital, this meant a continuous focus on bed utilisation and timely discharge; in CRT, this meant ongoing preoccupation with demand management.

Understanding between acute and community services was uneven. The orthogeriatric ward had strong social world understanding with primary care doctors, community nurses, and CRT therapists. They shared institutional structures, and largely understood the roles, professional logics and working constraints of their community counterparts. By contrast, its relationship with social care services, which operated within local authority structures and was governed by different regulatory standards, was more distant.

Transition Infrastructure

The socio-material arrangements for coordinating home discharge were complex and fragmented across service boundaries. Each interface with a community provider had its own infrastructure. The primary care interface was mediated by a paper-based Discharge Notification Proforma, typically completed by a ward resident doctor, which enacted the patient as a transition object focused on medication management. The community nursing interface was coordinated via a central hub. Ward nurses submitted requests for specific interventions, enacting the patient as a referral object. Requests were routed to the appropriate service by a call operator and screened by a team leader. A structured letter from nurses, outlining care needs, was given to patients on discharge to enact the patient for transition.

The hospital-CRT interface involved a formal referral process and pre-discharge screening. Referrals were faxed using a form which served two purposes: gatekeeping – ensuring patients met reablement criteria (e.g. motivation, independence potential, suitable cognition) (see Chapter 12, p. 231) – and enacting the patient into CRT therapists' and social carers' objects of practice. Immediately before discharge, all accepted referrals were screened by a CRT nurse – working with a standardised checklist – to confirm understanding of needs and readiness for home. As noted in Chapter 8, Jenolan's nursing admission documentation included the Unified Baseline Assessment – a proforma designed to enact the patient into social care objects of practice. Although it had a limited impact on coordinating ward nurses' work in the preoperative period, its completion was a prerequisite for CRT referral and pre-discharge screening.

A key component of transition infrastructure was the Joint Equipment Service (JES), a shared resource between the health board and two local authorities. It enabled hospital-based OTs to order standard equipment directly to patients' homes via a unified electronic system. However, it only served patients within the health board area; discharges outside of this footprint required separate arrangements with local authority equipment services.

While each infrastructure aimed to generate a detailed understanding of the patient for its respective service, they were not configured to ensure trajectory coherence. Despite the complexity and interdependencies of discharge arrangements, no formal document captured the overall plan. Within the acute sector, discharge tasks were distributed across the orthogeriatric team. Frailty nurses oversaw the process, but as plans crystallised, relational intricacies were bracketed off, and the focus shifted to high-level safety- and time-critical tasks. On discharge day, nurses coordinated activity using a checklist. There was no in-person handover with community services and no formal home care plan to share with patients, families, or providers which might have acted as a boundary object to mediate transition.

Transition Objects

As described in Chapter 11, object formation in postoperative orthogeriatric care encompassed broad concerns: the person's hopes, functional capacity, home affordances, social support networks, and the intricate infrastructural arrangements required for safe discharge and continued recovery. Trajectory narratives enacted the patient as a collective object of practice for discharge planning. Regularly rehearsed and revised during thrice-weekly board rounds, these emergent narratives entailed dynamic sensemaking and synthesis. More than the sum of their parts, they produced an interdisciplinary understanding of the patient that was held in common but not formally documented in the patient record.

At the hospital–community interface, transition involved translation of the patient into multiple separate objects of practice, each aligned with the institutional logics of individual services. For primary care, the object focused on medication, for community nursing, on discrete clinical interventions, and for CRT, on allied health and social carer roles, and home safety. In all cases, however, the patient was enacted as a concrete, stable, and specifiable technical object (Rheinberger, 1997).

Reconfiguring the patient from the unstable collective object of orthogeriatric practice into the stable technical objects of discrete community services was a complex translational task. It involved decoupling the comprehensive ward-based understanding and re-enacting the patient in alignment with the specific concerns and institutional logics of individual providers. It also required, fixing emergent trajectories. As discharge plans progressed, the detailed, interdependent narrative constructions of the earlier recovery phases gave way to more fragmented organisation. The patient was increasingly enacted as a technical object focused on the key time-critical tasks of discharge, which were inscribed in the Patient Status as a Glance Whiteboard (see Chapter 11) and the Jenolan discharge checklist.

Transition Processes and Practices

Transitioning from hospital to home involved assembling the individual's care infrastructure, translating the patient from a collective orthogeriatric object of practice into discrete community-based objects of practice, and coordinating arrangements on the day of discharge. The following sections examine these interrelated processes. First, it describes how the home care infrastructure – personal care, rehabilitation, medication, and the physical environment – was organised. Next, it examines the work of aligning care infrastructure interdependencies. Finally, it considers the organisation of transition itself – how transfer of care was enacted, how patients were reconstituted within community services, and how infrastructural arrangements were stabilised post-discharge.

Organising the Home Care Infrastructure

The hip fracture home care infrastructure comprised three pillars: community-based supportive care and rehabilitation, configuration of the physical environment for independent living, and medication administration. Responsibility for these arrangements was distributed: the ward occupational therapist managed home adaptations, equipment, and assistive technologies; the physiotherapist provided mobility aids; resident doctors prescribed medications and liaised with primary care; ward nurses coordinated community nursing referrals and enacted patients for social care; CRT liaison was typically led by frailty nurses or the occupational therapist.

Conditioned by unpredictable recovery and uncertain home environments, care infrastructures were complex and fragile. Progress was monitored during board rounds led by frailty nurses. Occasionally, unforeseen circumstances required adjustments or revised discharge plans, keeping the team's understanding of the patient open and evolving. However, as plans stabilised and discharge approached, this understanding became progressively more fixed and concrete.

Organising Care and Rehabilitation

Discharge following hip fracture typically required ongoing CRT support to assist with daily activities and promote independence. Formal referrals, led by frailty nurses or the occupational therapist, were mediated by a proforma designed to translate the patient into the objects of practice of allied health therapists and social carers. For therapists, this included concerns related to mobility, transfers, toileting, walking, swallowing, and nutrition. For social carers, it covered daily living needs – medication management, hygiene, meal prep, shopping, and home maintenance. The form also required information on the patient's prior functional fitness, current capacity, and long-term goals, along with a section on rehabilitation potential and limiting factors, reflecting CRT's reablement model.

While the orthogeriatric team understood the professional concerns of community healthcare therapists, object formation for social care was more challenging. It first required completion of the Unified Baseline Assessment in the Jenolan Admission Proforma. Ward nurses found this process onerous – primarily due to the translational burdens it imposed. These stemmed from the sheer volume of information required, lack of guidance on form completion, the differing jurisdictions of hospital nurses and social carers, and the uncertain impacts of the home environment in mediating patients' care needs. Frailty nurses, who understood the form's intent, sometimes intervened to expedite the process but lacked the patient-specific knowledge necessary for satisfactory completion of the form.

Social Worker: 'It might say "mobile with assistance of one", but we need more detail than that. What kind of assistance do they need, can they get out of a chair and how is this going to be affected by the new context they are moving to? [...] Staff nurses really know the patients, but they don't have time to complete the UAs (Unified Assessment) so the frailty nurses try to do them, but they do not know the patients that well'.

Referrals were screened at the daily CRT allocation meeting to assess eligibility. A key challenge for acute sector staff was timing. CRT was known to be overextended and operating a waiting list, prompting early referrals to avoid delays. Owing to recovery uncertainty, however, referrals were often rejected as premature, requiring repetition before discharge planning could commence.

DA:	How do you know when someone is ready for CRT referral?
Occupational Therapist:	'From our point of view, it is when the patient is safe to go. If they have the potential to improve, we can keep them here, but of course the aim of CRT is to ensure they improve too. So, it can be difficult to judge. CRT has a waiting list so we are referring sooner rather than later and that carries the risk that they may turn round and say the referral was premature'.

Social carers had a limited scope of practice, and many patients also needed community nursing input. Community nurses provided discrete clinical interventions – wound care, catheter care, injections – for patients unable to attend primary care. Referrals were made by ward nurses through the central hub, where non-clinical call handlers entered the details into the system.

Call handler described her function:	'We are a messaging service – that's all we are. Any medical terms they must spell out as we are not clinically trained'.

The referral information was the only detail available to community nurses before their first visit, and its quality was a frequent frustration.

Community Nurse:	'The information we get is diabolical. It's run by people who are totally non-clinical. [...]. Allergies are rarely filled in; alerts (lone worker safety) are rarely filled in'.

Referrals were screened by the team leader. Like CRT, community nursing was over-extended, but unlike CRT, it did not operate a waiting list.

Community Nurse:	'There is no cap. They just keep adding them. In hospital you get to thirty patients and its full, but they just keep adding to us and something gives'.

Screening was an opportunity to renegotiate unnecessary requests or seek additional information if details were unclear. For example, vague requests such as 'check a wound' were often interpreted as defensive practice – 'the hospital just covering their back'. In such cases, the team leader would contact the ward to confirm concerns. If there were none, she would ask staff to check the wound before discharge and provide the patient with contact details for follow-up if needed.

Both social carers and community nurses operated within delimited scopes of practice, and patients often had needs which fell outside the remit of both services. In such cases, families were often enrolled to bridge the gap. One observed example involved a patient requiring thickened fluids due to swallowing difficulties – a task not classed as a nursing intervention and prohibited for social carers. The issue was resolved by the patient's wife agreeing to feed him.

> Doctors are discussing the challenges of discharging the patient requiring thickened fluids. Orthogeriatrician evidently did not manage to persuade the senior social worker to reverse the decision to refuse to allow social carers to do this and it has been agreed that his wife will feed him.

Unlike hospital care, home care was intermittent. Outside scheduled visits, patients had to manage independently or rely on family. As described in Chapter 11, ward-based trials assessed patients' ability to cope with this discontinuity. Yet there is an inherent tension between the unpredictability of bodily needs and the rigid structure of scheduled care, which often requires interventions to bring the two into alignment. Discharge planning thus became an exercise in disciplining bodily functions to match the rhythms of community care. Continence was a common issue that threatened to destabilise discharge plans, and bladder and bowel training frequently became part of discharge preparation.

> *Orthogeriatrician*
> *(to nurse):* What are her bowel movements like? Can we monitor them please? If she is predictable – say after her porridge – then we can organise a package.

> In one case there is a query about whether the nurses are using the 'flick-flack' on a patient's catheter. Orthogeriatrician explains to the nurse that the woman has a very small bladder capacity, and this needs to be increased if they have any prospect of getting her home.

For some patients, urinary catheterisation was the only option.

The team are talking about the need to support a patient in becoming ready for discharge. The patient can only have four times a day care package and is unable to get to the toilet outside these times. The ward nurses are concerned because she is requesting the bed pan more frequently than this.

Orthogeriatrician: 'She'll need to be catheterised; it's the only way she can go home if she's not transferring.'

These examples underscore that discharge planning was not just about medical fitness and matching services with need, but also about preparing bodies to fit within the constraints of care schedules. Patients and families sometimes faced difficult choices – accepting interventions that might not be clinically necessary, or even desirable, in order to enable home discharge. In such cases, bodily adjustments became the currency through which the aspiration for returning home was realised.

Organising the Physical Environment

Patients discharged home following hip fracture surgery usually require assistive technologies and home modifications to support everyday living. Most were discharged with a walking aid, typically a frame. Certain types of surgery – where the hip had been replaced by a prosthesis in whole or in part – required restricted movement for three months to enable healing and prevent dislocation – no hip flexion beyond 90 degrees, no twisting or crossing the legs. In practical terms, this meant no baths, no driving, no bending, and sitting at the correct height.

To accommodate these restrictions, temporary adjustments to the home or living arrangements were often necessary. If stairs were unmanageable, a bedroom had to be created on the ground floor. Beds might be raised or repositioned to allow entry leading with the unoperated leg. Other adjustments included raising sofas, armchairs, and toilets, or providing commodes where access was limited. More independent patients were equipped with perching stools, grabbers, and long-handled aids for personal care. Some cases required physical modifications, such as installing handrails or key safes for carer access.

Working with the physiotherapist, the Jenolan occupational therapist played a central role in organising discharge resources. This involved tailoring interventions to mediate the relationship between the person's functional capacity and the affordances of the domestic environment – rearranging furniture, installing devices, or modifying bathrooms. Solutions were individualised but constrained by institutional provision. Therapists worked with a limited equipment menu – frames, stools, commodes, grabbers – which they adapted to each patient's needs and environment. The following examples are illustrative: in one case, a patient was provided with a different walking frame to access a narrow bathroom doorway;

in another, where toilet access was impossible with a frame and the patient could not manage without one, a commode was provided as an alternative solution.

> We saw our patient returning from the bathroom. Physiotherapist observed that he had now been given a narrow Zimmer frame because the entrance to his bathroom at home was tight.

Occupational Therapist:	So, we have got to think about the bed coming downstairs so we can set her up from a discharge point of view. The toilet is too small for her to get in there with a frame.
Son:	There are rails in there.
Physiotherapist:	She needs a walking frame, but we might be able to get around that. It might be that she needs a commode or both – perhaps for at night when your dad is upstairs.

Except for mobility aids, which were the responsibility of the physiotherapist, the occupational therapist organised all equipment, assistive technologies and home modifications. For patients resident within the health board footprint, this entailed placing an order through JES; for out of area patients, this entailed navigating a complex ecology of providers and services.

> Occupational Therapist talked about the challenges of Mountain Local Authority patients. 'It seems to be such a complex system, and I am never sure whether they will accept a referral. There's always a delay in sorting things out. My heart sinks when I find out it's a Mountain Local Authority patient'.

Occupational Therapist:	'What it takes time to learn is what services are available and what you can get from where. It's just trial and error basically'.

Resources took time to arrive. Given the inherent uncertainties in recovery trajectories, the modus operandi was to order everything that might be needed to cover all contingencies. This approach was not always welcomed by patients and as described in Chapter 12, could result in mismatched provision, but last-minute decisions about additional support needs could create delays.

> Occupational Therapist notices the daughter has arrived on the ward and we take her the equipment – this includes two toilet raisers and a perching chair. I helped carry them.

Patient is not hugely impressed.

Patient:	What's *that*?!
Occupational Therapist:	It's a perching chair, let me show you.
Patient:	I don't need that I've got a couple of stools.
Daughter:	It might be handy for you.

Patient acquiesces.

The occupational therapist also worked closely with families, who had a key role in preparing the home for discharge. She advised on reorganising living space, sourcing additional assistive technologies beyond standard provision, and installing equipment.

Occupational Therapist:	Lose rugs, you'll need to get rid of all those and you might need to move the furniture a bit so she can get around with the frame. If you're purchasing a bed, the mattress needs to be twenty inches from the top to the floor. Do you need any help to move furniture?
Son:	No, we're fine.
Frailty Nurse:	So, we need the bed to be in place and the commode.
Occupational therapist:	I'll order all the bits.

Occupational Therapist is at the desk, leafing through a set of notes when she is approached by the daughter of the patient we saw this morning. As far as Occupational Therapist is concerned the assessment has been completed and the orders and referrals made. The daughter is concerned as the patient 'has no lap' and will be unable to access the dining room as there is a step up. She has come to establish whether she can be provided with a table. Occupational Therapist explains that she cannot provide this kind of equipment but makes suggestions as to where the family might purchase an inexpensive table: Argos, Ikea, The Range.

Occupational Therapist takes the daughter into the bathroom to demonstrate how to fix the toilet raiser to the pan. She tells her to 'tighten these up so it's nice and firm; so, it gives her another couple of inches. It needs to be very solid because what she does is this – she pushes her hand behind her bum'.

These interactions underscore the practical and organisational complexity of preparing the home for discharge. While occupational therapists worked within equipment and service constraints, their role involved assembling resources tailored around each patient's spatial, functional, and social context. This required not only technical and local service knowledge, but also negotiation with families, and attentiveness to the contingencies of post-discharge recovery.

Organising Medication Management

All patients were discharged with medications, commonly referred to as 'TTHs' (to take home). Some received a limited hospital pharmacy supply; others required blister packs – pre-packaged doses arranged by time of day to support adherence. Blister packs were essential for patients on multiple medications or with cognitive impairment, and necessary when social carers were involved in their management, as they could prompt patients to take medications only from blister packs, not individual containers. Since the hospital pharmacy did not dispense blister packs, these had to be prepared by community pharmacies, requiring advance orders.

Families were routinely involved in medication management. Because social carers could not administer 'as required' medications, families often filled this gap. Many patients were also discharged on Clexane, a post-surgical anticoagulant injection. While self-administration was possible, it was often impractical. Given the 30-day course and limited community nursing capacity, the hospital had a policy of training family members to administer it.

Ward nurses coordinated discharge medication arrangements. When families agreed, nurses taught injection techniques. They also worked with resident doctors to ensure prescriptions were correctly formatted and ready on discharge day. Nurses educated patients and carers – typically through verbal instruction, or, in complex cases, by completing a 'green form' to guide ongoing medication use.

Aligning Infrastructural Arrangements

The orthogeriatric team engaged in continuous tinkering (Mol, 2008; Pols, 2008) with the evolving discharge infrastructure, adjusting arrangements to align bodies, needs, materials, and home environments. Seemingly minor issues or mundane elements often had disproportionate impacts on discharge feasibility, and unanticipated challenges frequently prompted major re-evaluations. For one patient, it was the difficulty of managing a continence pad without assistance that jeopardised the plan:

Patient explains to Orthogeriatrician:	'The problem I have when the carers are not there is when I need to go to the toilet. I wear pads and I manage to get on the toilet but when I get up, I struggle to get round there to pull the pad up'.

For another, it was the unpredictability of stoma functioning. The patient wished to return home but lacked the dexterity and eyesight to manage the stoma independently.

Orthogeriatrician:	The problem is with the stoma bags. We don't know whether carers will manage them, and we don't know when it (the stoma) will work. Carers come at certain times and it's no good if it works after they have gone. If the carers can't come in, I am not sure whether the district nurses have the resources. So, these things need clarifying.

The patient says her daughter would be able to help.

Orthogeriatrician:	It's a big undertaking. If the carers will take it on, we have a chance but if not, we may need to think about a care home. It depends where you would be happy. In an ideal world where would you be happiest?
Patient:	Home.
Orthogeriatrician:	Let's look at the options for getting home and give it a really good go, and we can practice the sort of care you would have at home here and see if it will work.
Outside the room, orthogeriatrician observes to the registrar:	She's going to really struggle at home.

This fieldnote, taken from a ward round, highlights both the team's uncertainty about community services' responsibilities and the challenges of responsively meeting needs with discontinuous provision. Though the patient expressed a strong desire to return home, the team privately doubted its feasibility.

The viability of many arrangements was dependent on family involvement. As discharge plans became more concrete, families sometimes reassessed their capacity to provide support. In one case, an acute episode of confusion led a daughter to withdraw her agreement to a home discharge:

Nurse:	Elizabeth Reynolds – we still do not know what's happening there. She was going home but the daughter has said 'no' as she's not walking.
Occupational Therapist:	We'll have a word with the daughter this afternoon. She can't walk alone.
Physiotherapist:	It depends on what she's expecting.

Occupational Therapist: She's having CRT.

Physiotherapist: It's still big chunk of day without anything and if the daughter feels she cannot cope.

Nurse: There was a problem yesterday with the buzzer or something as when we went in to her, she had been incontinent of faeces and was covered. It was everywhere, all over her, all over the chair, in her hair…

Physiotherapist: She has episodes of not knowing what is going on but are they treating her for a UTI (urinary tract infection) or anything? I don't blame her daughter if that's the case. She's got her husband to care for as well and she is probably concerned that she cannot do a good job. If she's lucid and just sat in her chair between calls that's fine, but if she's getting up and about then it's not feasible.

In another case, the patient was to be discharged to her son's home, with the living room repurposed as a bedroom. But the house was small, and the daughter-in-law expressed concern about the wider impacts of these plans.

Nurse: Donna Davis – she's supposed to be going home, but apparently her daughter-in-law is not happy about setting things up for her downstairs […] I think she has reasonable concerns. It's a small house and she's concerned about the logistics – it's a big thing to lose the living room.

These examples show how discharge planning transforms the home into more than just a space for recovery – it becomes a site of logistical coordination, emotional negotiation, and ethical tension. As family members are cast as central agents in ongoing care, their willingness and capacity may shift in response to clinical developments, practical constraints, and uncertainty. The boundaries of care – who provides it, where, and under what conditions – are constantly being renegotiated.

Many hip fracture patients had previously relied on family support, but hospital admission often exposed concerns about its sustainability. In one case, a patient with a long history of falls had been supported by her niece. A pattern of cancelling community services had shifted the burden of care onto the family, becoming untenable. During a discharge planning meeting, the niece spoke at length about the cumulative toll of repeated admissions. Only when directly asked by the doctor did she explicitly state that she could no longer continue.

The niece and her husband are the main carers [...] Doctor invites the niece to offer her perspective on the situation. She describes a long history of multiple admissions to hospital with discharge back home. There have evidently been previous attempts to provide carers who have been rejected after a short period of time with much of the burden of ensuring the aunt's well-being falling on the niece. The niece talks in detail about the features and circumstances of each hospital admission. Reference is made to arthritis, falls, cardiac issues, long term pain.

Niece:	Each time she is discharged they allocate a social worker and a package of care, but you have to pin her down to agree to it and then you get her home, and she cancels it.

[...]

Resident Doctor:	I know this will sound like a horrible question, but if you could, would you rather walk away and not be involved in her care?
Niece:	To be honest I would walk away now.

At this point the niece becomes tearful.

Resident Doctor:	I know it's horrible to say but it's better to be honest about these things.
Frailty Nurse:	It's more helpful for planning.

As described in Chapter 11, board rounds were the primary mechanism for coordinating action and decision-making within the orthogeriatric team. A collective understanding of each patient was constructed through collaborative care trajectory narratives. While discharge plans remained unsettled and arrangements were still evolving, these narratives functioned as epistemic objects – marked by indeterminacy, disagreement, and ongoing development (Knorr Cetina, 1997). As plans crystallised, these emergent constructions stabilised into boundary objects (Star and Griesemer, 1989), flexible but more settled understandings, which enabled individual team and family members to progress their respective responsibilities. However, as the discharge approached, these enactments shifted again – this time towards reductionist, task-oriented concerns – transforming the patient into a technical object of practice focused on time-critical discharge tasks. This shift is evident in the following exchanges.

Frailty Nurse:	Lorna Jones.
Orthogeriatrician:	She's doing amazingly.
Frailty Nurse:	For CRT.

Orthogeriatrician:	[...]
Frailty Nurse:	Can I tick her as medically fit?

Here, a positive but open-ended narrative judgment about progress ('doing amazingly') is rapidly translated into an institutional category – medically fit. Enacted through the ticking of a box, the patient is configured as a technical object, mediated by standardised discharge criteria.

Orthogeriatrician:	Christine Williams.
Frailty Nurse:	This lady's waiting for a commode.
Nurse:	They wouldn't accept a referral from the physio.
Orthogeriatrician:	She can go today.
Nurse:	Can she go before the commode's delivered? Does she need two because she can't do the stairs?
Physiotherapist is looking in the notes and reads:	'The plan's for home, bed downstairs. So, she needs the commode before she can go.'
Frailty Nurse:	Can you chase?
Occupational Therapist:	I will chase in a moment.

In this exchange, the patient is enacted primarily through her equipment needs. While the broader discharge plan remains implicit, professional attention is directed to a discrete logistical problem. Coordination of care becomes oriented around a single task, with each actor contributing to the resolution of that immediate constraint.

Organising Transition

Once discharge plans were agreed and infrastructural preparations underway, trajectory mobilisation involved enacting patients as multiple transition objects across community services, coordinating the hospital-to-home transfer, and stabilising the socio-material arrangements for ongoing care. This section examines these processes in detail.

Object Formation for Discharge

Discharge required translating the patient from the collective object of orthogeriatric practice into discrete transition objects aligned with CRT, primary care, and community nursing services.

As discharge approached, the CRT screening nurse contacted the ward by telephone and used a structured proforma to generate a transition object.

The aim was to assess the safety and readiness of the discharge plan and gather information relevant to CRT practice. As noted in Chapter 12, CRT did not have access to the full acute care patient record, making the screening documentation an important source of background information for the discharge visit.

The proforma reflected the distinct clinical and occupational logics of therapists, home carers, and formal safety protocols. It comprised 25 questions, aligned with the objects of practice of social carers (personal care needs, meal preparation, oral hygiene, toileting, medication management, and continence care) and CRT therapists (mobility, transfers, walking, sleeping arrangements). Cognitive functioning – relevant across all provider groups – was also assessed along with practical questions about home infrastructure (entry, key safe, equipment, community alarm, food), staff safety considerations, and the involvement of other agencies.

Knowledge necessary to enact a CRT transition object was distributed across the orthogeriatric team. There was no shared proforma in the patient's medical record to systematically detail discharge plans. The CRT screening proforma was not available on the ward, where it could have functioned as a coordinating and accumulating device (Berg, 1997). Screening calls were unscheduled, and the ward representative often lacked the necessary information to answer all questions. This could result in inaccuracies in object formation, or delays in the process while gaps and uncertainties were addressed.

CRT Therapist: 'If you screen you get three stories: one from the patient, one from the nurses, and one from the therapists'.

When I suggested making the CRT proforma available to the orthogeriatric team, participants underlined the importance of the conversation in generating a shared understanding of the patient. Nevertheless, although shared sensemaking is a powerful mechanism for constituting transition objects, these particular arrangements were most likely a legacy effect of earlier practices when CRT staff screened patients in-person – a resource-intensive approach discontinued because of capacity issues.

Object formation for primary care and community nursing was hospital-led and less complex. Resident doctors completed the Discharge Notification Form – an A4 carbonated document producing four colour-coded copies: yellow (for pharmacy), pink (for the consultant), blue (for the case notes), and white (for primary care). It included diagnosis, procedures, and TTH medications (dose, frequency, route), but had limited space for inpatient care details. As noted in Chapter 11, medications were often adjusted during admission to manage falls risk or initiate osteoporosis treatment. Yet, the form lacked space to explain these changes – which was critical information for primary care.

CRT Nurse: 'I had a very angry GP whose patient's medications had been changed in hospital. She said that they had no idea of how hard they had worked to get her (medications) sorted out before she was admitted'.

The Discharge Notification Form was designed to meet a range of institutional requirements – clinical, administrative and legal but, as Bowker and Star (1999) note, multi-purpose documents often fail to meet specific user needs. The result was a form both overloaded and underspecified: sufficient for pharmacy and hospital use, but inadequate for conveying clinical reasoning to GPs.

Ward nurses enacted patients as transition objects for community nursing. In addition to submitting information to the central hub, they prepared a 'district nurse letter', which was given to the patient at discharge. This was a loosely structured document, which enacted patients in alignment with the delimited concerns related to the reason for the referral, for example, wound management, medications administration, and catheter care.

*

While the complexity of transition infrastructures varied, all faced challenges with information quality. The primary care interface relied solely on the discharge form. There were limited opportunities for joint sensemaking with community nursing. CRT nurses valued the screening conversation, but its effectiveness depended on the ward representative having access to the required information

Organising the Transfer of Care

While discharge planning was distributed across the orthogeriatric team, ward nurses coordinated arrangements on the day. As one frailty nurse explained:

> 'It takes somebody to focus on getting everything they need to get them out safely, because nobody thinks it's their responsibility – 'I'm the doctor, I sorted that out, do their prescription,' and the nurse will go, 'Well, I'll refer to community nurses,' but someone just to pull all that together is often needed […] for making sure that process is safe'.

This work was mediated by a Discharge Checklist – a single A4 sheet itemising tasks to be signed off. Like all checklists, it black-boxed (Latour, 2005) the considerable labour required to reach the point of discharge. Intended for use in all discharges, it brought together logistical, clinical, and safety-related tasks, including:

- confirmation of the discharge date and that the patient and family had been informed
- assurance that the patient had a key or someone available to provide home access
- timing details for residential or nursing home discharges and ambulance bookings
- medication arrangements, including whether the patient could self-medicate or required blister packs
- occupational therapist confirmation that equipment was in place and, if needed, that a second Zimmer frame had been arranged for upstairs use
- installation of community alarms and key safes
- assessment of pressure-relieving and continence needs
- community nursing referrals, including confirmation that referral letters had been completed.

On discharge day, additional checks included medical approval, therapy completion, cannula removal, wound assessment, and if Clexane was prescribed – completion of a Community Medication Chart and provision of a Sharps Bin for needle disposal.

Activity was intense. The following extracts illustrate the pressures on staff. In the first, a staff nurse is finalising documentation after the patient has already been moved to the Discharge Lounge – a facility intended to free up acute beds by providing care for patients awaiting transport. In the second, a relatively inexperienced staff nurse is managing three discharges simultaneously and becomes visibly stressed when one patient reports, at the last minute, that they require ambulance transport.

> Nurse is currently doing the documentation for a patient who is being discharged today.
>
> *Nurse:* I was told this was done in handover and it's not been done. I am mopping up the bits that have to be done. It is very time consuming.
> *DA:* Is the patient ready to go?
> *Nurse:* They're in Discharge Lounge!
>
> I asked what documentation was involved.
>
> *Nurse:* The Clexane documentation and community drugs chart.
>
> A few minutes later, I observed Nurse working through the discharge checklist, ticking things off. She pauses, 'She's still got a cannula in!'. (To frailty nurse):This is what happens when you take them before I am done!

Staff Nurse makes a phone call to Discharge Lounge and asks if they will check her patient and whether they are able to remove the cannula for her.

Nurse (Northside) has returned and has a deflated expression:	Now [name] says he has no transport and can he have an ambulance!
Senior Nurse:	Where does he live?
Nurse:	I don't know.
Senior Nurse:	Don't panic, let's go and look. It might be he can go on [name of patient]'s ambulance.
Nurse:	Three discharges!!!! I am not having any admissions!

As described earlier, discharge marked a shift from the patient as a narrative object – attuned to the intricacies of life and recovery – to a technical object reduced to checklist tasks. Despite the interdependent and fragile nature of these arrangements, there was no integrated discharge plan or in-person handover at key interfaces. There was no collective enactment of the patient as a transition object – only a sequence of tasks to be ticked off.

Stabilising Infrastructural Arrangements

Planning discharge was inherently uncertain due to the complexity of home environments, evolving patient needs, and fragmented community services.

Hospital Occupational Therapist:	'It's positive risk taking. Which means three "Hail Marys" and keeping your fingers crossed'.
CRT Occupational Therapist:	'With the best will in the world, the hospital can't always predict what they are going to be like at home. [...] But when they are at home, we see things from a different perspective'.
CRT Occupational Therapist:	'The trouble is though there can be a gap between referral and patient transferring. For our part, we don't know what we're dealing with until we see them'.

Despite the hospital's extensive efforts, stabilising home care arrangements was a necessary component in the management of transition. Most cases required action on the part of community services to ensure safety and integration. Community nursing was 'never just about the task' but entailed invisible work to (re)organise arrangements to ensure safe care; without which many discharges would have failed. And as we saw in the previous chapter, a significant proportion of CRT work involved 'sorting things out', both in response to evolving patient need, but also in the immediate management of transition. Discharge visits were significant events, intended to enact patients for CRT work, but also to ensure the safety of arrangements. Spanning all three pillars of discharge plans – care organisation, material arrangements and medications management – stabilising interventions ranged from tinkering and adjustments to finesse arrangements, modifications and remedial actions designed to address safety risks and bridge gaps in provision, through to significant revisions of the original plan.

At discharge, arrangements were largely untested. Home visits pre-discharge was rare because of resource constraints, and planning relied largely on reported information. Equipment was a recurrent problem. CRT staff noted frequent problems with inappropriate or excessive equipment.

CRT Therapist: 'We did an audit on whether equipment had been appropriately provided [...] and there were lots of problems'.

While discharge plans were personalised, they were negotiated within institutional constraints, such as delivery schedules, and stock availability. Therapists often ordered every conceivable item to avoid delays, even when relevance was uncertain. For example, Andrea's bedroom could not accommodate both a commode and walking frame. Although manageable in her case because of the proximity of the bedroom and toilet which obviated the need for a commode, such limitations could significantly impact the feasibility of discharge arrangements. Gaps in provision, was another recurrent issue. Andrea had not been provided with risers to increase the height of her sofa and bed. Unclear whether these had not been ordered or undelivered because of an early discharge, the therapist improvised with blankets and towels to raise the sofa and an additional mattress to bolster the bed.

Families were integral components of home care infrastructures, and there could be misplaced assumptions about their ability to help a person's on-going care. Willing caregivers could later struggle with fulfilling their part in the network of relations, leading to crises.

Nurse 1: 'When they see a family member on the ward for an hour, they might think they seem OK but then it turns out that they are forgetful and can't help'.

Infrastructures had to be aligned with individual need, yet predicting how patients would manage at home was difficult. Functional assessments conducted within the controlled hospital setting did not always translate to the home environment. As illustrated in the previous chapter, Geoff's care arrangements had to be revised when he was unable to manage the stairs. In that scenario, the occupational therapist found a temporary solution, but such adjustments were not always feasible, threatening the discharge viability.

I learned of several cases where, despite formal ward-based assessments, patients proved unable to manage.

CRT Occupational Therapist: [name] one has got to back in. He's ninety-two, on his own, a double hander (requires two carers to mobilise). He's got to go into respite.

CRT Physiotherapist: We had one like that before. They knew it was difficult discharge, but he presented quite differently on the ward. When he got home, he was disoriented in time and place, couldn't mobilise or access the bed or the toilet. So, he went back in.

Both acute sector and community professionals recognised that hospital assessment and planning could only go so far in anticipating the real-world challenges a patient faced once home. While the goal was to support patients in the least restrictive setting, these decisions carry risk and must be continually revisited in response to the dynamic, often unpredictable, nature of post-discharge care. The CRT discharge visit was a critical checkpoint for ensuring the safety and sustainability of care arrangements.

Medication management was a 'massive issue' for the CRT and closely attended to during discharge visits. Andrea's medications were straightforward, but Geoff's were more complex. He was discharged with medications provided by the hospital pharmacy: Warfarin, which is taken in a variable dose depending on the patient's INR (blood clotting) results, and Paracetamol and Gaviscon, both taken as required for pain relief and heartburn respectively. He had also been prescribed regular medications, dispensed in blister packs by the community pharmacist. A significant proportion of Geoff's visit was spent making sense of these arrangements and explaining them to the family.

Occupational Therapist: Have you got any tablets?

Geoff: Yeah.

Occupational Therapist: Have you got blister packs?

Daughter: They should be here today. Something was delivered last week I don't know what these are.

She leaves the sitting room to locate them, and while she is gone, the therapist asks the patient about his weight and appetite.

Daughter:	This is what was delivered' (hands blister pack to Occupational Therapist).
Occupational Therapist:	It's not normal to deliver so early. We should wait to see what is delivered today and then take that one back to the pharmacy.

They look closer at the blister pack, and the daughter informs Occupational Therapist that these were delivered a day after the patient went into hospital for the surgery. So, they are clearly a repeat prescription.

[...]

Occupational Therapist:	OK. So, you are taking Warfarin. That won't be in the blister packs as it is a variable medication. Are you OK to take your medications?
Geoff:	I have been. The hospital wasn't sure if I would be OK. But they don't explain anything they just say take these home and put them all in the bag and hand it to you!

Occupational Therapist looks at the bag of medications the patient has returned with from hospital. It includes a blister pack which has been started.

Occupational Therapist:	Are these the medications you went in with?
Geoff:	I didn't go in with any.
Occupational Therapist:	In here there is Warfarin, Paracetamol and Gaviscon. The Warfarin is variable, so it means taking what is in the blister pack and what he's on. It should be on here (she shows the son the yellow Warfarin booklet).
Social Care Manager:	We can help with that.
Daughter:	The medications should be the same as before unless they have changed.
Geoff:	I just don't know. I had two hours' notice that I was going home. They didn't discuss them; they just put them in the bag. They don't tell you anything.
Occupational Therapist:	I suggest you ring the ward or the GP.

Together the son, daughter and occupational therapist are trying to work out what the current Warfarin dose is – they scrutinise the yellow booklet together.

Occupational Therapist (pointing to the test): I think it's telling you that he has got to take two milligrams those days then he'll need a blood test. There's a letter there, so the district nurse is coming in. So tomorrow two milligrams.

Daughter: I would take it then that he's had today's.

Occupational Therapist: I couldn't tell you. You'd better call the ward.

Daughter: OK I'll do that.

[...]

Occupational Therapist empties the medications out of the bag.

Occupational Therapist: There's a yellow booklet there which tells you what Warfarin to take but you need to call the ward to see what he has had today, painkillers which can be taken two every four hours but not to exceed eight in twenty-four hours (she is reading from the bottle), there is Gaviscon for heartburn, and the rest will be in blister packs. There is [name] for your bowels.

Patient says he stopped taking this yesterday.

[...]

Occupational Therapist (to son): That is the letter for the GP and so if that is a new prescription then, the sooner they get this then the better.

The son is still confused about the Warfarin.

Son: So, he gets the Warfarin in the blister packs, but the hospital has given it.

Occupational Therapist: No. It's not in the blister packs because it is a variable drug.

Son: So, he hasn't taken any today?

Occupational Therapist: I don't know.

Son: I'll call the hospital then.

Geoff's medication management was complex: it involved variable dose Warfarin, as required medications, and regular blister pack prescriptions.

Complications arose because the hospital included an old blister pack in his discharge medications, while a new one – clearly a repeat prescription – had been delivered to the home during his admission. As Geoff's case illustrates, when people are discharged with medications dispensed by the hospital, they enter a preconfigured world, which is not accounted for in discharge planning. My conversations with community services staff indicated this was a recurrent issue.

> *CRT Nurse:* 'I had to go in and see a couple who were taking their own medications from blister packs, and I went in, and it was only Tuesday and the whole weeks' worth was gone. Part of the problem is that pharmacy don't collect the old ones, they just deliver the new ones. So, they don't know if they have not been taken'.

Beyond medication management, advice and information were central to ensuring the coherence of discharge arrangements. Yet, conspicuously absent from the discharge checklist, responsibility for this work was distributed across the orthogeriatric team, often delivered incrementally and informally. As a result, key details could be overlooked, leaving community providers to fill the gaps. Geoff had been given a frame to place over the toilet, but the family appeared unaware of its purpose. Written instructions from the physiotherapist on stair use with crutches were also present, but neither Geoff nor his family referred to them during the failed stairs assessment.

> As this is going on I noticed some printed instructions for using crutches to go up the stairs and come down. These include instructions on which leg to lead with and whether to put the crutch on the stairs first or second. In addition, there are instructions to the family about supporting the patient to walk, which include drawing attention to the fact that he has a tendency not to place all his foot on the stair tread. Outside in the hall, these instructions are not being followed. Someone has found a 'stair crutch' but nobody seems to know what to do with it and when I went into the hall to see how he was managing, Geoff was coming downstairs without crutches but holding on to the banisters. Progress is slow and Geoff is obviously tired.

While all discharge arrangements were finely balanced, some were especially fragile – colloquially referred to as 'Ker-plunk plans'. Borrowed from the children's game, the metaphor captures the precariousness of arrangements where the removal of a single element can trigger a cascade of failure. Ensuring safety in such cases required more than minor adjustments; it demanded full reconfiguration of the care infrastructure. Yet, this was made difficult by fragmented information and the absence of a shared, integrated plan.

The following example illustrates these challenges. During a CRT discharge visit, a patient was found to be disoriented and unable to manage her medication. The team determined she needed support from social carers, which required medications to be dispensed in blister packs. Although community nurses do no typically manage medications, they agreed to assist temporarily until the blister packs were available. However, the GP refused to prescribe the necessary drug, citing inadequate information in the discharge letter. Eventually, a community consultant intervened.

Nurse 1: 'Only last week we had an issue with a lady who was one hundred and three and it took us four days to sort out. She was discharged home from hospital having been admitted with shortness of breath [...] She was sent home on a diuretic – a new one – I can't remember what it was. She didn't have blister packs but after her stay in hospital she was bit disoriented and so I phoned the GP and asked if he could prescribe the diuretic for the district nurses to give over the weekend, until we could sort out the blister packs. He refused. He looked at the discharge letter and there was nothing on there about why she was discharged with the drug. I looked on the clinical portal and she had an Echo (echocardiogram) suggesting heart failure. He still refused. So, we did all the groundwork with the district nurses who said they would do it, but we had to ring the ward and find the doctor who had discharged her and ask whether she could go without over the weekend. He said "no". Then I spoke to the consultant in the community team who wrote the drug chart, and I went and picked it up and gave it to the district nurses to do at the weekend. It shouldn't be up to us to sort all this out'.

It is uncertain whether the hospital failed to order blister packs or whether the patient's disorientation emerged only after discharge. What is clear is that the GP's refusal to prescribe the medication – based on inadequate documentation – stood in stark contrast to the flexibility shown by community nurses and the CRT's efforts to find a solution. This case illustrates the fragility of discharge arrangements and how minor changes – or the (in)actions of key individuals – can have significant consequences.

Transition and the Trouble with Unstable Objects

Organising home care infrastructures was inherently complex and uncertain. Patients transitioning from hospital to home were not stable or settled entities, but unstable objects – with shifting needs, capacities, and environments. Yet, the transitional arrangements designed to support discharge sought to translate them into technical objects, aligned with the discrete institutional functions of community services: immutable mobiles – fixed, stable, and recognisable across organisational boundaries (Latour, 1987). While this translation was administratively expedient, it obscured the contingent and relational nature of recovery and overlooked the interdependence of infrastructural arrangements that shape and sustain care across settings.

These tensions were not limited to the moment of discharge itself but reflected deeper systemic issues embedded in the design of transition infrastructures at the acute–community interface. Discharge represents a critical juncture in the care trajectory – one that demands responsiveness and adaptability. Yet, the system was structured around assumptions of stability, distributing responsibility across multiple providers and, in doing so, decentring the patient. This mismatch between the organisational demands of transition and the rigidity and fragmentation of infrastructural arrangements undermined integrated care. In this context, the CRT's role in stabilising discharge was not ancillary but central.

This tension between unstable objects and inflexible structures also had significant implications for capacity. The unpredictability of recovery trajectories meant that CRT staff deliberately delayed screening until a few days before discharge, aware that patients' conditions could shift rapidly. As one nurse explained

> We are full this week. There's one slot or two per day and more patients waiting than we can fit in. If I screen today, the situation can change, and I won't achieve anything by screening for next Monday. One week is a long time – particularly with the elderly who can fluctuate. You get a phone call on the day of discharge to say that they are not well.

Even though last-minute cancellations were common, the system lacked the flexibility to routinely escalate new cases and reallocate discharge visit slots, negatively impacting both CRT and hospital capacity. On one day during fieldwork, two available slots went unused – one due to a patient becoming unwell the day before, the other to equipment delays. The following day, a further slot was cancelled.

> Today has been a frustrating day for the team. Two of the slots available to support hospital discharge have been wasted. One was cancelled yesterday as the patient became unwell, and it was too late to fill the slot.

> We got back to base about midday, and I went to get some lunch from the shop, returning to the CRT office. Here it was decided that I would follow the occupational therapist to do a discharge visit this afternoon. Four had been on the whiteboard this morning. One was home care only, and one of the three full team visits had been cancelled. This is another wasted slot.

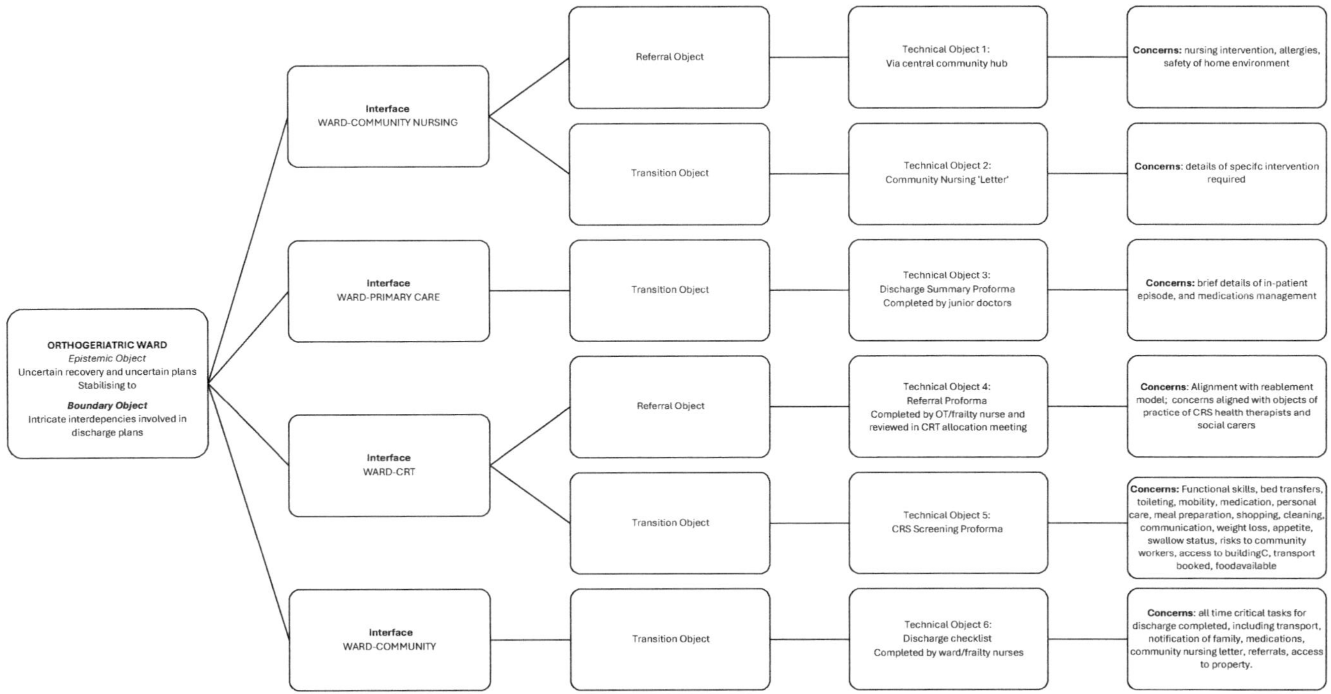

FIGURE 13.1 Transition arrangements in the recovery assemblage.

These observations may reflect a particularly difficult period for the service. However, even within a limited window, the frequency of unused discharge slots stood out as a striking inefficiency. In a context of constrained capacity and high demand, the system's inability to accommodate patients as mutable mobiles resulted in wasted resources and increased pressure on both hospital and community services.

In Wales, policy promotes new discharge pathways which aim to reduce hospital stays by shifting assessment and care planning into the community (NHS Wales Delivery Unit, 2021). As this study has shown, predicting patient requirements in the home environment from the hospital setting is inherently challenging, but assembling arrangements de novo at the point of discharge, presumes that services have both the capacity and the systems in place to support agile and responsive approaches. It also assumes clarity around the roles and responsibilities of community providers and the availability of informal support – particularly from family members – whose contributions are often taken for granted but remain critical to the viability of home-based care. While there have been investments in community provision in Wales since this study was undertaken, in the absence of integrated planning mechanisms that can accommodate the instability of patients in recovery and the unpredictability of discharge trajectories, there is a risk that policy aspirations will continue to outpace the practical realities of care.

Summary

This chapter examined the transition from hospital to home within the recovery assemblage, focusing on the challenges of enacting the patient as a transition object to ensure safe, integrated and efficient discharge. While acute and community services shared overlapping concerns, differing orientations to risk produced a gap between the emergent collective objects of practice on the orthogeriatric ward and the stabilised objects required by community services at the point of discharge.

Discharge infrastructures were designed to render patients as stable, transferable cases - immutable mobiles. Yet, patients in recovery were mutable – they had evolving needs. This mismatch between the fluidity of patients-as-objects and the rigidity of institutional processes fragmented the patient across acute and community sectors and complicated the organisation of integrated care.

Although healthcare–community interfaces were relatively well understood, the relationship between acute care and social services remained distant, further complicating object formation. No formal mechanisms existed to guarantee trajectory coherence. While outright discharge failures were rare, most cases required remedial community interventions to stabilise arrangements. Figure 13.1 summarises transition arrangements in the recovery assemblage.

Discharge visits demanded significant community resource investment, yet frequent cancellations and the absence of an agile and flexible infrastructure to reallocate visits in real time impaired both hospital throughput and community service capacity. In this context, the CRT's role in stabilising discharge was not ancillary but central.

References

Berg, M. (1997). 'Problems and promises of the protocol'. *Social Science & Medicine* **44**(8): 1081–1088. https://doi.org/10.1016/s0277-9536(96)00235-3
Bowker, G. and S.L. Star (1999). *Sorting Things Out: Classification and its Consequences*. Cambridge, The MIT Press.
Knorr Cetina, K. (1997). 'Sociality with objects: social relations in postsocial knowledge societies'. *Theory, Culture & Society* **14**(4): 1–30.
Latour, B. (1987). *Science in Action: How to Follow Scientists and Engineers through Society*. Cambridge, Harvard University Press.
Latour, B. (2005). *Reassembling the Social: An Introduction to Actor-Network-Theory*. Oxford, Oxford University Press.
Mol, A. (2008). *The Logic of Care: Health and the Problem of Patient Choice*. London, Routledge.
NHS Wales Delivery Unit (2021). *Delivering Home First: Hospital to Home Community of Practice: Key Learning and Practice Examples*. https://www.gov.wales/sites/default/files/publications/2021-08/hospital-to-home-community-of-practice-key-learning-and-practice-examples.pdf
Pols, J. (2008). 'Good care: enacting a complex ideal in long-term psychiatry'. *Medische Anthropologie* **20**(1): 73–89.
Rheinberger, H.-J. (1997). *Towards a History of Epistemic Things: Synthesizing Proteins in the Test Tube*. Stanford, CA, Standford University Press.
Star, S.L. and J.R. Griesemer (1989). 'Institutional ecology, 'translations' and boundary objects: Amateurs and professionals in Berkeley's Museum of Vertebrate Zoology, 1907–39'. *Social Studies of Science* **19**(3): 387–420. https://doi.org/10.1177/030631289019003001

SUMMARY OF PART 4

This part of the book has examined the recovery assemblage, focusing on object formation and the mobilisation of care across the postoperative work of the orthogeriatric ward, the social world of the Community Resource Team (CRT), and the organisation of transitions home. This phase of the hip fracture trajectory was complex and expansive. Object formation widened beyond the biomedical to encompass recovery and rehabilitation, personal futures, identity, and home. These extended concerns were reflected in the broadening of the orthogeriatric team and the increased visibility of patients and their families in shaping decisions about care and discharge.

Understanding of the patient was distributed, and recovery trajectories were uncertain. Discharge planning unfolded through an emergent process, accomplished through epistemic organisation. Initial enactments of the patient – open and indeterminate – gradually stabilised into boundary objects as discharge plans crystallised. More than the sum of their parts, these narratives combined an understanding of the person's unfolding recovery with the equivocal and complex dimensions of their lifeworld – elements not captured in the patient record.

While discharge arrangements varied, this analysis has focused on home discharge. Unlike transfers to institutional settings, home discharges required care infrastructures to be assembled in situ, as part of the management of transition. These arrangements were delicately balanced and highly contingent, assembled through intricate negotiations between individual needs, the material constraints of the home, standardised forms of provision, and family and supporters. Aligning a person's functional capacity with their domestic environment, social networks, and available services required careful calibration – small changes in one domain could destabilise the entire arrangement.

DOI: 10.4324/9781003475019-24

Managing transition involved complex translational processes. The narrative understanding of the patient as a collective object of practice of orthogeriatric work was progressively decoupled and reconfigured into multiple technical objects required by different community services. Documents were central actors. Burdensome to complete and only loosely coordinative of action, they were expected to perform significant translational work across divergent social worlds. Discharge infrastructures attempted to render patients as immutable mobiles – fixed and recognisable across organisational boundaries – but patients in recovery were mutable, with evolving needs. This mismatch fragmented the patient across sectors and complicated the organisation of integrated care. Despite the acknowledged intricacies and instabilities of discharge plans, transition infrastructures decentred the patient and lacked mechanisms to carry narrative knowledge forward or articulate collective understanding across institutional boundaries. Community services bore the burden of stabilising care arrangements post-discharge, often without direct involvement in earlier planning.

Misalignment of the transition infrastructure and transitional interfaces hindered discharge processes and impacted capacity across hospital and community services. Community services' demand for stability introduced delays. The system's limited responsiveness meant that cancelled discharge slots could rarely be reallocated, creating inefficiencies that reverberated across hospital and community settings.

Part 4 has traced the expansive and contingent nature of recovery, revealing how patients were reconfigured as care was mobilised across the orthogeriatric ward, the CRT, and the home. The analysis highlights both the limits of institutional coordination and the socio-material arrangements required to sustain care across settings. These findings now feed into the concluding chapter, which synthesises insights from across the hip fracture assemblage and considers their implications for integrated care.

PART 5

Conclusion

Trajectory Assemblage Synthesis and Implications for Service Improvement and Research

14

BEYOND PATHWAYS

Making Coordination Work

This book has explored how patients, care, and treatment are organised across the hip fracture trajectory, aiming to provide theoretically informed empirical foundations for understanding the persistent challenges of coordination in contemporary care systems. Drawing on ideas about patient trajectories, concepts from Translational Mobilisation Theory (Allen and May, 2017), and assemblage thinking (Deleuze and Guattari, 1987), the study moves beyond the normative prescriptions of the pathways metaphor to attend to everyday practices in the wild.

Taking object formation as my focal point, I have examined how activity is mobilised within and between services across the length of the trajectory, and the formal and informal mechanisms that enable concerted action. Studying these practices revealed diverse modes of organisation – from proactive structured coordination to responsive articulation and situational tinkering – surfacing the interplay between visible and invisible work. It also showed how trajectories are shaped by wider service demands and the shifting concerns through which patients are enacted. These dynamics gave rise to three distinctive temporal-spatial configurations within the hip fracture assemblage: unscheduled care, acute care, and recovery care – each with its own organising logics, socio-material relations, and collective objects of practice.

To the best of my knowledge, no previous research has examined the organisation and mobilisation of an entire patient trajectory. While the empirical chapters each offer stand-alone insights, this concluding chapter synthesises the findings from this unique, trajectory-wide perspective, and considers their broader implications for service improvement and future research.

DOI: 10.4324/9781003475019-26

Advancing Trajectory Assemblage Understanding

This section reflects on what can be learned from examining the whole trajectory. It compares the shifting shape of the assemblage, the influence of contextual constraints on mobilisation, and the interplay of diverse organisational modes and mechanisms. It explores object formation in professional practice and how these enactments both shape and are shaped by organisational priorities. It also examines the conditions that structure transitions and their implications for managing care transfers.

Scale and Complexity

Examining the full trajectory revealed how the hip fracture assemblage reconfigured over time and across organisational settings. Care expanded in both scale and complexity as it moved through unscheduled, acute, and recovery phases, each introducing new logics, relations, priorities, and objects of practice.

In unscheduled care, the assemblage was compact and linear. The patient's status remained provisional, and mobilisation through Emergency Medical Services (EMS) and the Emergency Department (ED) involved a limited number of actors following a sequential pattern. Activity focused on managing diverse cases and reaching a disposal decision amid high uncertainty, demand pressures, and time constraints.

Following diagnosis, the patient's status became definitive, marking a shift in the temporal and spatial configuration of the assemblage. In acute care, activity is centred on planning and delivering the surgical intervention, extending over days rather than hours, and drawing in a broader range of actors from Trauma and Orthopaedics (T&O), Anaesthetics, Orthogeriatric, and Operating Department services.

In recovery, the patient's status became distributed. This was the most complex and expansive trajectory phase, spanning months and involving a dispersed network of actors, including acute and community professionals, families, social networks, and the home environment. Concerns broadened beyond the biomedical to encompass social and biographical concerns and the contingencies of everyday life.

Together, these configurations show how care trajectories are shifting assemblages, each generating distinct institutional priorities and coordination demands as care progresses.

Object Formation and the Enactment of Patients

Pathways thinking assumes a stable patient progressing immutably through care systems. In this study, I have treated the patient as an organisational artefact – continually constituted through professional practices and institutional processes as a means of getting things done. Comparing object formation across the trajectory, reveals the diverse ways patients are enacted, the shifting matters of concern prioritised within the evolving assemblage, the qualities and affordances of these enactments, and their implications for organising activity. It also shows how object formation is embedded in professional practice, how different understandings of the patient coexist across the trajectory, and how these patterns shape concerted action.

Object Concerns

Studying object formation across social worlds illuminated the institutionally significant concerns in hip fracture care and how these shifted as the trajectory evolved. In unscheduled care, object formation centred on prioritisation, disposal decision-making, and patient flow. In acute care, the patient was enacted through the standardised medical, corporeal, and procedural concerns of surgical work. In recovery, the focus broadened to include home, family, identity, and the life-world.

Comparing these configurations shows that what is 'centred' in hip fracture care varies with service priorities and institutional pressures. Only the recovery assemblage could be described as genuinely patient-centred – at least in the conventional sense – given its focus on individual needs. In contrast, unscheduled care was primarily organisation-centred, and acute care was largely intervention-centred.

Tracing how patients are enacted across the trajectory challenges the notion of a stable or universally patient-centred orientation. Instead, it reveals how care is shaped by context-specific concerns – such as flow, procedure, or biography – and the organisational logics that in a given moment determine which concerns are prioritised and which are set aside. This analysis suggests moving beyond asking whether care is patient-centred to interrogating which concerns are centred, for whom, and to what effect across different phases.

Object Formation Processes

Studying how patients are constituted across the hip fracture trajectory exposed the diversity and complexity of object formation. Patients were enacted into multiple professional objects of practice, each serving distinct clinical purposes. While patients often expressed frustration at repeating their stories, professional logics are nuanced: different disciplines interpret and use the same information in distinct ways (Goodwin 1994). For example, both resident doctors and the ward pharmacist asked about medications, but with different concerns – doctors focused on preexisting conditions and inpatient prescriptions, while the pharmacist prioritised medication management and falls risk. Similarly, orthogeriatric staff inquired about social circumstances, but occupational therapists conducted more granular assessments critical for discharge planning. Community-based therapists went further, producing situated understandings that contrasted with the abstracted views formed in hospital settings.

Object formation typically began with an initial assessment – a discrete institutional process documented in the patient record. In the hospital, nursing admissions included standardised risk assessments and care plans; in medicine object formation entailed a formal clerking process; and physiotherapy, pharmacy, and occupational therapy followed systematic 'carding'. In the community resource team, formal tools translated the patient into a collective object in a joint discharge visit, followed by enactment into distinct professional objects by health therapists and social care workers.

Documentary enactments of the patient accumulated across the trajectory, distributed across professional records, forms, and systems. A striking finding was how practitioners selectively used others' documentation for their own purposes. ED staff drew on EMS Patient Care Records; on the orthogeriatric ward, the Hip Fracture Clerking Template became a shared resource; PACU nurses engaged with OD records to reassemble the patient for ward transfer; and community teams used referral and screening tools to build provisional understandings of the patient ahead of discharge meetings. Resident doctors also relied heavily on preexisting medical records during clerking.

These were not random searches: documents actively entered into professional sensemaking, with practitioners accessing specific records for specific clinical purposes. In addition to revealing the singular practices of object formation in professional work, this analysis highlights the infrastructural knowledge underpinning object formation – not just how to navigate and interpret records, but where information is located, how it was produced, its trustworthiness, and how it might be interpreted in context. This forms part of a wider ecology of information practices (Nardi and O'Day, 1999), in which documentary resources are selectively drawn upon, repurposed, and made meaningful within the practical concerns of particular roles and settings. Rather than producing a unified view of the patient, these ecologies support multiple, coexisting enactments, each responsive to different professional logics and purposes. Understanding these dynamics has important implications for digital patient information systems, which must support the heterogeneous, practice-based ways records are engaged with and the interpretive and relational work through which clinical practice is accomplished.

Object formation in EMS and OD work was distinct. Due to the time-sensitive and dynamic nature of these settings, object formation was tightly intertwined with care interventions. Documentation simultaneously enacted the patient as both an object *and* an account of professional practice. In both cases, the patient record was highly structured and granular, designed for completion under time pressure. Information was recorded in a reductionist format, and both EMS and OD staff expressed frustration that documentation failed to capture the hermeneutic sensemaking central to their clinical work.

Objects in and for Professional Practice

Tracing object formation across the hip fracture trajectory reveals tensions between institutional enactments of the patient for accountability and the situated enactments that emerge through practice. Chapter 8 highlighted the gap between formal nursing care plans – which constituted patients as technical objects aligned with standardised problems – and bedside care and trajectory management, which relied on embodied and situated knowledge to address individual needs. Similarly, occupational and physiotherapy practices required formal enactments through 'carding' or database entries – seen as bureaucratic, time-consuming, and disconnected from hands-on care, and often delegated to support staff. Notably, while there was no institutional requirement for nurses to document formal care needs assessments, none of the participants expressed concern about this omission. These examples reflect a broader pattern in which institutional norms of accountability and professional expertise are often decoupled from everyday clinical work. While these parallel enactments rarely created direct conflict, formal object formation consumed significant time and, being largely performative, added little value to service processes or patient experience.

Some professions – physiotherapy, occupational therapy, pharmacy, and social care – enacted patients primarily through the ontological logics of their own practice. Others were also drawn into institutional and administrative concerns. EMS professionals, for example, enacted patients as both clinical and trajectory objects, aligning with ED priorities for flow. In ED, nurses enacted patients as clinical, triage, allocative, and trajectory objects to balance acuity-based prioritisation with throughput. Junior doctors, following a disposal decision, generated distinct objects to secure specialist referrals. In PACU and the orthogeriatric ward, clinical and trajectory objects were closely coupled in nursing work, reflecting their central role in the mobilisation of care.

Studying object formation thus illuminates how professional groups are positioned within institutional structures, with some carrying significant organisational responsibilities alongside their clinical roles.

The Distribution of Objects

Foregrounding object formation in care organisation reveals how multiple versions of the patient coexisted across the assemblage. As Mol's (2002) work on ontological multiplicity highlights, if reality is differentially performed through practice, then decisions must be made about which versions of an object prevail. Different enactments may coexist, moreover, but what matters analytically is whether they compete, are kept apart, or persist in parallel – and how this coexistence is managed. In this study, as I have described, formal, accountability-oriented enactments often coexisted with more situated, practice-based versions within professional groups. Beyond these internal variations, however, diverse patterns of coexistence emerged across the trajectory.

In unscheduled care, the patient was enacted sequentially through EMS and ED structures. At any one time, understanding was largely confined to the perspectives of EMS crews or ED teams, layered and integrated as care progressed. Focused on immediate needs and disposal decisions – rather than long-term planning – this delimited scope of object formation enabled rapid mobilisation in fast-paced environments.

Acute care was marked by a clear divergence between orthogeriatric and OD objects of practice. Coexistence was managed through conscription, aligning patients with surgical requirements, and bracketing, which temporarily suspended other aspects of care. As patients transitioned back to the orthogeriatric ward, these bracketed elements were reassembled through narrative reconstruction, restoring a more integrated object to guide trajectory mobilisation.

The recovery phase was marked by a multiplicity of professional objects of practice across hospital and community services. Patients and families also played a more active role in object formation. Trajectory progression depended on integrating these diverse understandings into a collective object of practice – beginning with negotiating recovery goals and discharge destinations and continuing through coordination of home care to support independence. Unlike earlier phases, where objects were enfolded or kept apart, recovery involved greater interference among perspectives, creating space for negotiation and disagreement. While decision-making was more complex and protracted, this plurality was essential for developing integrated, sustainable plans – although the complexity of these processes or the time they entail is rarely acknowledged in policy debates on delayed discharges.

These shifting patterns of coexistence show that coordination is not simply about information transfer or role alignment, but about actively managing the enactment and mobilisation of the patient across professional and service boundaries. Attention to object formation reveals the organisational work required to sustain coordination as trajectories evolve – and the investments needed to support it.

Object Qualities

Beyond highlighting the diversity and complexity of object formation, this study also draws attention to the distinct qualities that characterise patients as objects of practice – situated, technical, narrative, and epistemic – and their implications for work organisation.

Situated objects were most evident in the work of nurses and the CRT, but they also characterised surgical work in the operating theatre. Centred on the immediate care arrangements and their interdependencies, situated objects were integrative, formed through embodied engagement with patients in context. Provisional and adaptive, they were oriented to shifting patient requirements and to the practical tinkering and relational alignment required to tailor activity and materials to the individual's circumstance.

Technical objects were reductionist, granular, and aligned with predefined criteria. Deployed through formal tools such as checklists, they black-boxed the preparatory and interpretive work that preceded their use. Designed to enact the patient as an immutable mobile (Latour, 1987), they enabled coordination by stabilising form across boundaries. While effective in acute care, technical objects failed to travel in unscheduled care due to widespread distrust of AMPDS technology, and their use in mediating discharge fragmented understanding of the patient in community care.

Narrative objects, by contrast, were evolving understandings of the patient's trajectory. Central to nursing practice, they articulated everyday activity and mobilised care. As mutable mobiles (Allen, 2015; Rolland et al., 2006), they were continuously refined in response to trajectory dynamics and adapted to the needs of diverse actors. Unlike technical objects, which retained their form, narrative objects were shaped through joint sensemaking and recipient design.

Epistemic objects were most visible in the recovery phase. These open-ended, emergent understandings of the patient's recovery served as shared focal points – inviting multiple perspectives, further inquiry, and knowledge generation. Whereas technical objects were fixed and narrative objects were flexibly stable, epistemic objects sustained productive indeterminacy, supporting coordination through deliberation, negotiation, and ongoing assessment.

While previous research has framed patients as boundary objects in healthcare coordination (Allen, 2015; Bishop and Waring, 2019; Middleton and Brown, 2005), it has not systematically analysed the distinct object qualities that emerge across contexts. This study advances understanding by showing how patient enactments – as situated, technical, narrative, or epistemic objects – both shape and are shaped by professional practice and institutional logics, with significant implications for the organisation and coordination of care. Some stabilise procedures, others guide practice in situ or enable transitions between settings. Many do not operate as boundary objects at all.

Organisation and Coordination

Examining the organisation of hip fracture care across the full trajectory reveals a more complicated landscape than standardised models or pathway-based planning suggest. Coordination practices varied across settings, shaped by distinct temporal rhythms, priorities, and organising logics. This section explores how coordination was achieved through diverse modes, mechanisms, and roles – highlighting how care was mobilised through a mix of formal tools, interpretive practices, and contingent responses. These variations expose the patterned yet heterogeneous ways organisational practices supported – or at times constrained – trajectory mobilisation.

Modes

While some aspects of hip fracture care aligned with linear, pathways-based thinking, these accounted for only a small fraction of activity. Coordination across the trajectory was not simply about aligning tasks or sequencing actions – challenging as that was – but also about responding to patients' evolving needs and shifting trajectories. This required more dynamic and generative forms of coordination, centred on synthesis, interpretation, and joint sensemaking. Indeed, this was the predominant mode of organisation.

Across the trajectory, two broad modes of organising activity can be distinguished: responsive and proactive.

Responsive organisation was grounded in the immediacy of practice – situated, contingent, and embodied – often unfolding in the moment and close to the patient. It included trajectory-focused *articulation*, where practitioners, particularly nurses, maintained awareness of the patient's evolving care and aligned activity in response to emerging contingencies. A second form, care-focused *tinkering*, was less concerned with forward movement and more attuned to the patient's changing condition, context, and comfort. Rooted in a logic of care rather than mobilisation, this mode demanded attentiveness, problem-solving, and responsiveness to small shifts in need (Mol, 2008; Pols, 2008). It was evident in both nursing work and the community resource team's efforts to stabilise care infrastructures at discharge as well as characterising cooperative activity in the operating theatre.

In contrast, **proactive organisation** involved anticipatory efforts to coordinate care in advance of need. *Rational-linear organisation* relied on formal mechanisms – treatment guidelines, protocols, and checklists – to sequence activities and discipline practice. Reflecting the logic of pathways thinking, it translated work into standardised prescribed steps, allocated responsibilities, and monitored compliance. It was particularly evident in surgical preparations within the acute care assemblage and in the assessment of risk across the trajectory. *Emergent-linear organisation*, while still oriented to a predefined path, was more interpretive and tailored to individual patients. It was evident in unscheduled care, especially in the work of EMS responders and nurses who rapidly mobilised patients with diverse needs through the ED, but also complemented rational-linear organisational processes elsewhere in the trajectory, such as the transition interface between PACU and the wards. *Epistemic organisation* represented a non-linear, collaborative mode of organisation, which aimed to generate understanding rather than deliver interventions. Professionals from different disciplines worked together to construct shared understandings of the patient's condition and needs. Rather than following a preset plan, this mode relied on collective sensemaking and negotiation, particularly in the recovery phase during discharge planning.

Taken together, these modes highlight how coordination in hip fracture care involved both formal, institutionally visible structures – such as protocols and checklists – and less visible, situated practices of interpretation, adjustment, and response. These forms of organising were not neatly separable; they overlapped, evolved, and were sometimes in tension, as practitioners navigated the intersection of planned, responsive, and emergent activity.

Mechanisms

Coordination in hip fracture care was achieved through a range of mechanisms varying in formality, visibility, and operation. These included formal tools such as checklists and templates, narrative mechanisms that sustained shared understanding across professional boundaries, and situated practices responsive to local contingencies.

Formal tools were pervasive across the trajectory, though their roles varied. In some areas – particularly surgical preparation – they were highly visible actors in care coordination. Elsewhere, they had become sedimented in local routines, operating as background structures. For example, the Hip Fracture Clerking Proforma and Initial Treatment Guideline disciplined the work of transient resident doctors, while in more stable teams like the ED and CRT, triage tools and risk assessments were less visible but still shaped how patients were enacted for institutional purposes.

Studying the breadth of organisational activity revealed both the strengths and limitations of formal coordinating technologies. In acute care, tools were used effectively: the Clerking Template and Treatment Guideline structured doctors' work, OD checklists managed theatre flow, and the WHO Surgical Safety Checklist – though sometimes ritualistic – coordinated practice at critical junctures across the patient trajectory.

Formal tools worked well when aligned with the prevailing mode of organisation and when patients were enacted as technical objects – standardised and specifiable – reducing the burden of completion. Their utility also depended on users' understanding of their purpose. For example, while checklist duplication between the orthogeriatric ward and OD might seem redundant, it functioned as a safety mechanism amid high staff turnover. Tool efficacy further relied on integration into broader working practices: frailty nurses monitored doctors' progress to ensure timely theatre preparation, and healthcare support workers informally ensured preoperative checklists were completed.

By contrast, tools designed to coordinate care across organisational boundaries were less effective. The Jenolan Admission Proforma placed a heavy translational burden on ward nurses, who were expected to enact patients for social care when discharge needs were still unclear. Its loose structure and unclear purpose undermined its coordinating function. Similarly, the CRT screening proforma – unavailable to acute staff – had limited agency at transition points, creating knowledge gaps at the point of completion. These examples underscore the need not only for well-designed tools and staff preparation, but also of deploying tools at the right moment within the care trajectory.

Elsewhere, narratives were the primary coordination mechanism. As evolving artefacts, they enabled actors to make sense of the patient's trajectory, translate information across boundaries, and orient activity over time. Narratives coordinated emerging trajectories, articulated care around contingencies, and enacted trajectory, interdisciplinary, and collective objects of practice. They allowed professionals to align perspectives, negotiate concerns, and construct shared, if shifting, understandings of the patient. Far from secondary to formal tools, narrative coordination was often the primary means by which care was held together.

Narrative coordination required ongoing effort. Maintaining trajectory awareness, constructing narrative accounts, and exchanging them across boundaries demanded cognitive and communicative labour. Though largely invisible to institutions, staff recognised narrative competence as a marker of professionalism.

A notable research finding was the absence of formal tools to support narrative and emergent coordination. Assessment unit nurses developed their own proformas to track evolving trajectories; ward nurses used handover sheets informally; frailty nurses adapted audit tools to support their work. While CRT screened discharge tasks, no shared document supported integrated care planning at the acute–community interface or ongoing coordination in the community.

Also significant was the limited use of formal team meetings. In the orthogeriatric service, weekly multidisciplinary meetings had been replaced by more frequent, operationally focused board rounds. In community settings, much decision-making occurred outside scheduled case reviews. These patterns reflect broader trends towards the intensification and acceleration of care, where coordination increasingly occurs in real-time interactions rather than structured events.

Roles

Different professional groups were enrolled in organisational processes across the trajectory, but nurses played a leading role. In the ED, they maintained trajectory awareness and mobilised action; on the orthogeriatric ward, they organised everyday care and managed discharges; and throughout the pathway, they acted as social worlds' representatives in managing transitions. Their responsibilities also extended to overseeing resident doctors, whose practice was often fragmented by interruptions and competing demands. While much of this work was taken for granted, its institutional value was reflected in the appointment of frailty nurses to support preoperative care and discharge planning – an adaptation to the difficulty ward nurses faced in balancing trajectory management with day-to-day care.

As previously argued (Allen, 2015), separating the clinical and organisational components of nursing fragments practice. This study further shows how different modes of organisation intersect in nursing work, with consequences for the division of labour and distribution of knowledge. Frailty nurses were effective in coordinating standardised, rational-linear tasks but lacked the embodied clinical intelligence of ward-based colleagues, making it difficult to fine-tune discharge arrangements. Here, structural separation disrupted the ecology of logistical and clinical knowledge, generating new organisational challenges.

Non-clinically qualified support staff were deployed in key roles throughout the trajectory. While valued team members, their work was tightly bounded by formal scopes of practice, introducing constraints into organisational processes. As described in Chapter 3, EMS call handlers' work was mediated by the AMPDS, requiring formal and informal workarounds that were only partially effective. Similarly, the limited jurisdiction of social carers posed challenges for discharge planning. When patients lacked informal networks to bridge service gaps, these constraints often determined whether they could return home or were diverted to institutional care. While deploying lower-cost staff may offer economic efficiencies, it reduces system adaptability, embedding inflexibilities most visible when care needs exceed narrow role definitions. Moreover, increased role specialisation adds coordination demands. More finely differentiated roles require additional effort to ensure coherent care across boundaries. As a result, apparent efficiencies gained through task shifting can generate burdens elsewhere in the system – particularly when patient needs do not align neatly with institutional categories of work.

Transitions

Examining a complete care trajectory enabled a systematic analysis of transitions. Aase and Waring (2020), in a recent review, note that research in this area often revisits the same issues and call for conceptual frameworks that better capture transition complexity. Building on previous work (Allen, 2015), this study conceptualised transition as an institutional status passage (Glaser and Strauss, 1971), involving the translation of the patient from one service's collective object of practice to another's. Analysis focused on three components: the interface between implicated social worlds, the infrastructural arrangements organising transition, and the enactment of patients into objects of practice for transfers of care.

In the unscheduled care assemblage, where there was reciprocal understanding of work processes, shared organising logics, and aligned collective objects of practice, EMS responders and ED nurses used narrative transition objects to enact patients as mutable mobiles – flexible, evolving understandings that supported trajectory mobilisation in a fast-paced environment. In contrast, services in the acute care assemblage worked with divergent collective objects of practice. Here, documents embedded in routine practice and supported by human actors coordinated activity around a shared logic of safety and efficiency. Translated into the standardised technical objects of OD practice, and bracketing off the broader clinical and social concerns of the orthogeriatric ward, the patient was enacted as an immutable and transportable object of practice aligned with OD work. Technical enactments alone were insufficient for managing transitions back to the ward, however. PACU nurses performed narrative reconstructions to reintroduce trajectory complexity and relational knowledge, restoring a more holistic object of practice for ward-based care.

Transitions in unscheduled and acute care occurred between preconfigured infrastructures. In the recovery assemblage, however, care infrastructures had to be actively configured to support the transition from hospital to home. As in acute care, documents were central actors, but here they operated alone – mediating the distal social worlds of hospital and community services, divergent collective objects, and misaligned logics. These documents attempted to enact patients as immutable mobiles – stable, knowable entities aligned with institutional requirements. Yet patients in recovery were mutable – their needs, capacities, and environments in flux. Designed to reflect the detailed concerns of home care planning, the documents were burdensome to complete, loosely coordinative of practice, and fragmented the patient into multiple objects across community services. With no formal integrating mechanisms, post-discharge stabilisation was required to ensure safe care. The transition infrastructure lacked the flexibility to accommodate trajectory contingencies, and this mismatch between patient fluidity and system rigidity had direct consequences for service capacity.

Taken together, these findings show that transitions are not simply handovers, but complex organisational accomplishments shaped by relationships, object formation, and infrastructure. Systematic comparison reveals that transition interfaces are conditioned by the degree of familiarity between services' social worlds, the alignment of their organisational logics, and the nature of their collective objects of practice. The effectiveness of transition infrastructures depends on their capacity to mediate these relationships and accommodate the enactment of patients as both mutable and immutable mobiles – as evolving, context-sensitive entities and as stable, transferable objects – across diverse care settings.

Intersecting Trajectories and Contextual Constraints

Scrutinising end-to-end care processes reveals how patient trajectories are shaped by intersections with other trajectories – clinical, organisational, and operational. Hip fracture care was delivered within services simultaneously responsible for patients following diverse and often competing trajectories. Unscheduled care services, among the most open and dynamic parts of the system, relied on triage and resource allocation tools to manage demand. EMS handled hip fracture cases alongside a wide range of calls, with response times shaped by overall system load. Transfers to ED and specialist care depended on bed availability, while timely surgery was contingent not only on patients' clinical readiness but also on theatre capacity. Home care relied on overstretched community services and family support, often resulting in delayed discharges. Taken together, these findings underscore how individual trajectories are continually negotiated within broader contextual constraints – where fluctuating capacity, demand, and social network availability directly shape service processes and patient outcomes. This complexity is rarely acknowledged in the care pathways literature.

Beyond these intersecting trajectories, staff capacity also conditioned trajectory mobilisation. As discussed earlier, resident doctors' work was fragmented and frequently interrupted, with ED and ward nurses mitigating these risks by overseeing trajectory progress. Due to the direct care demands on ward nurses, frailty nurses were appointed to support discharge coordination – though this introduced challenges around knowledge fragmentation. Similarly, physiotherapy pressures led to early withdrawal of inpatient care or delays in post-discharge rehabilitation. Service pressures had led to a reduction in home-based occupational therapy assessments, increasing the risk of misaligned care infrastructures when patients returned home. In-person CRT screening had been discontinued due to resource constraints, heightening the risk of knowledge gaps and poorly integrated discharge plans.

These findings suggest that improving service integration requires more than technical fixes. Without addressing the deeper structural conditions that shape coordination in practice, even the most sophisticated policies and systems risk falling short of their intended impact.

*

Tracing the evolving network of socio-material relations that organise patients, care, and treatment shows that the hip fracture trajectory does not follow a fixed pathway, nor can quality and safety be ensured simply by aligning the right person, in the right place, at the right time. Instead, the shape, scale, and complexity of the assemblage shift over time and space in response to institutional priorities and contextual constraints. These shifts generate different modes of organisation and object formation and determine what is centred in care work.

Studying organisational activity across the trajectory reveals where formal coordinating artefacts added value, where they did not, and where organisation relied on human actors – along with the varying visibility of this work. These findings also prompt reflection on the object qualities of patients that facilitate trajectory mobilisation, how systems can be designed to support these processes, and the institutional investments that are required.

Service Improvement

This book has had a long gestation, during which health and social care systems have undergone profound and accelerating change. The lasting effects of COVID-19, growing workforce shortages, and rising demand, have placed immense pressure on organisations, prompting rapid adaptation and ongoing service reconfiguration. Many of the specific structures and processes described herein no longer exist in their original form. Yet while the empirical details may have shifted, and will undoubtedly continue to do so, the study's core contribution lies in its alternative framing of the coordination problem. This section considers its implications for service improvement.

From Patient-Centred to Concern-Centred Care

The pathways metaphor is often used to promote patient-centred care. While rhetorically powerful and reassuring to providers, users, and families, it can obscure the system-level constraints that shape how care is actually delivered. By placing object formation at the centre of analysis, this study surfaces the institutional concerns that are prioritised – and rendered actionable – at different points along the trajectory. This framing invites system architects and service managers to critically reflect on which concerns are centred in formal processes, and what is at stake when care is organised around them.

A concern-centred approach foregrounds the variable priorities, pressures, and organising logics through which patients are enacted across the trajectory. Rather than assuming a fixed notion of the 'patient' or a universal ideal of patient-centredness, it recognises that what is centred in care is variable and context-specific. Attending to these dynamics reveals when patients need to be 'Taylored' to the organisation, and when the organisation must tailor care around the patient – along with the socio-material arrangements required to support these reconfigurations.

This framing also clarifies the relational, institutional, and infrastructural investments that make coordination possible. It creates space for more transparent conversations with patients and families about how care is organised and managed. In the context of rising demand, workforce shortages, and ongoing post-pandemic pressures, a concern-centred approach offers a fresh entry point into the coordination problem and the limits of patient-centred care as a universal good. By focusing on what concerns are centred – how and why – it provides a framework for critically examining the contingencies of coordination, the organisational commitments they require, and their implications for practice.

Objectification is often critiqued for its dehumanising effects, but it can be understood more neutrally as a routine and necessary part of organising care. Patients must be represented in particular ways to act on their needs, allocate resources, and coordinate activity. From a concern-centred perspective, the issue is not whether objectification occurs, but what forms it takes, what meanings it acquires, and what consequences it produces at different stages of care. Whether objectification is experienced as alienating or enabling depends on how institutional concerns align – or misalign – with the lived realities and expectations of patients and families (Timmermans and Almeling, 2009).

Coordination, Complexity, and Capacity

This study has shown that coordination in healthcare is not a discrete task or function, but a distributed accomplishment emerging through embedded, often invisible practices. By tracing how coordination is accomplished across services, professions, documents, and tools, the analysis highlights the importance of attending to both formal infrastructures and the everyday activities and improvisations that underpin care. These insights are especially relevant as services adapt to growing complexity, constrained resources, and rising expectations.

Any quality improvement initiative must begin with a grounded understanding of the processes it seeks to change. Yet, organisation is never neutral; improvement efforts must engage with a social world already shaped by institutional logics and structuring mechanisms. Everyday activities are often poorly understood; workers themselves may not fully recognise how their actions contribute to the broader system (Nardi and Engeström, 1999) or may describe their work in officially sanctioned rather than realistic terms (Dourish, 2001). As a result, many initiatives are driven by top-down 'work-as-imagined solutioneering' (Shorrock, 2022), rather than close attention to how work is actually done. While this critique may now seem axiomatic, it remains salient precisely because it is so often overlooked. A similar tendency exists in academic discourse, where scholars highlight healthcare complexity – often through intricate conceptual diagrams – yet offer limited guidance for engaging with that complexity in actionable ways.

The conceptual framework developed in this book supports analysts in making the familiar strange and examining organisational processes from a fresh perspective. It encourages attention beyond formal systems to the diversity of organisational practices and the socio-material arrangements that sustain them. It shows how formal tools and artefacts function not in isolation, but through their embeddedness in relationships, practices, and infrastructures. It also foregrounds the role of informal artefacts – developed by staff in response to unmet needs – as indicators of infrastructural gaps and signposts for where formal coordination mechanisms are lacking or misaligned. The framework further underscores the importance of recognising when delegation to less qualified staff or technological systems is appropriate, and when it risks diminishing returns – highlighting where clinical expertise is essential for managing ambiguity and enabling agile, context-sensitive coordination.

As healthcare systems face chronic workforce shortages and rising demand, there is growing pressure to reconfigure the division of labour – often by introducing new roles and relying more heavily on technology. These trends suggest that the coordinative demands on frontline staff will only intensify. In this context, the framework developed here offers a way to engage more meaningfully with these pressures – not by prescribing universal solutions, but by supporting grounded analyses of how care is actually organised and the investments required to sustain it.

New Collaborative Technologies

Historically, medical records followed a narrative format, reflecting the working knowledge of everyday practice. In modern healthcare, they have become fragmented across specialties, forms, and digital platforms – mirroring the distributed nature of care and the growing role of documentation in organisational accountability, but also undermining interdisciplinarity, trajectory awareness, and holistic clinical judgem ent. Today's record is a dense mix of checklists, reports, charts, care plans, proformas, risk assessments, and free-text entries, which functions primarily as an information repository (Fitzpatrick, 2004). Digital systems often worsen this fragmentation by favouring structured fields and automated data capture over narrative and contextual reasoning. Designed mainly for administrative and audit purposes, early electronic records were poorly aligned with clinicians' cognitive and organisational needs (Coiera, 1997; Pine and Mazmanian, 2014).

Digitisation and AI are widely promoted as solutions to coordination challenges. Shared electronic records and interoperable systems are seen as key to improving communication, especially across organisational boundaries. Yet, if coordination is treated as mere information transfer, these technologies risk falling short. This study demonstrates that coordination involves situated work – negotiation, interpretation, and collective sensemaking – that cannot be reduced to data availability. Digital tools must be designed with insight into how care is actually organised – or with a clearly articulated model of any practice changes they are designed to support.

In hip fracture care, collaboration at key points in the patient trajectory involved epistemic organisation around indeterminate objects of practice. Existing technologies poorly supported this process, resulting in system inflexibility at discharge. Visualisation tools – adapted from fields like architecture (Ewenstein and Whyte, 2009) – may help stabilise shared reference points while preserving the fluidity needed for collaborative sensemaking and problem-solving (Henderson, 1991). Generative AI also holds promise – not as a substitute for judgment, but as a means of synthesising disparate data and presenting it in ways that support shared understanding and timely decisions. This may be especially valuable when teams must interpret evolving situations and align around uncertain goals. When designed with insight into real-life care practices, such tools could help bridge organisational boundaries and support the expert, relational coordination on which safe, adaptive care depends.

Implications for Research

This final section considers the implications of the study for future research, highlighting the importance of rich description, the value of comparative trajectory studies, and opportunities for theoretical and methodological development.

Rich Description

Rich description is central to ethnography (Atkinson, 1990; Geertz, 1973), yet often undervalued in health services research, where funding priorities favour interventions, evaluations, and demonstrable impacts. In the pursuit of solutions, there is frequently a rush to implement interventions without a grounded understanding of the problem or the mediating effects of context (Berg, 1997). While implementation science has advanced recognition of contextual influences and promoted systematic approaches to change, it often begins with the intervention as the focal point, rather than with a deep exploration of the problem it seeks to address. As previously argued, growing recognition of healthcare complexity in quality improvement has not been matched by methods that deepen our understanding of that complexity. Descriptive research helps bridge this gap by uncovering the practices, relationships, and situated processes that shape healthcare delivery. Far from avoiding action, a commitment to description is a necessary step towards interventions that are sustainable, responsive, and contextually grounded. To support such inquiry, however, robust theoretical frameworks are essential.

Theory

Originally developed to analyse emergent organising in fluid, networked contexts (Castells, 2009), TMT served as a valuable starting point for examining care trajectories and the coordination work that sustains them. In this study, it was first adapted to create a theoretical framework that guided the analysis, with inductively derived concepts foregrounding object formation and the organisation of transitions (see Chapter 3, Figure 3.1). Taking object formation as the entry point into service organisation, and comparing processes across the assemblage, the analysis revealed a heterogeneous mix of organisational modes – responsive, proactive, linear, and emergent. These findings led to the formalisation of a typology of organising modes, which has since been incorporated into the trajectory assemblage framework. This final configuration – summarised in Figure 14.1 – enriches the original framework by enabling comparison of how different organisational forms shape coordination.

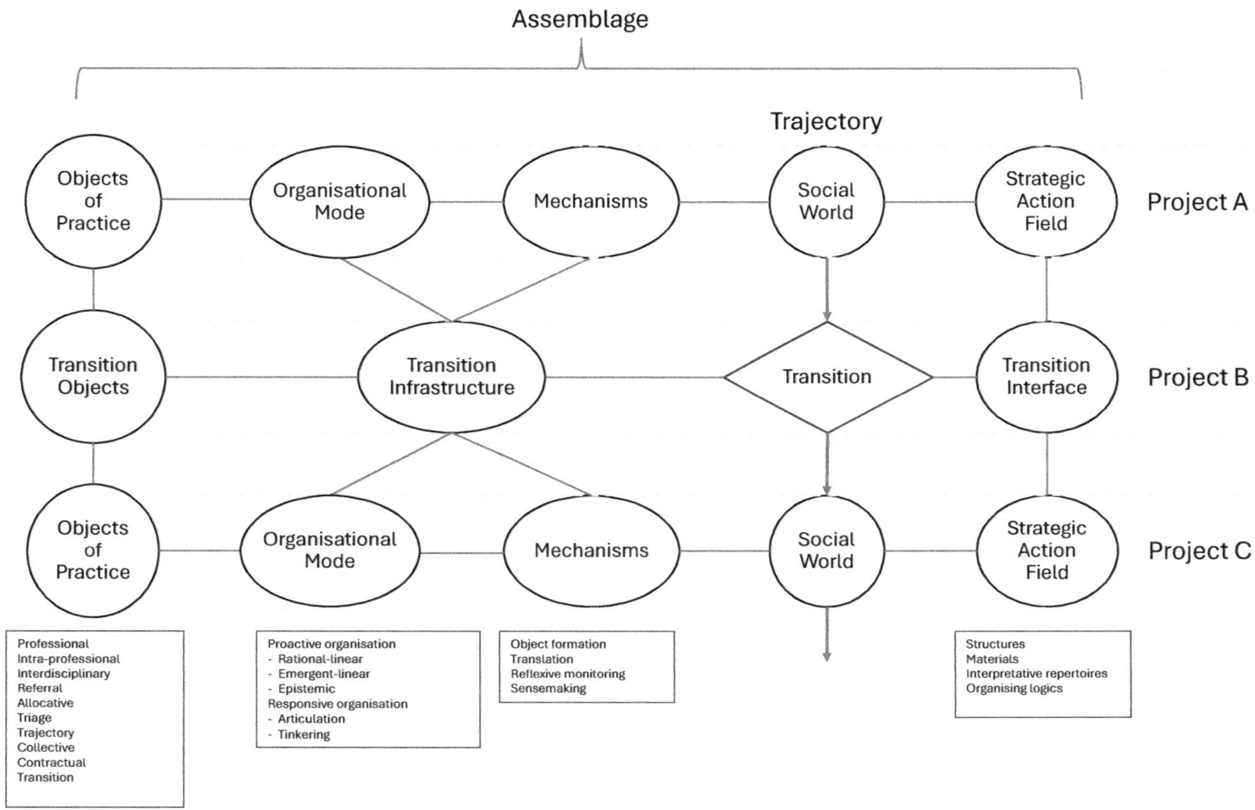

FIGURE 14.1 Trajectory assemblage framework: final configuration.

Beyond TMT, other theoretical resources can further enrich trajectory analyses. Assemblage thinking, for instance, enables fine-grained attention to how human and non-human elements shape care processes. In this study, mundane components – continence care, medication regimes, social support – had outsized influence on discharge trajectories. In other contexts, different elements (e.g. genes, symptoms, emotional states, diagnostic artefacts) may play central roles. Tracing such effects may reveal opportunities for new technologies and service interventions.

While this study focused on practices, future work could incorporate the perspectives of staff, patients, and families. Assemblage approaches attuned to emotion (Müller, 2015), affect, and lived experience would offer additional depth and help further ground care trajectories in the complexity of everyday life. These conceptual resources also open up new possibilities for comparative research. The following section outlines how trajectory studies can build on this foundation to explore variation across care configurations.

Trajectory Studies

While hip fracture provided a rich and instructive case, it represents just one assemblage within a broader ecology of service processes. To support cross-trajectory learning and advance theory, there is value in developing a programme of comparative studies. Such work could offer practical insight into what is – or should be – 'centred' in different care settings, on the trajectory of object formation, and how coordination is enacted or breaks down across diverse clinical and organisational contexts. Future studies might explore contrasting assemblage configurations, such as:

- *Acute-onset with variable recovery* – Sudden events (e.g. stroke, major trauma) requiring intensive early intervention and long-term, non-standardised rehabilitation.
- *Chronic progressive with episodic deterioration* – Long-term conditions (e.g. heart failure, COPD) marked by stability punctuated by exacerbations.
- *Degenerative with increasing dependency* – Gradual decline and growing reliance on services (e.g. dementia, neurodegenerative diseases).
- *Planned interventions with anticipated recovery* – Structured treatments (e.g. surgery, cancer care) spanning preoperative, acute, recovery, and survivorship phases.
- *Lifelong conditions with transition points* – Congenital or paediatric-onset conditions (e.g. cystic fibrosis, type 1 diabetes) requiring continuity across developmental and service boundaries.
- *Crisis-driven with uncertain stabilisation* – Acute episodes (e.g. mental health crises, substance use) demanding rapid, often repeated interventions.
- *Protracted diagnosis with evolving sensemaking* – Unexplained symptoms requiring extended investigation and iterative interpretation.
- *Abrupt diagnosis with immediate mobilisation* – Sudden diagnoses (e.g. advanced cancer) that reconfigure care priorities and trigger urgent coordination.

Attending to variation across trajectories can reveal what concerns are centred, how coordination is organised, patterns of object formation, and the qualities of transitions. The longer term aim is to develop a typology of assemblage configurations, clarifying the socio-material arrangements and institutional investments needed to support coordination under varying conditions. Rich description, grounded in a clear theoretical focus, enables analysts to trace these dynamics across diverse assemblage configurations.

Methods

While ethnography remains the preferred method for studying real-world practices, it is resource intensive. This study was made possible by a fellowship that provided the time and flexibility for research at this scale. Even with prior experience in healthcare ethnography, the work was demanding.

Although full ethnography may not always be feasible, the conceptual framework developed here offers a way to embed ethnographic sensitivity into other methods – such as interviews, focus groups, and surveys. Depending on study aims and resources, these can be used alone or alongside observations and document analysis. The key is to focus data generation on what people do and how. These methods also offer opportunities to explore participants' perspectives on organisational arrangements – something this study could only touch on. In service improvement contexts, this could support inquiry into how actors imagine alternative organisational arrangements and the conditions under which they might be realised.

*

By foregrounding rich description, grounded in robust theoretical frameworks, and embracing comparative inquiry across diverse care configurations, future studies can deepen our understanding of coordination as a situated, socio-material accomplishment. The trajectory assemblage framework developed here offers a flexible yet analytically powerful theoretical resource for tracing how care is mobilised, where it falters, and what institutional investments are required to sustain it. In doing so, it supports a mode of inquiry that is not only descriptive but generative – opening up new possibilities for theory, method, and practice in the pursuit of safe, adaptive, and contextually responsive care.

Conclusion

This book set out to move beyond the dominance of pathways thinking to offer a fresh perspective on the challenge of coordination. Through a detailed examination of the hip fracture trajectory, it has shown how care assemblages evolve across time and space, how roles, technologies, and organising logics interact to enact patients, and how these enactments shape outcomes.

By placing object formation at the centre of the analysis, it has introduced new ways of understanding the organisation and delivery of services. Reframing patient-centredness – not as a fixed ideal, but as something enacted through the evolving concerns and priorities that emerge across the trajectory – and bringing into view the diversity of formal and informal organisational processes through which care is mobilised across and between settings over time. Together, these insights underscore the need for more context-sensitive approaches to organising within care systems – approaches that account for both planned and emergent activity.

As the first study to follow a complete care trajectory in real time, the book offers a unique empirical foundation for understanding how coordination is accomplished across institutional contexts and boundaries. As care systems face growing pressures – from demographic shifts to workforce shortages and technological change – understanding these dynamics is essential. Not only to identify the conditions under which formal tools like pathways succeed, but also to recognise where alternative approaches have value and the relational, material, and temporal resources that underpin them.

This book offers both an empirical foundation and a conceptual framework for future trajectory studies and service design. In doing so, it invites a shift – from designing systems around imagined pathways to organising care in alignment with the realities of service delivery.

Afterword

Writing this book has been both intellectually demanding and personally confronting. What began as an investigation into organisational processes in the hip fracture trajectory soon revealed deeper systemic issues – not only in how care is organised, but in what is neglected. The study necessarily began after the hip fracture injury had occurred, yet it was impossible to ignore the absence of preventative measures that might have altered the trajectory entirely.

Among the most troubling findings was the routine neglect of older women with a history of fractures who had not been screened for osteoporosis – a stark reminder of the gendered inequalities that persist in healthcare. This neglect is compounded by the legacy of misleading messaging around hormone replacement therapy (HRT), which has scared many women away from a safe and effective treatment for maintaining bone health. Following publication of the Women's Health Initiative study (Rossouw et al., 2002), which overstated risks such as breast cancer and cardiovascular disease, HRT use plummeted, and prescribing patterns shifted dramatically. Although subsequent analyses have clarified that the risks were small and context-dependent, the damage was done: many women missed out on a treatment that could have significantly reduced their fracture risk (British Menopause Society and Women's Health Concern, 2023).

Despite robust evidence and updated clinical guidelines that support HRT as a viable option for osteoporosis prevention – particularly in younger postmenopausal women and those with premature ovarian insufficiency (National Osteoporosis Guideline Group, 2021) – regulatory caution and public confusion have contributed to a persistent treatment gap. This stands in stark contrast to repeated governmental ambitions to shift healthcare from cure to prevention, ambitions that remain largely unrealised.

These moments of injustice were not the central focus of this study, yet they surfaced repeatedly in the course of the inquiry and over the process of writing this book. They serve as a reminder of the wider implications of how care is materially and socially organised. While the primary aim of this study was to offer foundational insights into the intractable problem of coordination, it also highlights the value of attending to the socio-material arrangements that shape care trajectories and the opportunities for reconfiguring them to prevent harm. Future trajectory studies could begin earlier, not only tracing how care unfolds, but exploring how it might be organised differently to reduce risk and support prevention.

References

Aase, K. and J. Waring (2020). 'Crossing boundaries: establishing a framework for researching quality and safety in care transitions'. *Applied Ergonomics* **89**: 103228.

Allen, D. (2015). *The Invisible Work of Nurses: Hospitals, Organisation and Healthcare*. London and New York, Routledge.

Allen, D. and C. May (2017). 'Organizing practice and practising organization: an outline of translational mobilization theory'. *Sage Open* **7**: 2. https://doi.org/10.1016/j.socscimed.2009.05.002

Atkinson, P. (1990). *The Ethnographic Imagination: Textual Constructions of Reality*. London and New York, Routledge.

Berg, M. (1997). 'Of forms, containers and the electronic medical record: some tools for a sociology of the formal'. *Science, Technology and Human Values* **22**(4): 403–434.

Bishop, S. and J. Waring (2019). 'From boundary object to boundary subject: the role of the patient in coordination across complex systems of care during hospital discharge'. *Social Science & Medicine* **235**: 112370. https://doi.org/10.1016/j.socscimed.2009.05.002

British Menopause Society and Women's Health Concern (2023). *Recommendations on Hormone Replacement Therapy in Menopausal Women*. https://thebms.org.uk/wp-content/uploads/2023/10/02-BMS-ConsensusStatement-BMS-WHC-2020-Recommendations-on-HRT-in-menopausal-women-SEPT2023-A.pdf (accessed 6/8/25).

Castells M. (2009). *The Rise of the Network Society*. Oxford, UK, Wiley-Blackwell.

Coiera, E. (1997). *Guide to Medical Informatics, the Internet and Telemedicine*. London, Chapman and Hall, Medical.
Deleuze, G. and F. Guattari (1987). *A Thousand Plateaus: Capitalism and Schizophrenia*. Minneapolis, University of Minneapolis Press.
Dourish, P. (2001). 'Process descriptions as organizational accounting devices: the dual use of workflow technologies'. *International ACM SIGGROUP Conference on Supporting Group Work*. Boulder, CO, September 30–October 3.
Ewenstein, B. and J. Whyte (2009). 'Knowledge practices in design: the role of visual representations as "epistemic objects"'. *Organization Studies* **30**(1): 7–30. https://doi.org/10.1177/0170840608083014
Fitzpatrick, G. (2004). 'Integrated care and the working record'. *Health Informatics Journal* **10**: 291.
Geertz, C. (1973). 'Thick description: toward an interpretative theory of culture'. *The Interpretation of Cultures C. Geertz*. New York, Basic Books; 310–323.
Glaser, B.G. and A.L. Strauss (1971). *Status Passage*. New Brunswick and London, Aldine Transaction.
Goodwin, C. (1994) 'Professional vision.' *American Anthropologist* **96**(3): 606–633.
Henderson, K. (1991). 'Flexible sketches and inflexible data bases: visual communication, conscription devices, and boundary objects in design engineering'. *Science, Technology and Human Values* **16**(4): 448–473. https://doi.org/10.1177/016224399101600402
Latour, B. (1987). *Science I Action: How to Follow Scientists and Engineers Through Society*. Cambridge, MA, Harvard University Press.
Middleton, D. and S.D. Brown (2005). 'Net-working on a neonatal intensive care unit: the baby as a virtual object'. *Actor-Network Theory and Organizing* B. Czarniawska and T. Hernes. Malmo, Sweden, Liber and Copenhagen Business School Press: 307–328.
Mol, A.M. (2002). *The Body Multiple: Ontology in Medical Practice*. Durham, NC, Duke University Press.
Mol, A.M. (2008). *The Logic of Care: Health and the Problem of Patient Choice*. London: Routledge.
Müller, M. (2015). 'Assemblage and actor-networks: rethinking socio-material power, politics and space'. *Geography Compass* **9**(1): 27–41. https://doi.org/10.1111/gec3.12192
Nardi, B. and R. Engeström (1999). 'A web on the wind: the structure of invisible work'. *Computer Support Cooperative Work* 8(1–2): 1–8.
Nardi, B.A. and V.L. O'Day (1999). *Information Ecologies: Using Technology with Heart*. Cambridge, MA: MIT Press.
National Osteoporosis Guideline Group (2021). *Clinical Guideline for the Prevention and Treatment of Osteoporosis*. https://www.nogg.org.uk/sites/nogg/download/NOGG-Guideline-2021-g.pdf (accessed: 6/8/25).
Pine, K.H. and M. Mazmanian (2014). 'Institutional logics of the EMR and the problem of 'perfect' but inaccurate accounts'. *CSCW '14: Proceedings of the 17th ACM Conference on Computer Supported Cooperative Work and Social Computing*, 283–294.
Pols, J. (2008). 'Good care: enacting a complex ideal in long-term psychiatry'. *Medische Anthropologie* **20**(1): 73–89.
Rolland, K., H.V. Hepsø and E. Monteiro (2006). 'Conceptualising common information spaces across heterogeneous contexts: mutable mobiles and side-effects of integration'. *Proceedings of the 2006 20th Anniversary Conference on Computer Supported Collaborative Work*, ACM.

Rossouw, J.E., G.L. Anderson, R.L. Prentice, et al. (2002) 'Risks and benefits of estrogen plus progestin in healthy postmenopausal women: principal results from the Women's Health Initiative randomized controlled trial'. *Journal of the American Medical Association* **288**(3): 321–333.

Shorrock, S. (2022). *Work-as-imagined Solutioneering: A 10-step Guide*, https://humanisticsystems.com/2018/06/03/work-as-imagined-solutioneering-a-10-step-guide/ (accessed 20/9/23).

Timmermans, S. and R. Almeling (2009). 'Objectification, standardization, and commodification in health care: a conceptual readjustment'. *Social Science & Medicine* **69**(1): 21–27. https://doi.org/10.1016/j.socscimed.2009.04.020

APPENDIX 1

APPENDIX 1 Data Summary

Site	*Fieldwork duration*	*Shadowing*	*Events*	*Audio-recorded interviews*
Emergency Medical Services Control Centre	17 hrs 30 mins	Call handlers x2 Dispatch operatives x2 Nurse (clinical desk) Paramedic (clinical desk)	Call management, clinical triage, dispatch processes	Duty Manager
Emergency Medical Services Responders	37 hrs	Paramedics x5	Care at scene, transfer to ED, transitions	
Emergency Department	47 hrs	Streaming Nurse ED Nurses Healthcare support workers ED Doctors	Bed allocation, triage, nursing admission, medical clerking, transitions	
Assessment Unit	8 hrs 30 mins	AU Nurses Doctors	Unit activity and transitions	

(*Continued*)

APPENDIX 1 (Continued)

Site	*Fieldwork duration*	*Shadowing*	*Events*	*Audio-recorded interviews*
Orthogeriatric Service	146 hrs	Doctors Ward nurses Frailty Nurses Occupational Therapist Physiotherapists Pharmacist Trauma & Orthopaedic Bed Coordinator	Board Rounds Clerking Admissions Processes Discharge Planning Meetings Multidisciplinary Team Meetings Nursing Handover Doctors' Handover Trauma and Orthopaedic Team Meetings Ward Rounds	Frailty Nurses x2 Ward Manager Associate specialist surgeon Consultant ortho-geriatrician x2
Operating Department	12 hrs	Health care support workers Operating Department Practitioners Anaesthetist Anaesthetic Assistant Post-anaesthetic recovery nurse	Transport of patient (ward to OD) Anaesthetic induction Operation Post-anaesthetic recovery Transitions	Clinical leader (T&O theatres) Anaesthetics Assistants x2
Discharge Lounge	7 hrs	Nurses Health care support workers St John's Ambulance Personnel	Care and transport of patients	
Community Coordinating Hub	7 hrs	Call handler Social worker Clinical lead	Call management	
Community Resource Team	19 hrs	Screening Nurse Physiotherapist Occupational Therapists	Allocation Meetings Discharge Visits Routine visits	
Community Nursing Service	27 hrs	Team manager Community nurses x2	Routine visits Handover	

(*Continued*)

APPENDIX 1 (Continued)

Site	*Fieldwork duration*	*Shadowing*	*Events*	*Audio-recorded interviews*
Social Services	13 hrs 30 mins	Ward Social Worker Administrative Officer		Social services home care managers x2
Primary Care				Academic General Practitioner

(Developed from Allen, 2024)

Reference

Allen, D. (2024). 'Why is hospital discharge so difficult? Reconsidering patient trajectories in theory and practice: Insights from an ethnographic study of transitions in hip fracture care'. *Social Science & Medicine* **347**: 116769. https://doi.org/10.1016/j.socscimed.2024.116769

INDEX

Pages in *italics* refer to figures.

actor network theory 20–21, 29
articulation 16, 20, 30, 130, 289, 296, *306*
assemblage thinking 21

care infrastructure 232–233, 258–269, 273–279, 296
care trajectories 15–16, 28, 58
care trajectory narrative 97, 108, 111, *143*, 144, 168–169, 187
concern-centered care 291, 302–303
coordination, the problem 5–6

hip fracture 25–26

institutional logics 7–8
interpretative repertoires 30, 45, 64, 78–79, 125–127, 150, 198–199, 233
invisible work 20–21, 56, 95, 130, 144–145, 186–187, 273, 289

match making 81, 221, 228
materials 30, 45–46, 62–64, 79–80, 150–152, 199, 232–233
methods 26–28, 40, 120, 192–193, 308

negotiated orders 16, 29

object formation 30–32, 290–293; anaesthetics 153–155; collective practice 136–137, 221–226, *227*, 228, 234–250, 252–253; community occupational therapist 250; community physiotherapists 251; discharge 269–271; emergency department medicine 87; emergency department nurses 81, 84–87, 93–97; emergency medical services call handlers 49–55; emergency medical services clinical support officers 55–56; emergency medical services responders 66–74; frailty nurses 218–221; orthogeriatric medicine 130–137, 201–205; orthogeriatric nurses 137–142, *143*, 144, 217; orthogeriatric occupational therapist 211–217; orthogeriatric pharmacist 206–209; orthogeriatric physiotherapists 210–211; Post Anaesthetic Care nurses 160–165; in professional practice 293; social care 251–252; surgery 156–160
object functions: boundary objects 32, 228, 268, 284, 295; immutable mobiles 105, 184, 280, 285, 295, 300; mutable mobiles 103, 115, 295, 299–200
object qualities 294–295; epistemic objects 32, 121–128, 136, 225, 228, 294–295; narrative objects 32, 102, 294–295; situated objects 32, 153–160, 217, 247–250, 294–295; technical objects 32, 46, 102, 114, 126, 130, 137, 217, 255, 258, 280, 294–295, 297, 299

objects of practice 31; allocative 46, 81; collective 19, 31, 46, 76, 165, 169, 186–187, 234, 258, 282, 285, 292; contractual 252, 254; distribution of 293–294; performative 107, 139, 164, 210, 217, 293; professional 66–67, 87–91, 93–95, 130, 138–141, 201, 250–252; referral 92–93; trajectory 66, 68–73, 95–97, 141–142, *143*, 144, 217, 221–226, *227*, 228; transition 46, 91, 102–103, 169, 257–258; triage 46, 84–87; intra-professional 31, 139, 218, 220; interdisciplinary 136, 221–228; unstable 279–280, *281*, 282
organisational mechanisms 297–298
organisational modes 295–297
organising logics 30, 44, 62, 78, 125, 148–149, 197–198, 231–232
osteoporosis 309–310

patient pathways 6–10
patient record 46, 62–63, 74, 79, 127, 150–151, 199
patients, as objects 18–19
policy context: acute care 119–120; recovery care 191–192, 282; unscheduled care 39–40
practice approach 20, 29
professional vision 66, 249
projects 30

reflexive monitoring 30, 78, 81, 108
research 305
rich description 305
risk assessment 31, 45–46, 57, 79, 93–94, *98*, 106, 124, 138, 162, 172, 174, 199, 217, 234, 236, 242, 249, 252, 274, 292, 297
roles 298–299

sensemaking 17, 29–30, 66–68
service improvement 302–305
social worlds theory 17
strategic action fields 18, 30

technologies 20, 44–45, 49, 56, 199
theoretical framework 28–32, *33*, 305, *306*, 307
tinkering 141, 184, 233, 265, 289, 296, *306*
trajectory assemblage 290
trajectory studies 307
transition infrastructure 31, 101–102, 168–169, 256–257
transition interface 31, 100–101, 167–168, 256; emergency department Assessment Unit-ward 110, *112*, 111; emergency department Majors-Assessment Unit 108–110; emergency medical services control centre-emergency medical services responders 103–105; emergency medical services responders-emergency department 105–108; operating department-ward 178–182, *183*, 184; orthogeriatric ward-community nursing 271; orthogeriatric ward-community resource team 259–262, 269–270; orthogeriatric ward-operating department 170–178; orthogeriatric ward-primary care 265, 270–271
transitions 19, 31, 100–113, 167–182, *183*, 184–185, 299–300
translation 30, 92, 109, 142, 167, 178, 184, 216, 224, 228, 258–259, 297, 299
translational mobilisation theory 29–30, 305

work 20; community resource team 233–234; emergency department 80; emergency medical services control centre 47–49; emergency medical services responders 64–66; operating department 152–153; orthogeriatric 129–130, 200–201

For Product Safety Concerns and Information please contact our EU representative GPSR@taylorandfrancis.com
Taylor & Francis Verlag GmbH, Kaufingerstraße 24, 80331 München, Germany

www.ingramcontent.com/pod-product-compliance
Ingram Content Group UK Ltd.
Pitfield, Milton Keynes, MK11 3LW, UK
UKHW022031090226
467856UK00010B/278
9781032756523

BEYOND PATIENT PATHWAYS

How is care coordinated when the course is uncertain, the work is distributed, and the patient is constantly redefined? In this detailed ethnographic study of the hip fracture trajectory, *Beyond Patient Pathways* challenges the dominant rational-linear logic of care pathways to reveal the complex, evolving assemblages that underpin everyday service delivery.

The book traces how coordination is accomplished within and across diverse settings – from the control centre and ambulance services, through the emergency department, hospital ward, and operating theatres, to community-based care. The first ever study to examine the organisation of end-to-end processes in real time, it offers unique insights into the changing shape of patient trajectories. Anchored in classic sociological ideas on patient trajectories and informed by Translation Mobilisation Theory, *Beyond Patient Pathways* reframes patient-centred care not as a fixed ideal, but as something enacted through shifting concerns, technologies, and institutional arrangements. It brings to light the diversity of ways in which care is organised, including the often-invisible work that sustains coordination across time and settings. In doing so, it offers not only a powerful conceptual lens but also a methodological foundation for studying care trajectories in ways that are sensitive to the relational intricacies and dynamic configurations of care work.

The complexity of care systems is increasingly acknowledged, but they are difficult to study systematically. This book provides both the empirical grounding and the theoretical tools needed to do so – making it an essential resource for a wide readership of researchers, medical sociologists, service managers, improvement scientists, and healthcare professionals with an interest in health services management, quality improvement, person-centred care, care planning, and interprofessional education.

Davina Allen is a professor of Health Service Organisation and Delivery at Cardiff University. A nurse and a sociologist, her work spans foundational ethnographic studies, applied research, and theory development. A Fellow of the Academy of Social Sciences, the Learned Society of Wales, and the Health Foundation, she has a longstanding commitment to the value of sociological inquiry to illuminate and address the practical challenges of contemporary healthcare systems.